ONCOLOGY NURSING REVIEW

W9-AWH-044

Jones and Bartlett Series in Oncology

For a complete list of our oncology titles see www.jbpub.com/oncology

ONCOLOGY NURSING REVIEW
FOURTH EDITION

Connie Henke Yarbro, RN, MS, FAAN

Adjunct Clinical Associate Professor
MU Sinclair School of Nursing
Editor, *Seminars in Oncology Nursing*
University of Missouri–Columbia
Columbia, Missouri

Margaret Hansen Frogge, RN, MS

Vice President, Corporate Strategy
Riverside Health Care
Kankakee, Illinois

Assistant Professor of Nursing
Rush University College of Nursing
Rush University Medical Center
Chicago, Illinois

Michelle Goodman, RN, MS

Oncology Clinical Nurse Specialist
Rush Cancer Institute
Assistant Professor of Nursing
Rush University College of Nursing
Rush University Medical Center
Chicago, Illinois

JONES AND BARTLETT PUBLISHERS

Sudbury, Massachusetts

BOSTON   TORONTO   LONDON   SINGAPORE

World Headquarters
Jones and Bartlett Publishers
40 Tall Pine Drive
Sudbury, MA 01776
978-443-5000
info@jbpub.com
www.jbpub.com

Jones and Bartlett Publishers Canada
6339 Ormindale Way
Mississauga, Ontario L5V 1J2
CANADA

Jones and Bartlett Publishers International
Barb House, Barb Mews
London W6 7PA
UK

Jones and Bartlett's books and products are available through most bookstores and online booksellers. To contact Jones and Bartlett Publishers directly, call 800-832-0034, fax 978-443-8000, or visit our website, www.jbpub.com.

Substantial discounts on bulk quantities of Jones and Bartlett's publications are available to corporations, professional associations, and other qualified organizations. For details and specific discount information, contact the special sales department at Jones and Bartlett via the above contact information or send an email to specialsales@jbpub.com.

Copyright © 2007 by Jones and Bartlett Publishers, Inc.

All rights reserved. No part of the material protected by this copyright may be reproduced or utilized in any form, electronic or mechanical, including photocopying, recording, or by any information storage and retrieval system, without written permission from the copyright owner.

The authors, editor, and publisher have made every effort to provide accurate information. However, they are not responsible for errors, omissions, or for any outcomes related to the use of the contents of this book and take no responsibility for the use of the products and procedures described. Treatments and side effects described in this book may not be applicable to all people; likewise, some people may require a dose or experience a side effect that is not described herein. Drugs and medical devices are discussed that may have limited availability controlled by the Food and Drug Administration (FDA) for use only in a research study or clinical trial. Research, clinical practice, and government regulations often change the accepted standard in this field. When consideration is being given to use of any drug in the clinical setting, the health care provider or reader is responsible for determining FDA status of the drug, reading the package insert, and reviewing prescribing information for the most up-to-date recommendations on dose, precautions, and contraindications, and determining the appropriate usage for the product. This is especially important in the case of drugs that are new or seldom used.

Library of Congress Cataloging-in-Publication Data
Yarbro, Connie Henke.
    Oncology nursing review / Connie Henke Yarbro, Margaret Hansen Frogge, Michelle Goodman. — 4th ed.
        p. ; cm.
    ISBN-13: 978-0-7637-5030-5 (alk. paper)
    ISBN-10: 0-7637-5030-1 (alk. paper)
    1. Cancer—Nursing—Outlines, syllabi, etc. I. Frogge, Margaret Hansen. II. Goodman, Michelle. III. Title.
    [DNLM: 1. Neoplasms—nursing—Examination Questions. 2. Neoplasms—nursing—Outlines. WY 18.2 Y26o 2007]
    RC266.Y366 2007
    616.99'40231—dc22

                                    2007002843

6048

Production Credits
Executive Publisher: Christopher Davis
Production Director: Amy Rose
Associate Editor: Kathy Richardson
Production Assistant: Amanda Clerkin
Marketing Manager: Katrina Gosek
Associate Marketing Manager: Rebecca Wasley
Manufacturing and Inventory Coordinator: Amy Bacus
Composition: Northeast Compositors, Inc.
Cover Design: Anne Spencer
Cover Image: © Kristin/Shutterstock, Inc.
Printing and Binding: Courier Stoughton
Cover Printing: Courier Stoughton

Printed in the United States of America
11 10 09 08 07   10 9 8 7 6 5 4 3 2 1

CONTENTS

O*ncology Nursing Review* is a comprehensive book and CD-ROM learning package to help you review content related to oncology nursing and cancer care. From the authors of the authoritative *Cancer Nursing Principles and Practice* (6th ed.), this text contains 1,100+ multiple-choice questions with accompanying answers.

Organization

The book is organized into eight chapters corresponding to the areas tested on the Oncology Nursing Certification examination. The chapters include

1. Quality of Life
2. Protective Mechanisms
3. Gastrointestinal and Urinary Function
4. Cardiopulmonary Function
5. Oncologic Emergencies
6. Scientific Basis for Practice
7. Health Promotion
8. Professional Performance

Each chapter represents an important content area in oncology nursing. The chapters are further divided into subsections to facilitate study of major topics within these areas.

How to Use the Book

There are two approaches to using *Oncology Nursing Review*. If you are just beginning to review the subject matter, you will probably want to spend more time with the book questions before you attempt the practice tests. If you are further along in your study, creating practice tests and the subsequent self-assessment can help you identify areas that need further review.

If you are just beginning to review, we recommend that you work through a small section at a time, reading the question and recording the answer. Then consult the correct answers and the explanations. Read the explanations both for the answers that you got correct and for those that you missed. You may find additional information presented that will augment your knowledge base and clarify points that you may have overlooked or misunderstood. If you answer a question incorrectly, consult *Cancer Nursing Principles and Practice* (6th ed.) and *Cancer Symptom Management* (3rd ed.) for more information.

About the Accompanying CD-ROM

The CD-ROM that accompanies *Oncology Nursing Review, Fourth Edition* is a useful learning tool that contains multiple practice tests along with instant feedback to identify areas where further study is required. You can customize a variety of practice exams, including random selection, by subject, or all 1,100+ questions.

To approximate the testing situation most closely, create a 200-question exam, randomly selected from all eight content areas, and allow yourself 3½ hours to complete it. Then check your answers. Your performance will give you a realistic idea of your knowledge of key content areas and your ability to function under time pressure. With this valuable comprehensive study package, you will have the most essential and up-to-date knowledge needed to master the challenges of oncology nursing.

Finding Out About Certification Requirements

If you want to obtain the Oncology Nursing Certification, it is important for you to contact the certifying organization, the Oncology Nursing Certification Corporation (ONCC)®. The ONCC® publishes a *Test Bulletin*, which we suggest you acquire. This bulletin provides important information about certification, including test dates, application deadlines, test center locations, eligibility criteria, and information about the test itself, as well as sample questions.

You can contact the ONCC through its website, *www.oncc.org*; via e-mail at oncc@ons.org; by telephone at (877) 769-ONCC or (412) 859-6104; by fax at (412) 859-6168; or by mail at 125 Enterprise Drive, Pittsburgh, PA 15275-1214.

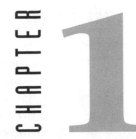

CHAPTER 1

Quality of Life

COMFORT

Pain

1.1 Mr. Allen describes his pain as a 7 on the verbal numeric rating scale. He has no evidence of tachycardia, hypertension, diaphoresis, or pallor. From these observations you conclude which of the following regarding Mr. Allen's pain?
   a. He is experiencing acute or intermittent pain.
   b. He is experiencing chronic pain.
   c. Because he does not appear to be in pain, further assessment is necessary before treating his pain.
   d. His pain medication is inadequate.

1.2 Poorly treated or unrelieved pain is a common problem for the individual with cancer. The primary reason for this is which of the following?
   a. Access to health care and appropriate treatment
   b. Reluctance of the patient to report pain
   c. Failure of the health care profession to routinely assess pain and pain relief
   d. Difficulty controlling cancer pain and expensive medications

1.3 Your patient recently began oral morphine therapy. He complains of nausea, vomiting, and itching. The best option(s) for managing these symptoms include which of the following?
   a. Change the dosing regimen or route of the same drug
   b. Switch to fentanyl or oxymorphone
   c. Add another drug that counteracts the adverse effects
   d. All of the above

1.4   Tricyclic antidepressants (TCAs) such as amitriptyline, desipramine, or imipramine are considered coanalgesics in pain management. Which of the following statements regarding the use of TCAs in pain management is (are) true?
a.   TCAs (low dose) are effective for the treatment of neuropathic pain.
b.   Concomitant use of opioid analgesics is not problematic because sedation and orthostatic hypotension are uncommon with low-dose TCAs.
c.   The use of regular-dose selective serotonin reuptake inhibitor antidepressants fluoxetine (Prozac), and paroxetine (Paxil) for concurrent depression is not contraindicated with TCAs.
d.   All of the above

1.5   Oral transmucosal fentanyl citrate (Actiq) is a solid oral dosage form of fentanyl incorporated into a sweetened lozenge on a handle. Which of the following accurately describes this novel approach to pain management?
a.   Only 25% of Actiq is absorbed into the oral mucosa.
b.   Actiq is indicated for the treatment of cancer-related breakthrough pain.
c.   Plasma concentrations peak approximately 10 minutes after the lozenge is consumed.
d.   All of the above

1.6   An example of counterirritant cutaneous stimulation is
a.   Subcutaneous administration of morphine
b.   Minor surgery
c.   Massage
d.   Imagery

1.7   Directing one's attention away from the sensations and emotional reactions produced by pain is known as
a.   Distraction
b.   Biofeedback
c.   Autogenic relaxation
d.   Hypnosis

1.8   The dimension of pain that encompasses the meaning that the pain experience has for a person is the
a.   Behavioral dimension
b.   Affective dimension
c.   Sensory dimension
d.   Cognitive dimension

1.9   Opiate-related daytime sedation is a known side effect of chronic pain management. Which of the following agents has *not* been shown to be an effective treatment for opiate-induced sedation?
a.   Lorazepam
b.   Methylphenidate
c.   Donepezil
d.   Dextroamphetamine

1.10   Which of the following is *not* a common obstacle to successful pain management?
a.   Inaccurate knowledge about pharmacologic principles
b.   A lack of basic assessment skills
c.   A lack of available knowledge in the field
d.   Legal impediments

1.11 Assessment of behavioral parameters in cancer pain includes an evaluation of
  a. The quality of the pain
  b. Associated psychologic problems
  c. The effect of pain on activities of daily living
  d. The duration of the pain

1.12 The presence of pain in cognitively impaired older adults is often difficult to assess. Which of the following would *not* be considered a pain cue in this population?
  a. Changes in appearance
  b. Changes in appetite
  c. Changes in overt behavior
  d. Changes in sounds

Fatigue

1.13 Fatigue associated with radiation therapy is most often associated with all but which of the following?
  a. An accumulation of cell-destruction end products
  b. Increased energy requirements to repair damaged epithelial tissue
  c. Age, diagnosis, or stage of disease at diagnosis
  d. Pain, depression, and weight loss

1.14 Ms. Clay has breast cancer and is currently undergoing chemotherapy and receiving an antiemetic regimen of granisetron, dexamethasone and lorazepam. Her white blood cell count is 3200/mm^3, hemoglobin is 11.2 g/dL, and platelets 72,000/mm^3. Her chief complaint for the week after her treatment is fatigue. She only begins to feel better just before her next treatment. Which of the following most appropriately addresses her complaint?
  a. Suggest that she increase her exercise to 20 minutes per day during the week after her treatment
  b. Evaluate her antiemetic regimen to determine which drugs might be causing her fatigue
  c. Suggest that she be started on darbepoietin alfa injections
  d. a and b

1.15 Research indicates that when compared to women who have no history of cancer, women who have completed their chemotherapy more than a year before participating in the study report which of the following concerning the symptom of fatigue and quality of life?
  a. Worse menopausal symptoms and poorer quality of sleep
  b. Excessive weight gain and lack of energy
  c. Increased psychosomatic complaints and depression
  d. Moderate to severe fatigue that is cumulative over time

1.16 Mr. James has metastatic prostate cancer, diabetes, and uncontrolled hypertension. He has mild congestive heart failure and is currently receiving two units of packed red blood cells for a hemoglobin of 8 g/dL. Your colleague asks why he is not given darbepoietin alfa rather than risk complications of a fluid overload. Your most appropriate response would be which of the following?
  a. Darbepoietin alfa injections take 2–6 weeks to be effective.
  b. Darbepoietin alfa is contraindicated in patients with uncontrolled hypertension.
  c. Darbepoietin alfa can potentially increase his severity of congestive heart failure and stroke.
  d. All of the above

1.17 Your patient has been receiving chemotherapy for some time and states that she has no energy to perform even the basic activities of daily living. Your advice to her is to do which of the following?
a. She needs to rest more because she needs to save her energy to resist infection.
b. Because it is possible that too much rest can exacerbate fatigue, she needs to be encouraged to establish an exercise program that is a balance between rest and activity.
c. She should be encouraged to take a sleep aid whenever she is unable to sleep.
d. a and c

1.18 According to research, which of the following nonpharmacologic measures is *most effective* in relieving fatigue?
a. Conservation of energy
b. Motivational strategies to increase self-efficacy beliefs
c. Increasing the number of hours resting or sleeping
d. Exercise

1.19 Prolonged or severe myelosuppression in elderly patients has been noted after chemotherapy and is thought to be primarily caused by which of the following?
a. There is an age-related decrease in the base number of myeloid cells.
b. Protein-calorie malnutrition can occur.
c. There is a failure to attenuate drug dosage based on chronologic age.
d. Drugs that bind to circulating red blood cells reach higher concentrations and therefore cause a greater toxic effect in elderly patients with anemia.

1.20 According to a national survey, which of the following best describes the oncologist's view of fatigue?
a. Fatigue is a result of chronic illness.
b. Fatigue is a sensation of tiredness.
c. Fatigue is a symptom of cancer.
d. Fatigue is a result of cancer treatment.

1.21 Based on modality of treatment, which of the following patients would you expect to have the most severe fatigue?
a. Joe, who is being treated with biologic response modifiers
b. Karen, who is undergoing chemotherapy
c. Martha, who has just had surgery
d. Thomas, who is undergoing radiation treatment

1.22 Which statement is true of individuals who have suffered from cancer-related fatigue once they have completed treatment?
a. Fatigue disappears almost immediately upon the conclusion of treatment.
b. Fatigue may gradually fade after the treatment is finished.
c. Fatigue absolutely should improve upon the completion of treatment.
d. The use of assistive devices and systematic planning of activities should be unnecessary upon completion of treatment.

Pruritus

1.23   Mr. Black presents to the physician's office with complaints of fatigue, loss of appetite, and generalized itching. Which of the following diagnoses is *least likely* to be associated with these presenting symptoms?
   a. Prostate cancer
   b. Multiple myeloma
   c. Small cell lung cancer
   d. Leukemia

1.24   Ms. Richards has metastatic breast cancer with extensive bony involvement. She is having an epidural catheter placed for pain control. Within a few hours of receiving epidural opioids she complains of generalized itching. Upon examination you see no evidence of a rash. Which of the following responses is most appropriate to manage her complaint?
   a. Itching is uncommon with epidural opioids, so it is probably related to another medication.
   b. Itching is a sign of hypersensitivity reaction and the opioids should be stopped.
   c. She probably has hypercalcemia, which is commonly associated with itching.
   d. Itching is a common precursor to a rash due to opioids and should be managed with pharmacologic therapy.

1.25   You are considering suggesting that your patient take diphenhydramine HCl 25 mg every 4–6 hours as treatment for her itching. While taking a drug history you learn she is taking other medications that are contraindicated with diphenhydramine HCl. Which of the following medications should *not* be given concurrently with diphenhydramine HCl?
   a. Monoamine oxidase inhibitors
   b. Opioids
   c. Hydroxyzine
   d. All of the above

1.26   Alex has undergone allogeneic bone marrow transplantation and is experiencing itching and burning of the skin, with skin involvement as a manifestation of graft-versus-host disease. With these findings, which of the following statements is true concerning his symptoms?
   a. These symptoms are indicative of acute graft-versus-host disease.
   b. These symptoms are indicative of chronic graft-versus-host disease.
   c. These symptoms are to be expected and are likely due to the multiple medications he is taking.
   d. These symptoms suggest an appropriate immune response.

1.27   After a sentinel lymph node mapping for breast cancer, a patient complains of generalized itching and a rash. What is *most likely* the cause of pruritus in this patient?
   a. Dehydration due to the surgical procedure
   b. Reaction to the pain medication
   c. Reaction to the local anesthesia
   d. An adverse reaction to the isosulfan blue dye used during the sentinel lymph node mapping

1.28   Pruritus frequently accompanies jaundice in patients with obstructive biliary disease. Which of the following best describes the mechanism of pruritus under these circumstances?
   a.   Itching is primarily due to dry flaky skin.
   b.   Itching is caused by irritation of the cutaneous sensory nerve fibers by accumulated bile salts.
   c.   Itching is due to poor body hygiene and the use of deodorant soaps.
   d.   Itching is due to the accumulation of cholestyramine.

1.29   Which of the following is *not* effective treatment for pruritus?
   a.   Meticulous skin hygiene
   b.   Oil-based lotions and antihistamines
   c.   Cholestyramine
   d.   Vitamins A, C, D, and B complex

1.30   During the initial history and physical the patient states that the most annoying symptom he has is constant itching and a burning sensation on the lower legs. These symptoms often intensify after consuming alcoholic beverages. Which of the following cancer diagnoses is *most often* associated with these symptoms?
   a.   Small cell lung cancer
   b.   Hodgkin's disease
   c.   Kaposi's sarcoma
   d.   Acute myelogenous leukemia

1.31   Mr. Marks has Hodgkin's disease. He has recently completed radiation therapy and chemotherapy. His chief complaints include pain, for which he is receiving morphine, and a generalized itching of unknown etiology. The itching is *most likely* due to which of the following?
   a.   A systemic symptom related to Hodgkin's disease
   b.   A side effect from opiate therapy
   c.   Dry skin due to radiation therapy
   d.   All of the above

1.32   Mr. Elliot presented to the outpatient ambulatory care center with a complaint of recent-onset generalized itching. This itching, or pruritus, could be related to which of the following?
   a.   Central nervous system malignancies
   b.   Hodgkin's disease
   c.   Occult metastases
   d.   a and b

1.33   Pruritus occurs in approximately 40% of patients with Hodgkin's disease and is *most often* associated with advanced disease.
   a.   True
   b.   False

1.34   Mr. Ely has recently been told he will be starting interleukin-2 therapy as part of a research protocol. Which of the following is *not* considered a side effect of interleukin-2 therapy?
   a.   Moderate hair loss
   b.   Moderate to severe itching
   c.   Rapid weight gain
   d.   Nausea, vomiting, and diarrhea

1.35 Which of the following measures is *not* therapeutic in the management of pruritus?
   a. Maintaining a warm and humid environment
   b. Cimetidine and diphenhydramine
   c. Moisturizing agents such as aquaphor, oil, and oatmeal baths
   d. Oral morphine as needed

Sleep Disorders

1.36 Research indicates that sleep deprivation following insomnia is associated with which of the following?
   a. Alterations in immune and neuroendocrine function
   b. Increase in attention deficit disorder
   c. Rebound hypersomnia
   d. No change in cognitive function

1.37 Which of the following is *not* considered to be a predisposing factor associated with sleep disturbance in cancer patients?
   a. Female gender
   b. Age
   c. A diagnosis of breast cancer
   d. A family history of sleep disorder

1.38 Which of the following agents is typically *not* associated with increased somnolence in cancer patients?
   a. Thalidomide
   b. Selective serotonin reuptake inhibitors
   c. Opioid toxicity
   d. Ketamine

1.39 Your patient, who is receiving radiation therapy for a malignant brain tumor, complains of increased daytime fatigue and somnolence. To help her understand what might be causing her symptoms, you could say *all but* which of the following?
   a. The incidence of sleep disturbances is 50% greater in people who receive radiation therapy to the brain.
   b. Radiation, regardless of the site radiated, commonly results in a decline in sleep efficiency.
   c. Higher levels of sleep disturbance occur in patients who are further along in their radiation treatment protocol.
   d. Her symptoms might be related to other medications she is taking, specifically corticosteroids.

1.40 Benzodiazepines are often not used to treat insomnia because of which of the following?
   a. Benzodiazepines tend to be addictive.
   b. They cause motor slowing.
   c. They cause cognitive difficulties.
   d. All of the above

1.41 Research into the incidence of sleep disturbances indicates that sleeping difficulty is reported by approximately what percentage of patients with cancer?
   a. 50%
   b. 40%
   c. 30%
   d. 20%

1.42   Your patient is receiving paclitaxel on a weekly basis. She commonly experiences nausea and is prescribed the antiemetic granisetron to take if she needs it. She complains that she is having trouble sleeping and often feels agitated at night. Which of the following is a logical explanation for her symptoms?
  a.   Her difficulty in sleeping is likely due to the decadron she takes to prevent hypersensitivity reactions to the paclitaxel.
  b.   She is probably feeling agitated due to the granisetron.
  c.   Adverse neurologic effects, including sleep disruption, are common in patients taking paclitaxel.
  d.   Insomnia and restlessness are common in anyone undergoing treatment for cancer.

1.43   Your patient experiences intense nausea and vomiting from chemotherapy and is given a prescription for lorazepam to take with her antiemetics at night. She wants to know why she is given an antianxiety agent when she does not feel anxious. Your explanation would include which of the following?
  a.   The lorazepam is given to increase the effectiveness of the antinausea pills.
  b.   She probably does not realize how anxious she really is and that it is important to suppress that anxiety before it contributes to her problem.
  c.   The lorazepam is given to induce sleep, which is an important strategy for preventing nausea and vomiting with chemotherapy.
  d.   All of the above

1.44   A patient is having trouble sleeping and wants to take a "natural" sleep aid rather than a prescription drug because she is afraid of becoming addicted to sleeping pills. Which of the following statements is *most accurate* concerning the use of herbal agents as sleep aids?
  a.   Herbal agents are perfectly safe, even if taken for extended periods of time.
  b.   Herbal agents, especially lavender, can be addicting.
  c.   Herbal agents often act by binding to benzodiazepine receptors and can increase daytime sedation.
  d.   Ginseng is an effective sleep aid and can safely be taken with monoamine oxidase inhibitors.

1.45   Benzodiazepines are commonly used sleep aids but have significant side effects. Which of the following statements concerning the use of benzodiazepine is *false*?
  a.   Benzodiazepines are primarily indicated for short-term treatment of insomnia.
  b.   Benzodiazepines are commonly prescribed because they are rarely addictive.
  c.   Benzodiazepines significantly increase sleep duration.
  d.   Benzodiazepines are associated with rebound insomnia once discontinued.

1.46   Early morning awakening, a form of insomnia, can be an important diagnostic indicator of depression.
  a.   True
  b.   False

1.47   Sleep aids are commonly prescribed to assist patients with insomnia to get to sleep and stay asleep. Which of the following statements regarding the newer nonbenzodiazepine sleep aids is *false*?
  a.   They suppress delta sleep, similar to traditional benzodiazepine sleep aids.
  b.   They have a shorter half-life compared with traditional sleep aids.
  c.   They are likely to cause less feelings of sedation after awakening.
  d.   They are less effective in maintaining a sleep state.

Dyspnea

1.48   In general, dyspnea most commonly occurs when which of the following is present?
a.   Physiologic parameters, indicating altered pulmonary function tests
b.   Chronic pain
c.   A decrease in the amount of respiratory muscles required to maintain adequate breathing
d.   An increase in respiratory effort necessary to overcome restrictive disease

1.49   Your patient is in Hospice. One of his primary complaints is that he cannot get enough air. Upon examination you learn he has a normal oxygen saturation, elevated blood pressure, and minimal pain, manageable by hydrocodone. Which of the following treatment scenarios would best address his chief complaint?
a.   Continuous pulse oximetry, low-dose oxygen therapy to treat his air hunger, and a benzodiazepine to treat anxiety
b.   Chest x-ray and arterial blood gases with pulmonary function tests to rule out pneumonia along with a benzodiazepine for anxiety
c.   Low-dose opioid therapy, a benzodiazepine for anxiety, position the patient upright, and provide a cool fan
d.   All of the above

1.50   Ms. Howe has persistent productive coughing, which, she says, is exhausting. Which intervention should *not* be used?
a.   Inspired air is warmed and humidified.
b.   Cigarette smoking is discouraged.
c.   Deep breathing and coughing techniques are taught and reinforced.
d.   Narcotic medications are used for cough suppression.

1.51   Mr. Smith has laryngeal carcinoma with regional recurrence. During a routine physical exam you notice he is experiencing stridor. This is *most likely* an indication of which of the following?
a.   Extrathoracic airway obstruction
b.   Intrathoracic airway obstruction
c.   Tumor
d.   a and c

1.52   Which of the following sclerosing agents are used to manage recurrent pleural effusions?
a.   Bleomycin
b.   Doxorubicin
c.   Tetracycline
d.   All of the above

1.53   Janis frequently experiences dyspnea due to recurrent pleural effusions. Her doctor has suggested that she have a more permanent device placed into her pleural space to make it easier to drain the fluid from her lung. Which of the following is an accurate description of this device?

    a. A pleuroperitoneal shunt can be inserted to divert fluid from the chest cavity to the abdomen.

    b. A pleural port can be implanted underneath the skin just below the ribs, with the catheter resting in the pleural space. The port is accessed with a 19-gauge Huber point needle whenever she complains of difficulty breathing.

    c. A small-bore catheter may be placed into the pleural space and allowed to drain through a one-way valve by gravity drainage.

    d. All of the above

1.54   Which of the following is the most accurate measure of dyspnea in the individual with cancer?

    a. Respiratory rate

    b. Oxygen saturation

    c. Arterial blood gas level

    d. Patient self-report

1.55   Mrs. James has recently started morphine sulfate to control her pain. She is concerned about the side effects. You assure her that within 1–2 weeks she will become tolerant of *all but* which of the following side effects associated with opioid administration?

    a. Constipation

    b. Lethargy

    c. Nausea

    d. Agitation

1.56   Which of the following is *not* considered appropriate first-line treatment for dyspnea?

    a. Morphine sulfate

    b. Benzodiazepines and oxygen

    c. Chlorpromazine

    d. Buspirone

1.57   As the gag reflex and reflexive clearing of the oropharynx decline, secretions accumulate in the oropharynx, and dyspnea becomes complicated. Which of the following measures is *most effective* to manage the accumulation of secretions often associated with the "death rattle"?

    a. Glucocorticoids to decrease swelling and secretions

    b. Benzodiazepines to sedate the patient and increase comfort

    c. Oral suctioning in the posterior pharynx to clear secretions

    d. Anticholinergic medications to dry secretions

1.58   Chest x-ray reveals that Mr. Stanton has a large pleural effusion contributing to his dyspnea and difficulty breathing. Once the fluid is drained, the physician instills a sclerosing agent into the pleural space. In preparing your patient for the procedure, you would be certain to mention *all but* which of the following?

    a. The purpose of injecting bleomycin into the pleural space is to kill any cancer cells that might be there.

    b. The procedure is painful, and therefore the patient will be given adequate pain medication before the procedure.

    c. If the fluid reaccumulates, it can be drained again.

    d. The sclerosing agent is given to obliterate the pleural space.

1.59 Dyspnea is often considered an early sign of cardiac tamponade. Which of the following statements best describes the symptom of dyspnea in a patient experiencing cardiac tamponade?
   a. Dyspnea is caused by an increased cardiac output.
   b. Dyspnea is caused by a decrease in lung expansion.
   c. Dyspnea occurs because of pulmonary congestion.
   d. All of the above

Fever and Chills

1.60 Your patient has lymphoma and has been tracking his fever for the past week. He has not recently had chemotherapy but does complain of a fever that has been low grade with only a slight spike without returning to normal. He is frequently tachycardic and tachypneic with some periods of extreme fatigue. Given these symptoms his fever pattern is probably indicative of which type(s) of infection?
   a. Disseminated fungal infection
   b. Viral infection
   c. Bacterial infection
   d. All of the above

1.61 Shortly after beginning treatment with a biologic response modifier your patient complains of intense chills and a headache. She informs you that she has been septic in the past and fears this may be happening again. Nursing action in this situation would include which of the following?
   a. Monitor her temperature and treat her symptoms with opiates/acetaminophen or benzodiazepines depending on the severity.
   b. Stop the infusion and notify the doctor because this could be a serious allergic reaction.
   c. Consider administering the dose in the evening so the patient can sleep through the worst of the symptoms.
   d. a and c

1.62 Rituximab is a monoclonal antibody used to treat patients with non-Hodgkin's lymphoma. During the initial infusion a patient begins to shake and complains of feeling very cold. Nursing management includes which of the following?
   a. Stop the infusion and administer diphenhydramine and acetaminophen as well as bronchodilators and epinephrine as needed.
   b. Resume the infusion at 50% of the previous rate once symptoms have resolved because the reactions are related to the infusion rate.
   c. Monitor the patient for cardiac arrhythmias because arrhythmias and angina have been reported with rituximab infusion.
   d. All of the above

1.63 Mr. Allen received high-dose methotrexate for sarcoma of his pelvis 6 days ago and is currently at home complaining of a low-grade fever, slight mucositis, and diarrhea (five to six times per day) for the past 2 days. His medications include prophylactic antibiotics and morphine sulfate for pain. Nursing management includes which of the following?
   a. Give imodium 2 mg orally with each loose stool, not to exceed 16 mg per day.
   b. Push fluids and oral hygiene. Slight mucositis and diarrhea are expected.
   c. Stop the antibiotics because they are probably causing the diarrhea.
   d. Get a stool specimen to test for *Clostridium difficile*, which is common in patients receiving prophylactic antibiotics. He is probably neutropenic.

1.64   Your patient received chemotherapy 6 days ago and has now called with a fever of 101°F and chills. She has a productive cough and, except for not being able to get warm, feels fine. You send her for a complete blood count and learn that her absolute granulocyte count is 500 cells/mm^3. You instruct her to come to the hospital to be admitted. Your decision is based on which of the following?
   a.   She is at risk for bleeding and severe anemia.
   b.   She probably has pneumonia and needs to be observed.
   c.   When the neutrophil count is 500/mm^3 or less, approximately 20% or more of febrile episodes have an associated bacteremia.
   d.   She is past her nadir, but cultures need to be done to determine the source of a possible infection.

1.65   Fever and chills are a common symptom associated with sepsis. What percentage of patients with severe sepsis present with fever and chills?
   a.   38%
   b.   55%
   c.   68%
   d.   95%

1.66   Your patient has a platelet count of 33,000/mm^3 and has had frequent nosebleeds. He is currently receiving his second platelet transfusion and is complaining of shaking chills and has a fever of 102.4°F. The cause of his chills and fever is *most likely* which of the following?
   a.   He has aspiration pneumonia from his nosebleeds.
   b.   He is having a transfusion reaction because of contamination of the platelet pack.
   c.   Unfiltered platelet concentrates accumulate high levels of cytokines.
   d.   His fever is most likely related to his pancytopenia.

1.67   Management of a febrile nonhemolytic transfusion reaction presenting as fever, chills, headache, hypotension, tachypnea, and dyspnea includes *all but* which of the following?
   a.   Stop the transfusion and maintain patent intravenous line with normal saline
   b.   Notify physician and administer acetaminophen for fever, meperidine for chills and rigors, and antihistamine for dyspnea
   c.   Place the patient in the Trendelenburg position and administer a fluid bolus
   d.   Continue the transfusion if symptoms are not severe

1.68   Mrs. Andrews has just begun her first dose of Herceptin. One-third of the way through the infusion she complains of feeling cold. She is experiencing a shaking chill and has a temperature of 101.4°F. Your interventions include *all but* which of the following?
   a.   Stop the infusion and notify the physician that the patient is having a reaction to the Herceptin therapy.
   b.   Monitor vital signs and administer diphenhydramine and acetaminophen as directed.
   c.   Inform the patient that people who react to the Herceptin the first time are more likely to react more intensely with each subsequent treatment.
   d.   Resume the infusion at a slower rate when vital signs are stable.

COPING

Spiritual Distress

1.69   Spirituality refers to that dimension of being human that
a.   Represents and expresses one's life principle
b.   Prompts individuals to make sense of their universe and to relate harmoniously with self, nature, and others
c.   Involves reflecting systematically about right conduct and how to live as a good person
d.   All of the above

1.70   Regardless of one's beliefs about religion, some individualized form of _____ prayer is known to be directly correlated with spiritual well-being.
a.   Petitionary
b.   Ritualistic
c.   Conversational
d.   None of the above

1.71   Helping patients find meaning in cancer through spirituality is best accomplished by which of the following?
a.   Helping patients to accept their diagnosis and prognosis
b.   Recognizing positive outcomes from negative experiences
c.   Counseling patients and families to find spiritual support
d.   Promoting religiosity among patients and families

1.72   Which of the following is *not* considered to be a central aspect of spirituality?
a.   An integrating energy
b.   Religiosity
c.   A life principle
d.   An innate human quality

1.73   Research into spirituality and death reveals many aspects of the relationship between spiritual issues and preparation for death. Which of the following assumptions regarding spirituality and preparation for death is *not* based in research and is considered to be false?
a.   There is a direct relationship between spirituality and imminence of death.
b.   The closer an individual gets to death, the more she or he will become aware of personal spirituality.
c.   Praying, having faith, and hoping are used as coping strategies equally among persons with advanced cancer and those with early-stage cancer.
d.   Religious faith or prayer are top-ranked coping strategies among over 80% of cancer survivors.

1.74   Although it is true that oncology nurses hold diverse perspectives about controversial issues such as physician-assisted suicide and active euthanasia, nurses' attitudes regarding end-of-life decisions are most significantly influenced by which of the following?
a.   Professional integrity
b.   Sanctity of life
c.   Personal religiosity
d.   Patient autonomy

1.75   Mr. Allen is distressed over his wife's apparent anger and rejection of God due to the recent discovery that her breast cancer has recurred. Your efforts to counsel him are based on which of the following cognitive strategies?
   a.   Individuals assume that traumatic events such as cancer strengthen one's belief that there is meaning and worth.
   b.   Individuals whose world is shattered will work to reconstruct their world view so that it includes a rationale for God's failings.
   c.   Individuals use strategies such as making comparisons to another situation to make the event meaningful.
   d.   The nurse helps to construct for the individual a possible meaning for this event.

1.76   Spirituality is best defined by which of the following components?
   a.   Meaning and motivation
   b.   Religious beliefs and dogma
   c.   Ethics and religiosity
   d.   Self-transcendence and beneficence

Financial Concerns

1.77   The widespread use of diagnostic-related groups, prospective payment, and increased out-of-pocket medical expenses for consumers have all combined to create which of the following demands in health care delivery?
   a.   A shift to a type of socialized medicine
   b.   A shift from hospital-based care to outpatient and home care settings
   c.   A shift of the responsibility for managing treatment side effects from the health care providers to patients and their families
   d.   b and c

1.78   Anna has worked as a clerk at a local grocery store for 12 years and has recently been let go because the owner states the cost of health care for all 11 employees is too costly. She has metastatic cancer and is afraid she cannot afford to pay for her own insurance. Your advice to her is based on which of the following?
   a.   She qualifies for protection from the Americans with Disabilities Act (ADA) and the Family Medical Leave Act (FMLA) and should apply for assistance.
   b.   She should apply for long-term disability and Medicaid.
   c.   She should sue her employer for discrimination.
   d.   The ADA and FMLA apply only to employers with more than 15 and 50 employees, respectively.

1.79   According to the Americans with Disabilities Act (ADA) the employer is required to do which of the following?
   a.   Change the individual's schedule to permit chemotherapy treatment.
   b.   Convert the individual's full-time job to a part-time job.
   c.   Provide insurance coverage for a period of 6 months after termination.
   d.   All of the above

1.80   Individuals with low annual incomes
   a. Are three to seven times more likely to die of cancer than those with high annual incomes
   b. Rarely experience a definable difference in survivorship or treatment outcome based solely on their economic status
   c. Are twice as likely to experience recurrence, treatment failure, or death as those with higher annual incomes
   d. None of the above

1.81   The differences in incidence, mortality, and survival among various ethnic groups has been studied, and it has been determined that poverty, not race, accounts for the lower survival rate. Poverty lowers the survival rate among the many ethnic groups by
   a. 5–10%
   b. 10–15%
   c. 15–20%
   d. 20–25%

1.82   A primary barrier to cancer care for many of the ethnic minority population is
   a. Inability to pay for services
   b. Language barrier
   c. Cultural differences
   d. Access to care

1.83   The growth of managed care and capitation have contributed to
   a. A dramatic drop in coverage of prevention-oriented services
   b. Driving the coverage of preventive services
   c. Reduced funding for immunologic studies
   d. Fewer elder care provisions

1.84   Rebecca's health plan committee at work has reviewed complaints from employees about their lack of ability to access care outside the present plan if they require a treatment found only in one of their city's two research hospitals. In response, the company switches to a plan that allows members to access out-of-plan providers but imposes strict utilization strategies. This is *most likely* a
   a. Point of service (POS) plan
   b. Health maintenance organization (HMO)
   c. Physician-hospital organization (PHO)
   d. Preferred provider organization (PPO)

1.85   Middle- and upper-class families with adequate health insurance and relatively secure jobs
   a. Can still be excessively burdened by out-of-pocket expenditures for deductibles and copayments
   b. Can expect no gaps in insurance coverage
   c. Represent the only segment of the population with no serious concerns about health expenses
   d. b and c

1.86   Nurses may use all of the following to justify needed resources *except*
   a. Feasibility studies
   b. Cost–benefit analysis
   c. Standards of quality care
   d. Cost-effectiveness analyses

1.87   The demand for charity care is steadily increasing at a time when many hospitals have negative operating margins. A significant reason for the increased need for charity care is
    a.   The dramatic growth in ambulatory, hospice, and home care
    b.   The number of people who are employed but not covered by employer health insurance
    c.   A trend toward reduced Medicare and Medicaid coverage for outpatient services
    d.   Changes in federal and state guidelines regarding reimbursement to physicians for charity cases

1.88   Along with the quantity and quality of care provided by alternative care settings, the other important factor that influences the selection of a care setting for the cancer patient is
    a.   Its proximity to the acute-care hospital
    b.   Its cost and the patient's financial resources
    c.   The professional training of its medical staff
    d.   Its policies relating to the multidisciplinary team approach

Emotional Distress

1.89   As you plan your interventions for assisting a family member who is grieving the loss of a loved one, you rely on which of the following truths regarding the grief process?
    a.   Denial can coexist and compete with awareness of the situation and may be a healthful coping mechanism.
    b.   The goal is to move quickly through denial to acceptance.
    c.   The grief process is linear, and the progression through each stage is predictable.
    d.   The absence of public expression of grief indicates possible denial.

1.90   In a discussion of the patient's prognosis for which the patient has requested, the patient and her husband begin to sob softly. Your nursing action would most appropriately be which of the following?
    a.   Ask them if you have said something that is upsetting to them.
    b.   To facilitate hope you encourage them not to cry because there are options available and describe what those are.
    c.   Stop talking, temporarily allowing them to express their grief.
    d.   Reschedule the appointment because they are not prepared for what you have to say.

1.91   A patient who has just been diagnosed with lung cancer denies the diagnosis and refuses to hear about it. The patient's denial behavior is
    a.   Adaptive
    b.   Maladaptive
    c.   Value neutral
    d.   None of the above

1.92   Two patients have the same stage II lymphoma diagnosis. One is 26; the other is 58. Younger patients report
    a.   Less confusion about prognosis and treatment options than their older counterparts
    b.   Fewer adjustment difficulties compared with their older counterparts
    c.   Greater adjustment difficulties compared with their older counterparts
    d.   a and b

1.93   In a recent article a colleague, Richard, writes about the emotional aspects of dealing with a unique patient he worked with last year. In describing the kinds of psychological boundaries he established with this patient, you notice that he has drawn a diagram in which his and the patient's boundaries are touching. You realize that his boundaries with this patient were
   a.   Rigid: the patient's boundary was not allowed to intersect, or overlap, with Richard's.
   b.   Clear: he was accessible but did not get mixed up with the patient's personal priorities or goals.
   c.   Diffuse: Richard became enmeshed with the patient and overinvolved.
   d.   Diffuse: his boundaries made a limited intersection with those of the patient, yet Richard managed to keep a "professional" distance.

1.94   A 68-year-old woman recently diagnosed with metastatic cancer confesses that she has no one to talk to and feels extremely depressed. She has a history of depressive disorder but is currently not taking any medication. Your nursing action is based on which of the following?
   a.   History of a previous psychiatric diagnosis increases the risk of developing depression after a cancer diagnosis.
   b.   Severity of disease is associated with poorer psychological adjustment.
   c.   Social networks have been found to increase psychological adjustment.
   d.   All of the above

1.95   Which of the following statements regarding decision-making in reference to treatment decisions is correct?
   a.   The majority of patients prefer to take an active role in making the final selection of treatment.
   b.   The majority of patients prefer to take a passive role, allowing the physician to make the final decision about treatment.
   c.   The majority of patients prefer to collaborate with the physician in making decisions regarding treatment.
   d.   None of the above

1.96   Ten-year-old Liza is to be assessed for possible acute myelogenous leukemia (AML) and acute lymphocytic leukemia (ALL). This proves to be quite a challenge because the two have similar symptoms. Liza has ALL and begins treatment with a combination of vincristine, prednisone, and L-asparaginase. The physician begins to express strong hopes for a remission, but Liza's mother takes you aside and says, "My husband's aunt died of AML at age 40—and she was very robust and athletic! What hope does a mere 10-year-old have? Liza's not exactly robust to begin with, and she's so young." Which of the following answers is correct?
   a.   The physician is aware that the prognosis is grimmer when ALL affects children but that psychosocial support for Liza can make a world of difference in survival rate.
   b.   Age and athletic ability have been shown to make no difference in the demographics of remission and survival rates in ALL.
   c.   Complete remission is achieved in 93% of children with ALL, as opposed to 70–75% in adults.
   d.   Remission rates in patients with ALL depend on etiology and stage of disease and are not reflected by age or activity levels.

1.97   Cancer patients who are *most likely* to exhibit psychosocial distress include all of the following *except*
    a.   Those who have been unsuccessful in resolving past stress situations
    b.   Those who are dealing with stressors simultaneously
    c.   Those who perceive minimal social support in the situation
    d.   Those who cope principally through adaptive defense mechanisms

1.98   An example of an emotion-focused nursing intervention that might be used to foster the coping response of a cancer patient is
    a.   Giving information to the patient about the subjective, environmental, and temporal features of diagnostic and treatment processes
    b.   Referring patients for more specialized or intensive therapy
    c.   Using role playing to help the patient understand the impact of personal responses on others
    d.   Practicing anticipatory socialization to expected life stressors and processes, such as loss and grief

1.99   Which of the following statements about psychosocial aspects of cancer care is true?
    a.   Denial or minimization may be an effective coping strategy, allowing individuals to assimilate the impact of the illness in manageable increments.
    b.   Psychosocial responses to cancer can be clearly identified as either adaptive or maladaptive.
    c.   A perception of uncertainty in a situation results in an appraisal of danger.
    d.   Distancing behaviors of health professionals are helpful in preventing overinvolvement.

Social Dysfunction

1.100   Your patient seems detached from decision making and tends to shy away from social situations. He says he is depressed regarding his diagnosis. After talking to him for a while about this you conclude that which of the following could be an appropriate approach to management?
    a.   Pharmacologic intervention for his depression is a logical approach.
    b.   Reassure him that depression is expected and will improve with time without medication.
    c.   Ignore his symptoms because talking about it could make it worse.
    d.   Encourage the doctor to place him on suicide precautions.

1.101   A patient who has finished treatment 6 months ago and is considered cured returns for a follow-up appointment. His major complaint is that he is distressed because he continues to experience symptoms related to his treatment, such as fatigue and difficulty sleeping. Your response is based on which of the following concerning psychosocial late effects in cancer survivors?
    a.   The persistence of late and long-term physiologic symptoms often contributes to psychologic distress.
    b.   Fatigue is not normal, and he should be evaluated for possible recurrence of cancer.
    c.   Depression is common regardless of the presence of comorbid conditions.
    d.   Quality of life before diagnosis is unrelated to quality of life after cancer treatment.

1.102 One dimension that is not as frequently represented in quality of life is _____ well-being.
   a. Psychological
   b. Functional
   c. Spiritual
   d. Social

1.103 The quality of life dimension of social well-being includes
   a. Family functioning and intimacy
   b. Religious practices
   c. Positive and negative moods
   d. All of the above

1.104 When patients are given higher rather than lower levels of information regarding their disease, which of the following is true concerning their coping abilities?
   a. Patients who know less about their illness experience less anxiety.
   b. Patients and their spouses who know little about the disease tend to make conclusions by conjecture.
   c. Patients and their spouses who know little about the illness tend to experience more denial and isolation as a couple.
   d. b and c

1.105 As an individual cancer patient faces imminent death, certain losses and changes are experienced. The individual's response to these losses and changes is usually to do which of the following?
   a. Search for immortality
   b. Search for meaning
   c. Search for acceptance
   d. Search for forgiveness

1.106 It is not uncommon for the spouse of a person with cancer to be unwilling to discuss his or her concerns with the person because of fears that it might be distressing to the patient. However, this need to "protect" can result in which of the following outcomes?
   a. Increased caregiver burden
   b. Decreased caregiver burden
   c. Increased denial, fear, and isolation
   d. a and c

1.107 During the initial family assessment in home care, which of the following is *least likely* to be considered during the evaluation?
   a. What is the pattern of authority at home?
   b. What is the functional ability of the primary caregiver?
   c. What are the social obligations of family members?
   d. What support mechanisms are available to the caregiver?

1.108 On conducting a family assessment, the home health care nurse identifies conflict among the family members caring for the patient. Upon inquiry, the nurse learns that the conflict is "not new" and has existed "for years." Using this information, the home health care nurse establishes a plan of care that
   a. Attempts to change the behavior among the family members because the patient is upset by the conflict
   b. Involves having psychological services counsel the "conflicting members"
   c. Schedules family meetings about how the conflict is affecting the patient and what can be done to resolve it
   d. Is sensitive to the feelings of the members in conflict but does not attempt to treat the causes of the conflict

1.109 The psychosocial dimension of cancer care focuses on both the unique needs of the individual at risk for or with cancer and the
   a. Unique needs of other individuals in society
   b. Clinical training of health care professionals
   c. Social groups affected by that individual
   d. Role of specific therapies in cancer treatment

1.110 Which of the following is *not* a strategy for family care?
   a. Family-level teaching with respect to the disease, treatment, rehabilitation, and/or prognosis
   b. Anticipatory guidance
   c. Mobilization of health care and/or community resources
   d. The provision of intensive family therapy to all families of cancer patients

Loss and Grief

1.111 Support of loss and grief in the person suffering from cancer is primarily concerned with which of the following?
   a. How to manage symptoms of cancer
   b. How to increase "masked grief"
   c. How to identify and become aware of losses
   d. How to use denial to cope with impending losses

1.112 Which of the following describes the major characteristics of grief?
   a. A reaction to serious loss
   b. A process dependent on an individual's perceptions of the loss
   c. A process that changes over time
   d. All of the above

1.113 Your patient has failed yet another treatment regimen and could benefit significantly from hospice care but his wife refuses to consent to hospice care. Your primary intervention to facilitate acceptance of hospice care is which of the following?
   a. Provide information to the husband and wife regarding response to therapy and the benefits of hospice care.
   b. Suggest a "drug holiday" to allow time to pass so she begins to see that hospice is the best choice.
   c. Point out that she is denying what is inevitable and that accepting hospice care is best thing for everyone.
   d. Refer the patient and family to a visiting nurse service.

1.114 Which of the following grief reactions of an elderly woman who has lost her husband of 40 years to lung cancer would prompt the hospice nurse to suggest counseling?
   a. She takes out 40 years' worth of photograph albums and wants to review her marriage and life with her deceased husband with the hospice nurse.
   b. She refuses to let her sister and brother-in-law into her home anymore, blaming them for buying her husband cigarettes "all those years."
   c. She plans her husband's funeral by herself, listens to all his favorite classical music pieces, and chooses passages from his Bible.
   d. She delegates all the responsibility for disposition of her husband's belongings to the children.

1.115 While describing her sadness about her husband's imminent death, the wife of your patient says, "I have never been able to accept the death of our son, and now my husband is going too." Which of the following is the *most appropriate* response?
   a. "Do you feel your husband is dying soon?"
   b. "What was it like for you and your husband when your son died?"
   c. "Losing your son and your husband must be so difficult for you."
   d. "At least your son and your husband will be together soon."

1.116 One year after the death of her husband, Mrs. Ely still cries and rarely goes out with friends. As part of bereavement counseling, you conclude which of the following?
   a. This is a normal grief reaction. She could benefit from being seen more often.
   b. This is an example of unresolved grief, which is associated with increased risk of suicide.
   c. Acute grief can last beyond a year, but Mrs. Ely could benefit from a support group.
   d. Grieving beyond a year is often associated with unresolved guilt about the death of a loved one.

1.117 Which of the following tasks is *not* considered crucial to the normal grieving process?
   a. Accepting the reality of the loss
   b. Experiencing the pain of grief
   c. Adjusting to a new environment where the deceased had never been
   d. Placing emotional energy in another relationship

1.118 Which of the following *excludes* a patient from meeting criteria for hospice care?
   a. The family prefers that the nurse not talk about dying around the patient.
   b. The patient explains that he wants to continue to receive the new monoclonal antibody because he is certain it will be curative.
   c. The doctor orders two units of blood to be given at home along with pamidronate.
   d. The patient explains they are not ready to look at funeral homes.

1.119 A typical reaction of an adolescent after the death of a parent is to
   a. Blame the remaining parent and/or other family members for the parent's death
   b. Shield the remaining parent from discussing distressing feelings
   c. Withdraw from family relationships during a protracted period of grieving
   d. Openly share information and feelings with the remaining parent and other family members

1.120 Deterioration in communication patterns between individuals with cancer and their children is *most* predictable under which of the following circumstances?
   a. When the cancer is first diagnosed
   b. When the individual is reluctant to discuss prognosis
   c. When the prognosis is poor
   d. b and c

1.121   The process by which a grieving person begins to work through part of his or her grief before the patient dies is termed
a. Final reconciliation
b. Grief premonition
c. Resolution of guilt
d. Anticipatory mourning

Anxiety

1.122   Which of the following symptom clusters has the strongest correlation with patients undergoing chemotherapy?
a. Fatigue and depression
b. Fatigue and insomnia
c. Insomnia and depression
d. Anxiety and depression

1.123   For the person with cancer who is experiencing anxiety, which of the following interventions is *most commonly* used?
a. Individual counseling based on the crisis intervention model
b. A prescription for an antianxiety agent
c. Relaxation tapes and exercises
d. Referral to a psychiatrist specializing in behavioral disorders

1.124   On his most recent visit your patient, who is suffering from lung cancer, appears anxious but denies difficulty breathing. He complains of inability to sleep and believes this is due to depression related to his illness. The *most appropriate* pharmacologic intervention for him might be which of the following?
a. Chlordiazepoxide (Librium)
b. Selective serotonin-norepinephrine reuptake inhibitors (SSNRIs)
c. SSNRI plus a short-acting benzodiazepine
d. Lorazepam (Ativan)

1.125   Which of the following symptoms is *least* diagnostic of anxiety in the person with cancer?
a. Anorexia
b. Distractibility
c. Worry
d. Restlessness

1.126   When standardized psychiatric interviews and research diagnostic criteria are used, the prevalence of anxiety among cancer patients is approximately which of the following?
a. 0.5–10%
b. 10–30%
c. 30–50%
d. 50–70%

1.127   Anxiety is defined operationally as an increased level of arousal associated with vague, unpleasant, and uneasy feelings that occur in response to a perceived threat. What is the source of this perceived threat?
a. A nonspecific external stimulus
b. A specific external stimulus, often a physical threat
c. A nonspecific internal or external stimulus
d. A specific internal stimulus, usually pain or inflammation

1.128 Empirical data suggest that anxiety is associated with selected patient outcomes. In one study, for example, women with high anxiety related to breast biopsy were found to have
a. A higher than average mortality rate
b. Elevated diastolic blood pressure
c. Recurrent nausea
d. Positively correlated critical thinking ability

1.129 Among the nursing interventions shown to be effective with cancer patients experiencing anxiety are all of the following *except*
a. Helping the patient learn new coping strategies through anxiety-reducing role playing
b. Helping the patient focus on the perceived threat and appraise the stimuli in a different way, thus reducing anxiety
c. Helping the patient identify stimuli that have resulted in a loss of self-esteem
d. Exploring perceived patient concerns and helping patients evaluate these concerns

1.130 Why are cognitive and behavioral techniques such as hypnosis, biofeedback, progressive muscle relaxation, or music therapy helpful in the treatment of anxiety related to cancer?
a. These techniques restore or enhance a sense of self-control.
b. They provide temporary emotional distraction from the reality of the situation.
c. Channeling anger makes it less threatening.
d. Cognitive techniques promote effective denial.

Altered Body Image

1.131 Women treated for gynecologic malignancy face a 50% or greater chance of sexual dysfunction due primarily to which of the following?
a. Changes in body image
b. Changes in sexual functioning
c. Fertility issues
d. All of the above

1.132 The latest population estimates of erectile dysfunction demonstrate which of the following to be the *most significant* independent predictor of erectile dysfunction?
a. Type and location of cancer
b. Heart disease and cigarette smoking
c. Age
d. Diabetes

1.133 Early-stage prostate cancer commonly involves surgery or radiation therapy. Diagnostic transurethral resection of the prostate (TURP) commonly causes retrograde ejaculation and may be associated with erectile dysfunction what percentage of the time?
a. 10%
b. 25%
c. 35%
d. 50%

1.134 Most empirical studies dealing with the relationship of cancer to self-concept have focused on
a. The total self-appraisal of cancer patients, both men and women
b. The effects of various treatments on relationships of cancer patients with significant others
c. Women with gynecologic or breast cancer or males with testicular or prostate cancer
d. The interaction of variables such as age, depression, and activity status on the psychosocial aspects of sexual health

1.135 Which of the following systemic treatments for breast cancer is *least* likely to cause impairment in sexual function?
a. Monthly goserelin injections
b. Monthly goserelin injections plus tamoxifen
c. Chemotherapy alone
d. Tamoxifen alone

1.136 Following four courses of chemotherapy, Albert shows you that his fingernails have developed transverse white lines or grooves. You explain to Albert that this symptom
a. Is a response to doxorubicin because pigmentation has been deposited at the base of the nail
b. Indicates a reduction or cessation of nail growth in response to cytotoxic therapy
c. Reflects a cytotoxic reaction to cyclophosphamide
d. Is a partial separation of the nail plate called onycholysis and is a reaction to 5-FU therapy

1.137 Because of the staging of her cancer, the size of the tumor, and a number of other factors, Marcia will undergo immediate breast reconstruction after her surgery. Her surgeon has explained that the procedure most likely to be used in her case is the TRAM flap. You explain to Marcia that this will involve removing tissue from her _____ and tunneling it to the mastectomy site.
a. Abdominal muscle
b. Latissimus dorsi muscle
c. Lower abdomen
d. Buttocks

1.138 Two basic nursing interventions for alterations in sexual health encountered by cancer patients are
a. Education and counseling
b. Screening and role playing
c. Affective therapy and role modeling
d. Enhancing reality surveillance and reinforcing personal power

1.139 Sexuality in the cancer patient may be affected by the following factors *except*
a. Psychosexual changes associated with mutagenicity
b. Physiologic problems of fertility and sterility
c. Psychologic issues such as loss of self-esteem and fears of abandonment
d. Changes in body appearance resulting from therapy

1.140 Mrs. Archer has recently had a radical cystectomy with resection of nearly one-third of the anterior wall of the vagina. She is approaching discharge and requires teaching regarding any changes she can expect in terms of her sexuality. It would be appropriate to include which of the following in your discussion?
a. The diameter of the introitus and the vaginal barrel may be compromised due to the surgery.
b. Intercourse may be restricted, even painful.
c. The clitoris may be injured or have compromised function because of scarring and fibrosis after surgery.
d. All of the above

1.141 Radiation is commonly used in conjunction with surgery as treatment for vaginal cancer. Patient education before discharge would include which of the following?
   a. Vaginal fibrosis and scarring can occur due to a loss of blood supply; therefore vaginal intercourse is to be minimized.
   b. Vaginal intercourse and the use of a vaginal dilator are encouraged to prevent narrowing of the vagina.
   c. Water-soluble lubricants or prescribed estrogen cream are effective measures to minimize functional loss.
   d. All of the above

1.142 Mrs. Parnell received a bone marrow transplant and total body irradiation as treatment for her leukemia. She is 2 years posttransplant and returns for a doctor visit complaining of vaginal dryness, dyspareunia, lack of energy, and loss of femininity. Your assessment and management of her complaints are based on which of the following?
   a. These symptoms are common following treatment for leukemia and are likely due to the radiation.
   b. Approximately 50% of women experience fatigue and lack of energy following transplant that is severe enough to interfere with sexual function.
   c. Most women experience depression and anxiety regarding sexual function following transplant, and she needs a referral to a psychologist.
   d. a and b

1.143 An individual's body image is affected by all of the following *except*
   a. Feedback from significant others and significant events
   b. What one perceives as an "ideal" body or image
   c. How one's body actually looks and functions
   d. The various elements that refer to psychological self

Alopecia

1.144 According to the World Health Organization's criteria for grading alopecia, the primary difference between a grade 3 and a grade 4 toxicity is which of the following?
   a. Grade 3 refers to patchy loss and grade 4 refers to complete hair loss.
   b. Grade 3 refers to complete hair loss and there is no grade 4.
   c. Grade 3 refers to complete but reversible hair loss and grade 4 refers to nonreversible complete hair loss.
   d. Grade 3 refers to patchy hair loss and grade 4 refers to nonreversible complete hair loss.

1.145 When documenting patterns of hair loss due to chemotherapy, it is important to include *all but* which of the following assessment criteria?
   a. Family history of male pattern baldness
   b. Length, texture, and curl/wave of hair
   c. Condition of the scalp
   d. Description of patterns of hair loss over entire body

1.146 Your patient has notified you that she has intense pain across her scalp 2½ weeks after her first dose of chemotherapy. Your advice to her would include *all but* which of the following management strategies?
   a. Referral to her doctor because this could indicate skin metastases
   b. Anti-inflammatory agents to decrease inflammation
   c. Massage the scalp
   d. Warm compresses to the scalp

1.147   Research concerning the use of Minoxidil to enhance hair growth in patients receiving chemotherapy has produced which of the following results?
   a.   Patients who used Minoxidil as directed experienced significantly less hair loss compared to those who did not use Minoxidil.
   b.   Patients who used Minoxidil as directed experienced a reduction in the period of time required for hair regrowth.
   c.   Patients who used Minoxidil as directed experienced significantly less hair loss with chemotherapy provided they also used hypothermia at the time chemotherapy was administered.
   d.   All of the above

1.148   The degree of hair loss varies depending on the area of the body exposed to radiation, the dose, and the radiosensitivity of the exposed structures. Which of the following describes the correct order of *decreasing* radiosensitivity?
   a.   Scalp, beard, eyebrows, eyelashes, axillary, pubic, fine body hair
   b.   Fine body hair, eyebrows, eyelashes, pubic hair, scalp hair, beard
   c.   Beard, eyebrows, scalp, pubic hair, fine body hair
   d.   All body hair is equally sensitive to radiation.

1.149   Albert is about to undergo chemotherapy that is known to cause significant hair loss. Which of the following will *not* be part of your patient education plan for Albert?
   a.   Chemotherapy-induced alopecia occurs slowly and may not occur for several months after the treatment.
   b.   Once chemotherapy is complete, regrowth is visible in 4–6 weeks.
   c.   Complete regrowth of hair may take 1–2 years.
   d.   In situations involving very high doses of alkylating agents, hair may not regrow.

1.150   A woman with breast cancer is being treated with six courses of oral cyclophosphamide for 14 days and methotrexate and 5-fluorouracil injections on days 1 and 8 every 28 days. She is very upset about the possibility of losing her hair. The *most appropriate* response to her concerns regarding hair loss would include which of the following?
   a.   Reassure her that although she will have significant hair loss, it will grow back.
   b.   Assure her that it is likely she will not lose any hair at all.
   c.   Inform her that hair loss is gradual over the next 2 months, and she will require a wig sooner rather than later.
   d.   Let her know that her hair will likely thin, but she will probably not require a wig.

1.151   Your patient asks whether there is anything he or she can do to prevent hair loss with chemotherapy. Which of the following would *not* be an appropriate response?
   a.   Minoxidil might be helpful to prevent hair loss.
   b.   Avoid washing or combing the hair for as long as possible.
   c.   High doses of vitamin E have been shown to help prevent hair loss with chemotherapy.
   d.   All of the above

1.152 A patient being treated with radiation to an abdominal field is concerned about hair loss that she expects to experience following radiotherapy. You can best reassure her by telling her that
    a. Hair follicles are relatively radioresistant due to their low rate of growth and mitotic activity.
    b. Radiation response is seen mostly in tissues and organs that are within the treatment field.
    c. Alopecia is permanent only when radiation is administered in low doses over an extended period of time.
    d. Alopecia is more closely associated with brachytherapy than with teletherapy.

1.153 Chemotherapy agents damage the hair most when it is in which phase of hair growth?
    a. Anagen
    b. Catagen
    c. Telogen
    d. Transitional

1.154 Which of the following chemotherapy agents is *least likely* to cause hair loss?
    a. Cyclophosphamide
    b. Docetaxel
    c. Vinorelbine
    d. Etoposide

Cultural Issues

1.155 Which of the following is the leading cause of cancer death in women in developing countries such as Thailand, Vietnam, and Colombia?
    a. Ovarian cancer
    b. Cervical cancer
    c. Breast cancer
    d. Gastrointestinal cancer

1.156 According to research, which of the following statements concerning breast health of African-American women of lower socioeconomic status compared to age-adjusted non-Hispanic white women is accurate?
    a. When offered free mammograms, African-American women obtained significantly fewer (17% vs. 60%) mammography screenings.
    b. Premature deaths from breast cancer is higher in African-American women (37% vs. 28% per 100,000).
    c. African-American women experience lower relative 5-year survival rates (73% vs. 88%).
    d. All of the above

1.157 In the Asian culture illnesses such as cancer are believed to be due to which of the following?
    a. An imbalance between *yin* and *yang*
    b. A curse by a spirit/spiritual imbalance
    c. An obstruction of *chi* (an essential life energy)
    d. All of the above

1.158   Respect for cultures other than one's own and for people's specific beliefs and behaviors that emanate from their cultural background is known as
   a.   Multiculturalism
   b.   Cultural sensitivity
   c.   Ethnoculturalism
   d.   Developing rapport

1.159   Strategies for designing effective culturally sensitive patient education programs include which of the following?
   a.   Consulting with key members of the cultural community in designing the program
   b.   Limiting involvement of members of the community in program development
   c.   Presenting the program to the community leaders for their support
   d.   Teaching educational programs in high school

1.160   The first line of treatment in Hispanic cultures is the use of
   a.   Home remedies
   b.   Prayer
   c.   Conventional Western medicine
   d.   Holistic medicine

1.161   Among the high-risk behaviors in the Hispanic population are
   a.   Obesity
   b.   Heavy over-the-counter and street drug use
   c.   Voodoo practices
   d.   All of the above

1.162   In Native American cultures, the singers are those healers who
   a.   Can transform themselves into other forms of life to maintain cultural integration at a time of great cultural stress
   b.   Diagnose the cause of disharmony and may indicate a cure; their primary interest is care for souls
   c.   Treat illnesses and disharmony by laying on of hands, massage, sweat baths, and the use of herbs and roots
   d.   All of the above

1.163   In a culture plagued by poverty, secondary prevention may be absent because of
   a.   A lack of insurance or inability to pay for service
   b.   A present orientation where survival needs take precedence over screening and early detection
   c.   Limited care access
   d.   All of the above

1.164   Helen is preparing to discuss options with a patient who speaks only Spanish. Helen speaks only English. If given a choice, Helen will probably want to choose the use of
   a.   A professional interpreter
   b.   A family member as interpreter because the family is an integral part of treatment delivery and involvement in most Hispanic cultures
   c.   A friend as interpreter because of the emotional support friends lend in a Hispanic extended-family social structure and because a friend is more likely than family to relay the complete message
   d.   Any of the above, as long as the interpreter is fluent in both languages

1.165 The basic unit of society is the
   a. Family
   b. Social structure
   c. Religious structure
   d. Relationship of ethnicity and culture to role assignment

Loss of Personal Control

1.166 According to the Common Sense Model, a person who experiences cancer-related symptoms processes information about these symptoms in which of the following ways?
   a. By evaluating the symptom and obtaining feedback
   b. Cognitively and emotionally
   c. Intellectually and socially
   d. By its presentation and controllability

1.167 Key principles in teaching self-care in symptom management include
   a. Consideration of the roles and needs of the family
   b. Consideration of what barriers and facilitators exist regarding learning
   c. Consideration of baseline educational needs assessment
   d. All of the above

1.168 Your patient expresses reluctance to return to work because he feels he is being discriminated against because of his diagnosis of cancer. Your advice to him would include *all but* which of the following?
   a. Consider legal action sooner rather than later
   b. Write down what occurred in an objective manner
   c. Talk to your supervisor or human resources manager
   d. Cite the law and get help from cancer survivor organizations

1.169 The most common means of reducing uncertainty for the patient is
   a. Providing preparatory information and education
   b. Referring him or her to a professional therapist
   c. Protecting the individual from all negative information
   d. a and c

1.170 One of the principal appeals of most alternative methods of treatment to the cancer patient is their
   a. Perceived absence of risks and side effects
   b. Ready availability and modest costs
   c. Level of acceptability to family and friends
   d. High degree of efficacy and safety

1.171 Which of the following reasons is *least likely* to explain a decision by a cancer patient to explore an alternative method of treatment?
   a. A desire for greater control over the treatment process
   b. Pressure from family and friends
   c. Valid data on the efficacy of the method
   d. Resentment toward an impersonal medical system

1.172 Which of the following "directions" provides patients who are at risk for loss of decision-making ability the *best* chance of having their health care wishes carried out?
  a. Power of attorney for health care
  b. Verbal instructions to the attending physician
  c. A living will
  d. A do-not-intubate/ventilate order on admission

1.173 The federal Patient Self-Determination Act, enacted in 1991, was intended to accomplish which of the following?
  a. Provide all patients with information about patient's bill of rights
  b. Enable health care agencies to provide patients with information about their right to accept or refuse treatment
  c. Enable health care agencies to provide ways to execute advance directives
  d. b and c

1.174 Marion performs breast self-examination on a regular basis; Ginny does not. Marion is more likely to have
  a. An external locus of control
  b. A low perceived susceptibility
  c. A high perceived benefit
  d. An internal locus of control

1.175 Which of the following is one of the key issues for adult children of cancer patients?
  a. Disruption of current family relationships
  b. Behavior problems
  c. Lack of involvement in decision making regarding the parent's illness
  d. Assuming the protector role and shielding parents from discussing feelings

Depression

1.176 Which of the following statements regarding risk factors for depression in the cancer patient is *inaccurate*?
  a. A history of substance abuse increases risk for depression.
  b. Adaptation to illness tends to be greater in younger persons than in older persons.
  c. Times of treatment failure and recurrence of disease increase risk of depression.
  d. Medications commonly prescribed for cancer patients have depression as a side effect.

1.177 When assessing patients for depression, it is important to be aware of certain myths regarding depression in the individual with cancer. Which of the following statements is a myth and unsubstantiated by empirical data?
  a. Depression is expected in cancer patients and occurs more commonly in cancer patients compared to other medical-surgical patients.
  b. Suicide is a logical choice for all cancer patients because of the debilitating effects of cancer.
  c. People with cancer who are depressed are not likely to respond to medical intervention because depression is a normal response to their situation.
  d. All of the above

1.178   When screening for depression in individuals with cancer, which of the following questions has the highest sensitivity and specificity for correctly identifying depression?
a.   "Are you depressed most of the day nearly every day?"
b.   "Have you lost interest in all or almost all activities?"
c.   "Do you often feel sad or low?"
d.   "Have you lost interest in sexual intimacy?"

1.179   What is one major reason that a diagnosis of depression among cancer patients is often complicated?
a.   Some cancer patients had preexisting depressive symptoms before the diagnosis of cancer.
b.   Instruments have yet to be developed to measure depression among cancer patients.
c.   Symptoms of depression are often identical to those of anxiety.
d.   The signs and symptoms of cancer are markedly different from those of depression.

1.180   With depression, responses to a perceived loss of self-esteem may be affective, behavioral, or cognitive. Which of the following is an example of a *behavioral* response associated with depression?
a.   Lack of energy
b.   Guilt
c.   Indecisiveness
d.   Suicidal ideation

1.181   The primary criteria for assessment of depression include all of the following characteristics *except*
a.   Characteristics that are a change from previous functioning
b.   Characteristics that are persistent
c.   Characteristics that were preexistent
d.   Characteristics that occur more days than not

1.182   A nursing intervention for the treatment of patients with depression that deals with the patient's *affective* responses is
a.   Negotiating goals for increasing independence in self-care and decision making
b.   Giving permission for expression of feelings
c.   Contracting short-term goals of care that the patient can achieve
d.   Encouraging physical mobility

1.183   Unlike anxiety and depression, which of the following statements is true of hopelessness as a response of patients to the cancer experience?
a.   It involves a combination of affective, behavioral, and cognitive responses.
b.   It has not been implicated in the development of cancer or in the quantity and quality of life after diagnosis of cancer.
c.   It can be clearly distinguished from other similar concepts using the accepted defining characteristics.
d.   It appears to wax and wane with perceived changes in the patient's life.

1.184 Which of the following statements most accurately describes the relationship between family responses to a diagnosis of cancer and the responses of patients themselves?
   a. Family responses are similar to patient responses.
   b. Responses of anxiety and depression are less common among family members than among patients.
   c. Responses of hopelessness and altered sexual health are less common among family members than among patients.
   d. Family responses generally are not similar to patient responses.

1.185 Fatigue may produce anxiety or depression in some individuals with cancer. Which of the following is the best explanation for this effect?
   a. Fatigue-induced electrolyte imbalances often trigger feelings of anxiety or depression.
   b. Fatigue, anxiety, and depression have the same etiology.
   c. Treatment-induced fatigue may force the individual to give up usual social roles.
   d. Anxiety or depression frequently forces individuals with cancer to expend too much energy.

Survivorship Issues

1.186 Research results concerning overall survival of women with breast cancer indicate for the first time that which of the following is true?
   a. Anastrozole is the first aromatase inhibitor to provide an overall survival benefit, compared with tamoxifen.
   b. Anastrozole decreases the incidence of recurrence of breast cancer by 50% in postmenopausal women treated for early breast cancer.
   c. Anastrozole reduces the risk of death by nearly a third in postmenopausal women treated for early breast cancer.
   d. All of the above

1.187 According to the National Comprehensive Cancer Network guidelines, the surveillance recommendation for carriers of hereditary nonpolyposis colon cancer–associated mutations include which of the following?
   a. Colonoscopy beginning at age 40; repeat every 2 years
   b. Transvaginal ultrasound and endometrial aspirate annually, starting at age 40
   c. Colonoscopy beginning at ages 20–25; repeat every 1–2 years
   d. Transvaginal ultrasound and endometrial aspirate every 2 years starting at age 30

1.188 Survival rates from cancer have only recently begun to improve. Which of the following *most accurately* depicts the percentage of persons surviving 5 years and beyond after diagnosis?
   a. Fifty percent of adults and 60% of children survive beyond 5 years.
   b. Sixty percent of adults and 77% of children survive beyond 5 years.
   c. Sixty-five percent of adults and 85% of children survive beyond 5 years.
   d. None of the above

1.189 Which of the following statements about employment among cancer survivors is correct?
   a. Approximately 40% of cancer patients return to work after being diagnosed.
   b. The work performance of cancer survivors differs little from others hired at the same age for similar assignments.
   c. "Job-lock" refers to the situation in which cancer survivors are reluctant to accept new jobs that might involve increased responsibilities.
   d. Most federal and state laws specifically include cancer survivors among the "handicapped or disabled."

1.190   Your new position in a cancer clinic gives you the opportunity to counsel cancer survivors. You are aware that the adult cancer survivor's ability to achieve optimal physical, social, and psychologic function can be most significantly affected by
    a.   Socioeconomic considerations
    b.   Disease trajectory considerations
    c.   Physical function and cosmesis
    d.   All of the above

1.191   The most powerful predictor of cancer survival is _____ at diagnosis.
    a.   Advanced disease
    b.   Changes in appearance or body function
    c.   Comorbid physical or mental conditions
    d.   a and b

1.192   Survival analysis is defined as
    a.   The probability that an individual will live with or without cancer for a specified period of time
    b.   A time interval without evidence of recurrence of disease
    c.   An observation of individuals with cancer and a calculation of their probability of dying over time
    d.   The length of time an individual with cancer survives with evidence of disease

1.193   According to research, the ability to conceive or father a child after bone marrow transplantation is *most likely* to be related to which of the following?
    a.   Age (older patients were less likely to reverse gonadal dysfunction)
    b.   Whether or not total body irradiation is used
    c.   The use of colony-stimulating factors
    d.   a and b

1.194   Your patient, Melissa, is beginning her treatment for osteogenic sarcoma and is concerned that the chemotherapy and radiation therapy might cause congenital abnormalities in her future offspring. An appropriate response would include which of the following?
    a.   Explain that what she should be thinking about is her own situation instead of dwelling on what might never be.
    b.   Explain that this is a legitimate concern and reassure her that research has found no higher incidence of congenital malformation in the children born of women who have had treatment for cancer than in the general population.
    c.   Explain that it is difficult to answer her question because there is a much higher incidence of miscarriage in women who have been treated for cancer.
    d.   Explain that you understand how she feels and refer her for genetic counseling.

1.195   The late effects of cancer treatment on the endocrine system result from damage to the hypothalamus pituitary axis and/or to
    a.   Target organs (e.g., the thyroid, ovaries, testis)
    b.   The cortical areas of the brain
    c.   The chemical structure of key hormones (e.g., insulin)
    d.   Epithelial tissue (e.g., blood vessel linings)

1.196   Growth impairment as a late effect of treatment for cancer occurs as the result of
    a.   Overproduction of thyroxine by the thyroid gland
    b.   Deficient growth hormone release by the hypothalamus
    c.   Primary hypothyroidism
    d.   A disruption in pituitary control of several target organs

SEXUALITY

Reproductive Issues

1.197 After 18 months of intensive chemotherapy, a 32-year-old woman with breast cancer reveals to you her concern regarding the effects of cancer chemotherapy on her future children. Your counsel to her would include which of the following?
   a. There has been an increased incidence of birth defects in the offspring of women previously treated with chemotherapy.
   b. There has been no increased risk of nonhereditary cancers among offspring.
   c. There has been an increased risk of hereditary cancers among offspring.
   d. a and c

1.198 Both chemotherapy and radiation therapy are known to have teratogenetic effects on the fetus, causing spontaneous abortion, fetal malformation, or fetal death. These complications are *most likely* to happen during which trimester?
   a. First
   b. Second
   c. Third
   d. The risk to the fetus is equal among the three trimesters.

1.199 Janie is 7 months pregnant and has recently had a lumpectomy for breast cancer. She is scheduled to begin chemotherapy followed by radiation. She is debating whether to start her chemotherapy or delay it until after she has her baby. She is concerned about the effect of the chemotherapy on her baby. Your comments and counsel are based on which of the following true statements regarding the effect of chemotherapy on a developing fetus?
   a. Chemotherapy during the second and third trimesters may cause premature birth or low birth weights.
   b. Chemotherapy during the second and third trimesters is not associated with a higher incidence of congenital abnormality compared with the normal pregnancy incidence.
   c. Alkylating agents and antimetabolites are most often associated with fetal malformations during the first trimester.
   d. All of the above

1.200 The fertility of which of the following patients is most likely to be affected by chemotherapy?
   a. Kevin, who is 7 years old
   b. Dan, who is 60 years old
   c. Elaine, who is over 30
   d. Pamela, who is 15

1.201 It has been suggested that women with breast cancer wait 1–5 years after the completion of adjuvant chemotherapy before attempting conception. The rationale for this recommendation includes *all but* which of the following?
   a. Many women require tamoxifen and should avoid becoming pregnant.
   b. Pregnancy shortly after completion of chemotherapy could potentially increase risk of recurrence.
   c. Time is needed for recovery of ovarian function.
   d. Recurrence is most likely within the first 2 years after cancer therapy.

1.202 Which of the following statements about pregnancy and cancer is *false*?
  a. Most cancers do not adversely affect a pregnancy.
  b. In general, pregnancy does not adversely affect the outcome of a cancer.
  c. Therapeutic abortion has been shown to be of benefit in altering disease progression.
  d. Treatment options should be evaluated as though the patient was not pregnant, and therapy should be instituted when appropriate.

1.203 Invasion of a cervical carcinoma into underlying tissue is found in a woman during the third trimester of her pregnancy. Which of the following treatments is *most likely* to be followed?
  a. Fetal viability is awaited, and appropriate therapy is given after delivery of the baby by cesarean section.
  b. Surgery or radiation therapy, without therapeutic abortion, is undertaken immediately.
  c. A radical hysterectomy and pelvic node dissection are performed and combined with radiation therapy.
  d. Therapeutic abortion is performed immediately and followed by standard treatment for advanced disease.

1.204 Evaluation of the placenta for evidence of metastasis to the fetus is *most likely* to be carried out under which of the following situations?
  a. When the mother has received combination chemotherapy during the third trimester of pregnancy
  b. When the mother has received low doses of radiation during the first trimester of pregnancy
  c. When the mother has breast cancer or invasive cervical cancer
  d. When the mother has a melanoma or lymphoma

1.205 Which of the following is *most likely* to involve risk to the fetus whose mother is being treated for cancer?
  a. Pelvic surgery on the mother during the second trimester of pregnancy
  b. Low doses of radiation associated with diagnostic x-rays
  c. Chemotherapy during the first trimester of pregnancy
  d. The use of anesthetic agents during surgery on the mother during the second trimester of pregnancy

1.206 In a support group you are conducting for expectant mothers with breast cancer, the following question is raised: "How likely is cancer to spread from the mother to the fetus?" You explain that only a few cancers spread from the mother to the fetus. Which among the following cancers mentioned by the group is *least likely* to spread from the mother to the fetus?
  a. Melanoma
  b. Non-Hodgkin's lymphoma
  c. Leukemia
  d. Breast cancer

Sexual Dysfunction

1.207 Your 55-year-old patient with lung cancer has completed his treatment, including three cycles of chemotherapy and radiation. He expressed some problems with erectile dysfunction and states his internist seems reluctant to address the issue. Which of the following is the most appropriate response to his concerns?
  a. Erectile dysfunction is common due to the paraneoplastic component of his illness.
  b. The chemotherapy and radiation are probably the cause, and it is not likely to improve.
  c. Attention to his erectile dysfunction by his internist is overshadowed by his history of cancer and treatment.
  d. Sexual dysfunction is to be expected in someone his age.

1.208 Using a battery of quality-of-life instruments tested for reliability and validity, researchers attempted to document the long-term effects of cancer treatment and consequences of cure on quality of life. They concluded that cancer survivors enjoy quality of life similar to their neighbors in *all but* which aspect of daily life?
   a. Energy level
   b. Sexual functioning
   c. Sleep
   d. Appetite

1.209 Advocates who claim that sexuality should be a routine part of every assessment for every patient diagnosed with a chronic illness propose which of the following benefits?
   a. Routine assessment decreases embarrassment on the part of the patient and practitioner if it is viewed as a normal aspect of health care.
   b. It gives the patient permission to mention sexual difficulties to the practitioner.
   c. It gives the practitioner permission to ask specific questions when there is reason to believe sexuality related side effects are present.
   d. All of the above

1.210 Mr. Crane is about to undergo a radical prostatectomy. He is concerned about his ability to be sexually active after his surgery. Your preoperative teaching of this patient is based on which of the following factors that promote sexual function after prostatectomy?
   a. Age less than 50
   b. Stage of disease
   c. Preservation of neurovascular bundles
   d. All of the above

1.211 For patients who undergo surgery for gastrointestinal cancer, possible organic sexual dysfunction is *most closely* associated with which of the following?
   a. Placement of a colostomy
   b. Removal of rectal tissue
   c. Changes in body image
   d. Responses by family and friends

1.212 Treatments for prostate cancer have the potential to alter sexual function, even though prostate cancer occurs mostly in older men. Permanent damage to erectile function with loss of emission and ejaculation is *most likely* to occur with
   a. Radical prostatectomy
   b. Transurethral resection
   c. Bilateral orchiectomy
   d. Transabdominal resection

1.213 Assessment of a patient's alteration in sexual function includes information regarding medical, psychologic, and psychosexual status. One method for assessing sexual dysfunction includes the use of the ALARM model. ALARM is an acronym for which of the following?
   a. Assess, Learn, Arousal, Relearn, Medical data
   b. Assess, Libido, Activity, Relearn, Meditation
   c. Activity, Libido, Arousal, Resolution, Medical data
   d. Arousal, Libido, Action, Resolution, Meditation

1.214 Which of the following side effects is *least likely* to occur as a result of radiation therapy?
a. Alterations in organ function (e.g., decreased vaginal lubrication)
b. Enhanced hormonal activity (e.g., overstimulation of the hypothalamus or pituitary)
c. General or psychologic side effects of therapy that can alter sexual function (e.g., diarrhea, loss of sexual desire)
d. Primary organ failure (e.g., ovarian failure)

1.215 A patient is about to receive radiation for prostate cancer. He is concerned about sexual dysfunction as a result. As part of your patient education plan, you tell him that radiation therapy can cause sexual and reproductive dysfunction through
a. Primary organ failure
b. Alterations in organ function
c. Temporary or permanent effects of the therapy itself
d. All of the above

1.216 Which of the following has been implicated in sexual dysfunction in both men and women receiving chemotherapy?
a. Depletion of the germinal epithelium
b. Treatment with estrogens
c. Combination chemotherapy, including an alkylating agent
d. Treatment with androgens

1.217 Marcia, a patient of yours, will be starting chemotherapy in 2 weeks. She asks you to explain to her the risks and side effects of chemotherapy. You tell her all of the following *except*
a. Chemotherapy can cause ovarian failure.
b. Irregular menses are a common side effect.
c. Sexual dysfunction is normal.
d. Hot flashes and night sweats are to be expected.

1.218 The traditional bilateral retroperitoneal lymph node dissection (RPLND) results in
a. The loss of antegrade ejaculation
b. Infertility from retrograde ejaculation
c. Impaired ability to experience a normal orgasm
d. a and b

SUPPORTIVE CARE

Dying and Death

1.219 You are working with Mr. Gunther and his family, who have just discovered not only that his lung cancer has recurred, but also that it is terminal this time. Which is *not* likely to be true regarding Mr. Gunther's psychosocial needs?
a. When coping with a difficult disease like lung cancer, it is the discovery of meaning in the disease that gives one a sense of mastery.
b. The recurrence of lung cancer can be a greater crisis than the initial diagnosis.
c. Often the fear of dying is not as profound as the fear of suffering in the process.
d. Patients who are allowed to indulge excessively in expressing their fears, concerns, and wishes regarding death are more prone to morbid depression.

1.220 Active euthanasia refers to
   a. The intentional taking of one's own life
   b. Direct intervention, causing death
   c. Letting a sufferer die by withdrawing life-sustaining care
   d. All of the above

1.221 The most frequently addressed factors contributing to cancer-related suicide or euthanasia are
   a. Pain and other symptom distress
   b. Advanced illness and poor prognosis
   c. Family history of suicide or personal suicide history
   d. Hopelessness and loss of self-esteem or control

1.222 The basic medical and nursing approach toward patients in a hospice program is
   a. Acute care
   b. Curative care
   c. Palliative care
   d. Euthanasia care

1.223 Which is preferable: the durable power of attorney or the living will, and why?
   a. The living will is preferable because it prevents more suffering.
   b. The durable power of attorney is preferable because it covers only terminal situations.
   c. The durable power of attorney covers not only decisions in a terminal situation, but also any treatment decisions, and therefore is preferable.
   d. The living will is better because health care providers are concerned about the ethical issues in active direct euthanasia.

1.224 The Patient Self-Determination Act provides for which of the following?
   a. The patient has a right to request euthanasia, provided it is in writing.
   b. The physician must by law inform patients of their right to determine the manner in which they will die.
   c. On admission to the hospital, all health care institutions receiving Medicare or Medicaid reimbursement must ask patients whether they have an advance directive.
   d. No patient admitted to a hospital that receives Medicare or Medicaid reimbursement may be denied terminal care at that institution.

1.225 The husband of a woman with end-stage breast cancer is concerned that his wife is sleeping more and is not even waking to eat or drink. The hospice nurse would explain to the husband that
   a. These are signs of approaching death
   b. The pain medication has reached a high blood level and needs to be reduced
   c. There is no reason to be concerned
   d. Her oncologist should be called to obtain some direction for her care

1.226 The hospice nurse may decide in the initial interview that patient criteria for hospice care will *not* be met because
   a. The patient's spouse expresses his wish to be involved in his wife's care.
   b. The patient has entered a clinical trial through the National Cancer Institute.
   c. The patient has expressed that she wishes to die without the use of narcotics.
   d. The patient does not wish to be resuscitated if she stops breathing at home.

1.227 The federal Patient Self-Determination Act requires hospices, hospitals, and other health care agencies to provide patients, on admission, with written information about which of the following?
   a. Their right to accept or refuse treatment
   b. Various ways to execute advance directives
   c. Information regarding living will and a durable power of attorney for health care
   d. All of the above

Local, State, and National Resources

1.228 Direct to Consumer Advertising (DTCA) is permitted in the United States but not in Canada, Europe, or Australian markets. Risks associated with DTCA include which of the following?
   a. DTCA increases cost of health care.
   b. Advertisements tend to overestimate drug benefits and underestimate risk.
   c. Advertisements tend to reinforce gender stereotypes.
   d. All of the above

1.229 Local and national efforts to curb smoking in public places has gained support due to research findings concerning lung cancer in never-smoking lung cancer patients. Which of the following statements regarding lung cancer incidence/survival in never-smoking lung cancer patients is *false*?
   a. The greater the exposure to second-hand smoke, the shorter the lung cancer patient's survival.
   b. Second-hand smoke is associated with worse survival among never-smoking lung cancer patients.
   c. Second-hand smoke increases risk of adenocarcinoma of the lung but not non–small cell lung cancer in persons who have never smoked.
   d. Lifetime never-smokers with lung cancer likely represent a genetically susceptible subgroup.

1.230 The primary purpose of the Health Insurance Portability and Accountability Act, or HIPAA, is to provide guidelines for which of the following?
   a. Methods to provide health insurance for the uninsured
   b. Measures to ensure each state honors insurance policies issued in other states within the United States
   c. Methods to describe how patient documents should be written and transcribed
   d. Measures to provide for electronic health care transactions and privacy

1.231 Effective cancer control is influenced *most* by which of the following?
   a. Government policy
   b. Routine chest x-rays
   c. Hygiene
   d. A low-fat diet

1.232 The goals of the Cancer Patient Education Network include which of the following?
   a. To increase cancer patient educators' access to the materials, services, and technical expertise of the National Cancer Institute's Patient Education Section
   b. To encourage networking and sharing of information among cancer patient educators
   c. To provide the patient educator with a direct link to the issues and concerns of cancer patients
   d. All of the above

1.233 Which of the following most accurately describes the philosophy of the National Hospice Organization?
   a. Patients can be made comfortable with alternative and complementary care.
   b. Euthanasia is an integral aspect of care if the patient requests it.
   c. Palliative management is centered around providing relief from suffering.
   d. Hospice is specialized care for the dying that is nonphysician-based care.

1.234 Which of the following is *not* a characteristic of the American Cancer Society?
   a. It is part of the National Cancer Institute with branches in nearly every state.
   b. It is a voluntary health agency.
   c. It sponsors several publications.
   d. It promotes advanced nursing education.

1.235 Which of the following does the federal government insist on before a drug can be marketed?
   a. The safety of the drug only
   b. The efficacy of the drug only
   c. The safety and the efficacy of the drug only
   d. The safety, efficacy, and long-term value of the drug

1.236 Guidelines for the handling of antineoplastic agents in the home are in accordance with those established by
   a. The Food and Drug Administration
   b. The Occupational Safety and Health Administration
   c. The American Nurses Association
   d. The Health Care Financing Administration

1.237 Which of the following does COBRA, a federal law passed in 1986, do?
   a. It offers extended medical coverage to those who leave jobs.
   b. It provides low-cost insurance to cancer survivors and other high-risk individuals.
   c. It provides free group health insurance to individuals not otherwise covered by medical plans.
   d. It prohibits employment discrimination against cancer survivors.

1.238 The primary function of the Cancer Information Service (CIS), sponsored by the National Cancer Institute (NCI), is to
   a. Perform diagnostic screening on large numbers of high-risk individuals
   b. Investigate suspected carcinogens in the workplace and home
   c. Set standards for potentially hazardous products
   d. Answer inquiries from the general public concerning cancer-related issues

Blood Products

1.239 Which of the following presents the best explanation for why blood-derived cells rather than bone marrow–derived cells are most often used for autologous transplantation?
   a. Bone marrow–derived cells are obtained by bone marrow aspiration, and it is more painful.
   b. Bone marrow can be contaminated by tumor cells.
   c. The procedure of obtaining cells from the bone marrow increases neutropenia.
   d. A shortened nadir period is found with blood cell transplant.

1.240 Under which of the following circumstances is administration of platelet concentrate from a single donor or human leukocyte antigen (HLA)-matched donor preferable to that of a random donor platelet concentrate?
a. When the patient is severely immunosuppressed
b. When cost is a major factor
c. When a patient's red blood cell antigens (ABO) are not known
d. When time is a major factor

1.241 Mrs. Ryan has metastatic cancer and develops fever, increased pulse rate, and flushing during her transfusion. As you are checking her vital signs, she experiences anaphylaxis. Mrs. Ryan's reaction is *most likely* due to
a. ABO incompatibility
b. Recipient antibodies against immunoglobulin in the plasma
c. Antileukocyte antibodies directed against the donor blood
d. Development of alloantibodies to transfused blood

1.242 Therapy for disseminated intravascular coagulation (DIC) often involves the administration of several substances. Which of the following is *not* a common treatment for DIC?
a. Heparin
b. Epsilon-aminocaproic acid (ACA or Amicar)
c. Vitamin K
d. Platelet replacement

1.243 A patient is to receive a blood transfusion of two units of packed red blood cells that have been irradiated. Which of the following explains the rationale for irradiating the blood?
a. To kill any possible cancer cells in the blood
b. To prevent the spread of the AIDS virus
c. To prevent graft-versus-host disease
d. To sterilize the blood

1.244 Providing leukocyte-depleted blood products to patients is intended to accomplish which of the following?
a. Prevent febrile nonhemolytic reactions
b. Prevent transmission of viral infections such as cytomegalovirus infection
c. Prevent alloimmunization to blood products
d. All of the above

1.245 Mr. Svensen, who is scheduled for surgery, expresses an interest in autologous blood donation. Which of the following parameters must be met to qualify?
a. He must be nonanemic.
b. He can donate no more than 6 units of blood before surgery.
c. The blood can be donated from 42 days to 72 hours before surgery.
d. All of the above

1.246 Ms. Daniels, who had an allogeneic bone marrow transplant, is about to receive a blood product. You must ensure that the blood has been specially treated to prevent graft-versus-host disease. This means you will check to be sure that the blood product has been
a. Exposed to alloimmunization and platelet refractoriness
b. Infiltrated with saline solution
c. Treated via plasmapheresis
d. Irradiated

1.247 Which of the following is *least likely* to be a cause of anemia in the cancer patient?
   a. Decreased red cell production
   b. Iron deficiency
   c. The primary disease process
   d. Radiation therapy

1.248 Stanley has lung cancer and is receiving chemotherapy every 3 weeks and erythropoietin subcutaneously on a weekly basis. He has been doing well but lately has begun to complain of headaches and occasional dizziness. These symptoms are *most likely* the result of which of the following?
   a. Metastatic disease in the brain
   b. Severe anemia
   c. Hypertension due to erythropoietin
   d. All of the above

Enteral and Parenteral Nutrition

1.249 Which of the following are considered contraindications to enteral nutrition?
   a. Severe diarrhea
   b. Mechanical obstructions
   c. Severe bleeding
   d. All of the above

1.250 Which of the following strategies is effective for managing regurgitation with gastrostomy feedings?
   a. Use large-bore tube
   b. Measure residuals and withhold feeding if more than 25–50 cc
   c. Consider drugs to decrease motility
   d. Place tube distally into jejunum

1.251 While receiving parenteral nutrition your patient complains of pain at the site of the catheter. Appropriate nursing action includes which of the following?
   a. Stop the infusion and assess for catheter patency.
   b. Irrigate the catheter with a small-diameter syringe.
   c. Slow the infusion and observe for swelling.
   d. Do nothing because slight discomfort is normal.

1.252 The most important role of the nurse in home parenteral nutrition (HPN) is to
   a. Keep records of times of infusion, intake, and output
   b. Deliver all supplies, equipment, and medicines to the patient
   c. Evaluate the patient, the home environment, and the family's ability to manage HPN
   d. Perform all infusion regimens at home

1.253 Total parenteral nutrition for prolonged periods or at home is indicated in *all but* which of the following situations?
   a. As a treatment for cancer cachexia
   b. Where enteral feedings are not feasible
   c. For patients with enterocutaneous fistulas
   d. For patients with acute radiation enteritis

1.254 Which of the following statements regarding enteral and parenteral nutrition is *not* accurate?
    a. Compared to parenteral nutrition, enteral nutrition is associated with more diarrhea.
    b. Compared to parenteral nutrition, enteral nutrition is associated with a higher incidence of metabolic imbalances.
    c. With enteral nutrition, normal enzymatic and mucosal activity is maintained in the gut.
    d. With parenteral nutrition, there is a higher incidence of infection.

1.255 Which of the following is considered to be a potential hazard of a macrobiotic diet?
    a. Protein deficiency
    b. Vitamin D and vitamin B_{12} deficiency
    c. Calorie and iron deficiency
    d. All of the above

1.256 Mr. Smith, who seems healthy, is scheduled for surgical resection of an esophageal lesion. Which route of administration of nutritional support do you predict is *most likely* to be appropriate for Mr. Smith immediately after surgery?
    a. Enteral nutrition
    b. Total parenteral nutrition for 7–10 days
    c. Home total parenteral nutrition
    d. None of the above

1.257 Which of the following patients would generally *not* be candidates for home parenteral nutrition?
    a. Those who are terminally ill and unable to drink fluids
    b. Those with severe enteritis due to radiation
    c. Head and neck cancer patients who have an upper airway obstruction
    d. Those patients with significant gastrointestinal malfunction

1.258 Mr. Cruz is receiving enteral nutrition every 4 hours and complains of diarrhea and cramping. The *least likely* cause of his discomfort is which of the following?
    a. The formula is probably too concentrated.
    b. The formula is probably too cold.
    c. The formula is probably infused too rapidly.
    d. The formula probably has too much fiber.

1.259 Your patient with esophageal cancer is undergoing surgery for placement of a feeding tube. The most logical explanation for using this procedure instead of parenteral nutrition is which of the following?
    a. Enteral feedings are more economical.
    b. Parenteral nutrition is associated with more metabolic complications.
    c. Enteral feedings maintain the normal stimulation of enzymatic and mucosal activity in the gut.
    d. Parenteral nutrition is indicated when the patient needs long-term nutritional support.

Rehabilitation

1.260 Which of the following points are included in the teaching plan for breast and prostate cancer patients receiving oral bisphosphonates?
    a. Oral bisphosphonates should be taken with food.
    b. The purpose of this treatment is to treat bone metastases.
    c. Oral bisphosphonates help to prevent and treat osteopenia due to hormone therapy.
    d. All of the above

1.261 Shortly after beginning therapy with an epidermal growth factor receptor inhibitor your patient experiences a macular papular rash over 25% of his body. Your nursing interventions would include *all but* which of the following?
   a. Inform the patient that this is an allergic reaction and the drug needs to be stopped.
   b. An antibacterial lotion would be appropriate.
   c. Steroid cream should be avoided.
   d. Wash the area with warm soap and water at least once a day.

1.262 Mrs. Howe is undergoing adjuvant therapy for breast cancer and asks you if it is a good idea for her to exercise while she is taking chemotherapy. Which would be the *most appropriate* response?
   a. Exercise can intensify her feelings of nausea, and she should avoid exercise for 3–4 days following her treatment.
   b. Research shows that exercise following meals relieves heartburn and is a good idea.
   c. Aerobic exercise is especially effective in relieving fatigue and is highly recommended for women undergoing adjuvant chemotherapy for breast cancer.
   d. Exercise can lead to dizziness, and she should consult with her doctor before engaging in any form of exercise.

1.263 Homeopathy is defined as a medical approach to care that emphasizes which of the following?
   a. Holistic care focuses on the whole person in their environment.
   b. Energy techniques correct physical problems with adjustments in energy flow.
   c. It is based on the theory of similars, which holds that a drug causing symptoms at full strength will cure those symptoms if it is diluted.
   d. Care of the individual and family in their own home using traditional herbal therapies is stressed.

1.264 Which of the following is considered an accepted means of communication for the person who has undergone a laryngectomy?
   a. Artificial larynx
   b. Esophageal voice
   c. Tracheoesophageal puncture
   d. All of the above

1.265 Six months after his surgery Mr. Fox, after participating in extensive speech rehabilitation, learns to speak by diverting exhaled pulmonary air through a surgically constructed fistula tract directly into the esophagus. This method of speech is produced through
   a. An artificial larynx made available immediately after surgery
   b. Esophageal voice therapy
   c. Surgical voice restoration or tracheoesophageal puncture
   d. None of the above

1.266 After surgery part of Ms. Eliot's rehabilitation process involves restoring the swallowing function, because aspiration during swallowing is one of the major complications following supraglottic laryngectomy. Initially, _____ will be the most difficult thing for Ms. Eliot to swallow without aspirating.
   a. Soft mashed foods
   b. Dry crunchy foods
   c. Liquids
   d. Hard bulky food boluses (especially meats)

1.267 After laryngectomy, heavy lifting is restricted because of the
 a. Lack of thoracic fixation
 b. Risk of aspiration
 c. Risk of hiatal hernia
 d. Reduction in cough effectiveness

1.268 A program that regards rehabilitation in cancer care as a dynamic rather than a passive process is *most likely* to emphasize both ongoing reassessment and
 a. Customary convalescence
 b. A hospital or community base
 c. Redefinition of goals
 d. Frequent nursing referrals

1.269 The overall goal of rehabilitation for the person with cancer is to
 a. Return to baseline performance before the cancer
 b. Anticipate and prepare physically for future debilitating effects of cancer
 c. Achieve optimal functioning within the limits of cancer
 d. Maintain an active busy life

1.270 Which of the following factors have been found to be *most closely* related to rehabilitation needs of the cancer patient?
 a. Medical and family history
 b. Type of treatment and side effects experienced
 c. Cancer site and stage of disease
 d. Severity or duration of disease

Vascular Access Devices

1.271 Following administration of cyclophosphamide and fluids via an implanted port, your patient complains of chills, which she states she has had in the past after her chemotherapy. You take her temperature and note a slight elevation. Subsequent nursing action would include *all but* which of the following?
 a. Let her go home and instruct her to call with any temperature elevation.
 b. Notify the doctor and prepare to draw blood cultures.
 c. Consider the presence of a septic thrombus at the catheter tip.
 d. Avoid vigorously flushing the catheter.

1.272 Which of the following skin disinfection solutions has been found to provide the best protection against central venous catheter colonization in hospitalized patients?
 a. 2% aqueous chlorhexidine
 b. 70% isopropyl alcohol
 c. 10% povidone-iodine
 d. Sterile water

1.273 Which of the following is a major advantage of the peripherally inserted central catheter?
 a. It does not require frequent flushing because of the one-way valve.
 b. Dressing changes are simpler and more cost-effective.
 c. It can be inserted at home by a certified nurse.
 d. It has a separate designated port for blood withdrawal.

1.274 The cause of extravasation in implanted ports is generally which of the following?
   a. The caustic nature of the drugs
   b. Misplaced or displaced needle
   c. Retrograde or subcutaneous leakage from percutaneously inserted catheters obstructed by a fibrin sheath
   d. b and c

1.275 Your patient has had an implanted port for 4 months. He is currently due for routine cisplatin and 5-fluorouracil. Following access with a Huber point needle, the port flushes easily with no evidence of swelling or pain. However, there is no blood return despite repositioning. The most appropriate nursing action would include which of the following?
   a. Avoid using the port if there is no blood return.
   b. Infuse fluids followed by chemotherapy as ordered.
   c. He probably has withdrawal occlusion and will benefit from a tissue plasminogen activator.
   d. b and c

1.276 An Ommaya reservoir is generally placed underneath the skin of the scalp overlying the cranium with the catheter extending to the ventricle of the brain. The purpose of this catheter placement is which of the following?
   a. Measurement of intracerebral pressure
   b. Sampling of cerebrospinal fluid for tumor cells
   c. A portal for injection of chemotherapeutic agents
   d. b and c

1.277 Which of the following statements concerning peripherally inserted central catheters (PICCs) is *not* correct?
   a. PICCs are excellent for long-term intermittent infusional therapy.
   b. PICCs can be inserted at the bedside by specially trained nurses.
   c. PICCs require sterile external site care and routine flushing.
   d. PICC lines are used for intravenous administration of antibiotics, chemotherapy, and total parenteral nutrition as well as for blood drawing.

1.278 Which of the following statements regarding use of the epidural implanted port is *not* correct?
   a. Epidural ports are used to administer intrathecal or epidural medications, including chemotherapy and analgesics.
   b. Only preservative-free medication is instilled or infused into the port.
   c. The port is flushed with preservative-free heparin after each use.
   d. A 24-gauge noncoring needle and meticulous sterile technique are used to access epidural ports.

1.279   Mr. Archer has had an implanted port for 4 weeks and recently complained of pain in his right neck and shoulder, just above the catheter insertion site. On examination you notice slight swelling over the neck, face, shoulder, and arm. He also complains that his arm is cold at times and there is some tingling in his arm and shoulder. What is the *most appropriate* action to take?
   a. These symptoms are normal following port placement and should resolve in 2–3 weeks. Have him return to the clinic in a week if he is not better.
   b. Flush the line with heparin to make sure it is not clotted.
   c. Notify the physician to examine the patient. A venogram will probably demonstrate a venous thrombosis.
   d. Notify the physician to obtain an order for a tissue plasminogen activator. The patient probably has a fibrin sheath formation around the tip of the catheter.

1.280   Ms. Charles needs a peripheral intravenous injection of doxorubicin, a known vesicant. When giving a vesicant,
   a. It is always better to have a blood return throughout the injection
   b. A smaller-gauge needle is preferable
   c. To patients with small veins, choose an angiocatheter that is thin walled with an over-the-needle cannula
   d. a and c

1.281   Which of the following factors should influence the choice of catheter used in the blood cell transplant (BCT) process for a patient?
   a. The patient undergoing BCT requires a catheter that is stiffer than the traditional central venous catheter used for autologous bone marrow transplant (ABMT).
   b. The stiff catheters used in ABMT are not necessary in BCT pheresis because there is a less rapid withdrawal of blood in BCT.
   c. High volume and pressure are needed during pheresis.
   d. a and c

Pharmacologic Interventions

Antimicrobials

1.282   Serious refractory infections occur in patients with cancer. Risk factors for development of refractory infections and sepsis include *all but* which of the following?
   a. Complex polymicrobial infections
   b. Infections lasting more than 21 days
   c. High serum albumin at the onset of symptoms of sepsis
   d. Shock associated with infection

1.283   Contraindications to ambulatory oral antimicrobial therapy for treatment of fever in neutropenia include which of the following?
   a. Hematologic malignancy
   b. Suspected pneumonia
   c. Hospital-acquired infection
   d. All of the above

1.284   After a long period of time Ms. Daniels, who had an allogeneic bone marrow transplant, develops recurrent varicella zoster virus. What is the *most likely* treatment approach?
a.   Cyclosporine
b.   Methotrexate
c.   Acyclovir
d.   Cyclosporine and methotrexate in combination

1.285   Patients with HIV and neutropenia who have received treatment with corticosteroids or who have had prolonged immunosuppression should be monitored for which of the following?
a.   Tuberculosis
b.   Second malignancies
c.   *Pneumocystis carinii* pneumonia
d.   Elevated CD4 lymphocyte count

1.286   Ribavirin is a synthetic guanosine nucleoside used to treat respiratory syncytial virus infection in blood and marrow transplant recipients. Special precautions are used when administering this therapy for which of the following reasons?
a.   Ribavirin is mutagenic.
b.   Ribavirin is gonadal toxic.
c.   Ribavirin is tumor promoting.
d.   All of the above

1.287   Which of the following measures has been found to be most consistently effective in preventing infection in the bone marrow transplant environment?
a.   Meticulous hand washing
b.   Scrupulous hygiene
c.   Protective isolation
d.   All of the above

1.288   Which of the following agents is used to prevent graft-versus-host disease in bone marrow transplant?
a.   Medroxyprogesterone acetate
b.   Cyclosporine
c.   Cyclophosphamide
d.   Dexamethasone

1.289   Risk factors for venoocclusive disease of the liver in bone marrow transplant include *all but* which of the following?
a.   Patients with hepatitis
b.   Antimicrobial therapy with acyclovir, amphotericin, or vancomycin
c.   Cytomegalovirus and fungi
d.   Chemotherapy and radiation therapy before transplant

1.290   Trimethoprim-sulfamethoxazole is generally the treatment of choice for *Pneumocystis carinii*. Which of the following is *not* usually a side effect of this drug?
a.   Nausea and vomiting
b.   Hemolytic anemia
c.   Hepatotoxicity
d.   Myelosuppression

1.291 A patient diagnosed with candida esophagitis is about to receive her first dose of amphotericin B. Which of the following is *not* a side effect of this drug?
a. Fever and chills
b. Nausea and vomiting
c. Hypertension
d. Bronchospasm

1.292 Prevention of acute side effects of amphotericin B includes *all but* which of the following?
a. Pepcid 20 mg intravenously
b. Intravenous meperidine
c. Hydrocortisone sodium succinate
d. Acetaminophen

Anti-Inflammatory Agents

1.293 The primary rationale for the use of corticosteroids in the management of arthralgias and myalgias due to taxane therapy is which of the following?
a. Corticosteroids decrease symptoms of inflammation.
b. Steroids decrease the fever associated with taxane therapy.
c. Steroids suppress muscle enzymes, which cause myalgias.
d. Steroids increase proinflammatory genes.

1.294 When patients are receiving biotherapy as their primary treatment for cancer, corticosteroids are generally avoided for which of the following reason(s)?
a. Corticosteroids mask a fever that is therapeutic.
b. Corticosteroids may block the effects of biotherapy on the immune system.
c. Corticosteroids promote prostaglandin synthesis.
d. All of the above

1.295 Nonsteroidal anti-inflammatory agents (NSAIDs) and acetaminophen are effective in pain management because they facilitate which of the following pharmacologic action(s)?
a. They are antipyretic.
b. They inhibit prostaglandin synthesis.
c. They facilitate the conversion of arachidonic acid to prostaglandins.
d. a and b

1.296 Corticosteroids and nonsteroidal anti-inflammatory drugs (NSAIDs) are commonly used in the treatment of patients with brain tumors. Which of the following are considered anticipated side effects of this therapy?
a. Hypertension and psychiatric reactions
b. Hypotension and hypoglycemia
c. Hyperglycemia and peptic ulceration
d. a and c

1.297 Elise develops graft-versus-host disease after undergoing allogeneic bone marrow transplant. Which of the following will probably *not* be part of Elise's treatment plan?
a. Systemic immunosuppressive therapy
b. Topical steroids
c. Nonsteroidal anti-inflammatory drugs
d. Fluoride therapy

1.298 James recently received chemotherapy as treatment for his bladder cancer. He asks what he should take if he gets a headache. Which among the following would be an appropriate response?
   a. Aspirin is discouraged because it can cause increased risk of bleeding.
   b. If his platelet count is below 130,000/mm^3, he should avoid taking nonsteroidal anti-inflammatory drugs.
   c. Acetaminophen does not interfere with clotting and is safe to use.
   d. All of the above

1.299 It is recommended that zoledronic acid be infused over not less than 15 minutes and that the dose not exceed 4 mg every 3–4 weeks. The rationale behind this recommendation is which of the following?
   a. Doses higher than 4 mg given in less than 15 minutes increase bone marrow suppression.
   b. Doses higher than 4 mg given in less than 15 minutes increase nausea and diarrhea.
   c. Doses higher than 4 mg given in less than 15 minutes increase renal toxicity.
   d. a and b

1.300 Which of the following drugs is *most commonly* associated with platelet dysfunction?
   a. Cimetidine
   b. Heparin
   c. Aspirin
   d. Estrogen

1.301 Which of the following *best* describes the effect that nonsteroidal anti-inflammatory drugs (NSAIDs) have on platelets?
   a. NSAIDs enhance the platelet secretory process.
   b. NSAIDs increase epinephrine-induced aggregation.
   c. NSAIDs inhibit platelet function.
   d. All of the above

1.302 Nonsteroidal anti-inflammatory drugs have been purported to prevent which of the following?
   a. Bladder cancer
   b. Breast cancer
   c. Colorectal cancer
   d. Prostate cancer

1.303 Nonsteroidal anti-inflammatory drugs (NSAIDs) are known to cause gastrointestinal (GI) side effects. The etiology of these GI effects is best explained by which of the following?
   a. NSAIDs cause GI side effects only in the presence of preexisting mucosal irritation, as would occur with chemotherapy.
   b. The increased release of prostaglandin increases GI side effects.
   c. The drugs directly irritate the GI mucosa, which is why they should be taken with an antacid.
   d. The loss of the cytoprotective effect of prostaglandin causes increased GI side effects.

Antiemetics

1.304 Aprepitant is indicated for the prevention of delayed nausea and vomiting with highly emetic chemotherapy. Which of the following statement(s) is(are) *true* in regards to its mechanism of action?
   a. Aprepitant acts to suppress all major neuroreceptors in the nausea and vomiting process.
   b. Aprepitant effectively blocks substance P, a neurokinin-1 receptor.
   c. To be effective, aprepitant must be given daily for 5 days with a serotonin antagonist.
   d. None of the above

1.305 Your patient returns for her third round of high-dose chemotherapy and states she had unrelenting nausea for a week. Which of the following factor(s) will most influence your approach to managing this problem?
   a. Neurokinin-1 receptor antagonist on days 1, 2, and 3 will help to manage delayed nausea.
   b. Serotonin levels are minimal in the delayed phase of nausea.
   c. Lorazepam is useful on days 1–4 to increase the effectiveness of other agents, and the sedation helps to decrease nausea.
   d. All of the above

1.306 The primary mechanism of action of granisetron and ondansetron as antiemetics is which of the following?
   a. Dopamine antagonist
   b. Serotonin antagonist
   c. Sedation
   d. Suppression of autonomic pathways

1.307 The primary mechanism of action of dexamethasone as an antiemetic is
   a. Anti-inflammatory
   b. Inhibits prostaglandin synthesis
   c. Dopamine antagonist
   d. Histamine receptor antagonist

1.308 Delayed nausea and vomiting occurs more commonly with which of the following agents?
   a. Carboplatin
   b. Mechlorethamine
   c. Cisplatin
   d. Vincristine

1.309 Dexamethasone is usually administered along with granisetron or ondansetron. The purpose of the dexamethasone is to do which of the following?
   a. To treat delayed nausea
   b. To prevent side effects of granisetron or ondansetron
   c. To potentiate the antiemetic effect of the granisetron or ondansetron
   d. To produce euphoria

1.310 Which of the following is *not* a side effect of the serotonin antagonists?
   a. Dizziness
   b. Constipation
   c. Extrapyramidal reactions
   d. Sedation

1.311   When highly emetogenic chemotherapy is to be administered, the patient generally receives a combination of antiemetics rather than a single drug. The rationale for the use of multiple antiemetics is which of the following?
   a.   A combination of different antiemetic agents permits the use of lower doses of each agent and is therefore more economical.
   b.   Drugs such as prochlorperizine and granisetron are synergistic in their action.
   c.   The vomiting center is directly activated by multiple pathways.
   d.   All of the above

1.312   The discovery of serotonin has greatly increased the efficacy of antiemetic protocols. Which of the following *best* describes the role of serotonin in nausea and vomiting?
   a.   Serotonin activates 5-HT$_3$ receptors on visceral and vagal afferent pathways.
   b.   Serotonin acts on dopamine receptors in the brain.
   c.   When serotonin levels are reduced by serotonin antagonists, the patient is more at risk for delayed nausea and vomiting.
   d.   Serotonin levels are increased when toxic substances such as chemotherapy drugs stimulate the parafollicular cells of the gastrointestinal tract.

1.313   Substance P/neurokinin-1 receptor antagonists are a new class of drugs. Which of the following is an example of these agents and their appropriate indication for use?
   a.   Aprepitant is used to prevent or reduce acute and delayed nausea and emesis with chemotherapy.
   b.   Atovaquone is used to treat taste alterations.
   c.   Dapsone is used to prevent or treat retrovirus, common in immunosuppressed patients.
   d.   Gabapentin is used to treat respiratory congestion in patients with end-stage disease.

1.314   Mrs. Levy is noticeably anxious as she waits for her chemotherapy to be administered. This is her fourth cycle of chemotherapy, including cyclophosphamide orally (days 1–14), and methotrexate and 5-fluorouracil intravenously on days 1 and 8. She states that she felt nauseated yesterday and still feels sick today. Which of the following best describes the etiology of her nausea and the appropriate nursing action?
   a.   Her symptoms are likely due to something she ate. She will benefit from prochlorperzine.
   b.   The cyclophosphamide is probably causing her nausea. Prochlorperzine each day and intravenous granisetron and dexamethasone with her chemotherapy injection are appropriate.
   c.   Anticipatory nausea and vomiting occur in roughly 60% of patients on CMF, and she will benefit from behavioral modification and lorazepam.
   d.   She should be referred to the psychooncologist for desensitization because her symptoms are psychological in origin.

Analgesic Regimens

1.315   Which of the following opioids is/are *not* recommended for cancer pain?
   a.   Demerol
   b.   Darvocet
   c.   Tramadol
   d.   a and b

1.316 Patients with metastatic disease to the bone who have little benefit from nonsteroidal anti-inflammatory drugs (NSAIDs) and steroids are *most likely* to benefit from which of the following systemic therapies?
   a. Mithramycin
   b. Zoledronic acid
   c. Saline hydration
   d. Calcitonin

1.317 Which of the following statements regarding the transdermal fentanyl system is *not* accurate?
   a. Twelve to 16 hours is needed after application of the patch to achieve a therapeutic effect and 18 hours to achieve a steady state in the blood.
   b. Fentanyl is equal to morphine in potency.
   c. Approximately 92% of the drug is absorbed into the systemic circulation by 72 hours.
   d. Chronic administration in the elderly can lead to toxicity due to saturation of storage sites.

1.318 The drug used to treat respiratory depression related to opioid analgesics is
   a. Naproxen
   b. Methadone
   c. Meperidine
   d. Naloxone

1.319 Which of the following is *not* a common side effect of opioids?
   a. Sedation
   b. Respiratory depression
   c. Increased motility
   d. Constipation

1.320 Antidepressants such as amitriptyline may be used to treat pain that is caused by
   a. Tumor infiltration of nerves
   b. Narcotic withdrawal
   c. Brain metastases
   d. Surgery

1.321 Mrs. Villegas experiences extreme sedation as a result of her course of opioid analgesics. There are no other central nervous system problems, and she is in severe pain when the opioid dose is lowered. _____ may be indicated.
   a. Antihistamines
   b. Steroids
   c. Biphosphonates
   d. Psychostimulants

1.322 Steroids are sometimes used in the management of pain related to
   a. Bowel obstruction
   b. Spinal cord compression
   c. Trigeminal neuralgia
   d. Tumor pressing on a vital organ

1.323   Scheduling of oral analgesics generally should be
    a.   At fixed intervals
    b.   Every 2 hours
    c.   As needed
    d.   Related to a patient's activity level

1.324   The nursing diagnoses for patients receiving intraspinal opioids would include *all but* which of the following?
    a.   Potential alteration in respiratory function
    b.   Potential alteration in comfort related to pruritus, nausea, and vomiting
    c.   Potential alteration in cardiac function
    d.   Potential infection at the catheter site

1.325   Which of the following statements regarding administration of morphine sulfate external release capsule (Avinza) is *not* correct?
    a.   Avinza is available in capsule form and is swallowed whole once a day.
    b.   Avinza uses the spheroidal oral drug absorption system technology to provide extended release.
    c.   If the patient is unable to swallow, the contents of the capsule may be crushed and administered via a nasogastric tube.
    d.   Avinza should not be used in patients taking monoamine oxidase inhibitors.

Psychotropic Drugs

1.326   When administering psychotropic agents along with opioid analgesics, it is important to counsel the patient's family concerning which of the following?
    a.   Psychostimulants can interfere with the therapeutic effect of opioid analgesics.
    b.   Psychostimulants may increase agitation and confusion.
    c.   Psychostimulants may increase complaints of fatigue and anorexia.
    d.   All of the above

1.327   While caring for a terminally ill patient who is receiving high doses of opioids you notice nocturnal myoclonus. Which of the following constitutes an appropriate therapeutic intervention?
    a.   The opioid dose should be reduced by 25%.
    b.   Naloxone should be given to reverse the opioid effect.
    c.   The dose of the opioid should be reduced by 50% and a benzodiazepine added.
    d.   a and b

1.328   Cannabinoids such as Marinol are generally used as second-line antiemetics. Which of the following is a side effect of cannabinoids?
    a.   Dysphoria
    b.   Disorientation
    c.   Impaired concentration
    d.   All of the above

1.329   The clinical efficacy of antidepressants in persons with cancer is thought to be caused by which of the following?
    a.   Antidepressants exert effects on the 5-HT neurotransmission system.
    b.   Antidepressants act as stimulants and promote wakefulness.
    c.   Antidepressants act to dull awareness of one's situation.
    d.   Antidepressants suppress serotonin and block serotonin receptor uptake.

1.330 Allison has shingles that was successfully treated, but she was instructed to take an antidepressant for approximately 2 weeks. Which of the following explains the purpose of the antidepressant?
   a. Treatment for postherpetic neuralgia
   b. Treatment for her depression
   c. To inhibit uptake of the neurotransmitters into nerve terminals
   d. a and c

1.331 Which of the following has been shown to increase toxicity from antidepressant medications?
   a. A history of liver dysfunction or liver failure
   b. Chronic alcohol use
   c. Isoniazid therapy
   d. All of the above

1.332 Patients with advanced cancer are at a heightened risk for suicide. Which of the following has been identified as a significant risk factor for suicide in these patients?
   a. Complaints of unmanaged symptoms
   b. Increasing need for physical and social support
   c. Increasing use of narcotics to manage pain
   d. Weight loss

1.333 Lorazepam is commonly used in combination antiemetic therapy. Side effects of this drug include *all but* which of the following?
   a. Addiction
   b. Drowsiness
   c. Amnesia
   d. Diarrhea

1.334 Mr. Goodie has complained of feeling more depressed over the last 2 weeks. He had been taking his Prozac faithfully but stopped taking it a week ago when he was started on a new antidepressant, Parnate, a monoamine oxidase inhibitor, which he started 3 days ago. He now presents with mental status changes, including severe agitation and insomnia. The best explanation for his current symptoms includes which of the following?
   a. He is experiencing normal reactions to the new antidepressant. These symptoms will subside over 3–4 days.
   b. The Prozac is still in his system and is causing a drug interaction.
   c. Once a patient is on a serotonin uptake inhibitor, a monoamine oxidase inhibitor is generally not sufficient to treat the depression.
   d. Most antidepressants must be taken for 2 weeks to reach therapeutic levels.

1.335 Methylphenidate (Ritalin) is commonly added to opioid analgesics when used to treat chronic pain. What is the purpose of the methylphenidate in this instance?
   a. To act as an antidepressant
   b. To counteract the respiratory depression of the opioid analgesics
   c. To counteract the sedation of the opioid analgesics
   d. To act on the cortex and reticular activating system to decrease awareness of pain

1.336   In the weeks before death many patients on opioid therapy experience agitation, confusion, and difficulty sleeping, especially at night. Which of the following medications is most therapeutic for patients experiencing these symptoms?
   a.   Amitriptyline, for its anticholinergic effect
   b.   Lorazepam, for its sedating effect
   c.   Promethazine, because it potentiates the analgesic effect of opioids
   d.   Haloperidol, to combat confusion and agitation

Growth Factors

1.337   Colony-stimulating factors act on the stem cells to specifically mediate which of the following steps in hematopoiesis?
   a.   Cellular proliferation
   b.   Cellular differentiation
   c.   Stem cell maturation
   d.   All of the above

1.338   Granulocyte and granulocyte-macrophage colony-stimulating factors
   a.   Increase febrile episodes
   b.   Decrease myelosuppression
   c.   Increase mucositis
   d.   Decrease anorexia

1.339   Overexpression of epidermal growth factor receptors has been found to correlate with a poor prognosis in which of the following?
   a.   Breast cancer
   b.   Bladder cancer
   c.   Glioblastoma
   d.   All of the above

1.340   Hematopoietic growth factors (HGFs) are given to prevent infection in potentially neutropenic patients. These injections achieve which of the following?
   a.   Decrease the time from the administration of the drug to the onset of the nadir
   b.   Decrease the activity of mature cell lineages, thereby preserving them for the period of neutropenia and infection
   c.   Enhance phagocytosis, antibody-dependent cytotoxicity, and chemotaxis
   d.   Enhance neutrophil regeneration

1.341   Which of the following is *not* considered a primary reason to administer colony-stimulating factors to patients receiving chemotherapy?
   a.   To permit administration of full doses of the chemotherapy agents
   b.   To decrease infectious complications
   c.   To shorten the period of febrile neutropenia
   d.   To prevent neutropenia in all patients receiving chemotherapy

1.342   Which of the following is considered to be the *most* potent stimulus for erythropoietin production?
   a.   Hemoglobin less than 9 g/dL
   b.   Hypoxia
   c.   Hematocrit less than 30 g/dL
   d.   Active bleeding

1.343 Procrit (epoetin alfa) is contraindicated in patients with which of the following medical conditions?
a. Chronic diarrhea
b. Renal insufficiency
c. Uncontrolled hypertension
d. Glaucoma

1.344 Granulocyte colony-stimulating factor is intended to accomplish which of the following?
a. Decrease the duration of neutropenia related to chemotherapy
b. Decrease the number of episodes of neutropenic fever
c. Decrease the number of hospital days in patients receiving chemotherapy
d. All of the above

1.345 Hematopoietic growth factors are used as supportive therapy for which of the following conditions?
a. A patient undergoing modified radical mastectomy
b. A patient with severe cachexia
c. A patient receiving myelosuppressive therapy or a bone marrow transplantation
d. A patient with iron-deficiency anemia

1.346 Hematopoietic growth factors approved by the U.S. Food and Drug Administration (FDA) include all of the following agents *except*
a. Granulocyte-macrophage colony-stimulating factors
b. Interleukin-2
c. Granulocyte colony-stimulating factors
d. Interleukin-11

1.347 Hematopoietic growth factors (HGFs) are administered not sooner than 24 hours after chemotherapy for which of the following reasons?
a. HGFs could increase cell kill of white blood cell precursor cells if given before 24 hours postchemotherapy.
b. Myalgias and arthralgias are enhanced when HGFs are given before 24 hours postchemotherapy.
c. HGFs are ineffective when given before 24 hours postchemotherapy.
d. All of the above

1.348 Epidermal growth factor receptors have recently been found to be an important prognostic indicator in breast cancer. Which of the following statements regarding the relationship between epidermal growth factor receptors and breast cancer is *false*?
a. The presence of the epidermal growth factor receptor means that a woman is most likely to be estrogen receptor (ER) and progesterone receptor positive.
b. The presence of the epidermal growth factor receptor means the patient has a poor prognosis.
c. Inhibiting growth factor receptors is therapeutic in women with breast cancer.
d. The presence of the epidermal growth factor has implications for selection of chemotherapy protocols.

Non-pharmacologic Interventions

1.349   In a large survey concerning use of complementary and alternative medicine therapies, patients indicate they employ which of the following non-pharmacologic approaches most frequently?
   a.   Massage
   b.   Relaxation
   c.   Prayer
   d.   Special diets

1.350   Cognitive Behavioral Therapy is based on which of the following principle(s)?
   a.   Cognitive reframing
   b.   How a patient perceives a situation affects their ability to control it
   c.   A patient's ability to control a situation can be improved by changing their perspective
   d.   All of the above

1.351   Your patient complains of being somewhat depressed and does not want to take the more traditional antidepressants. She states she would like to try St. John's Wort. Your most appropriate response would be which of the following?
   a.   In studies of persons who were severely depressed St. John's Wort was not proven to be superior to placebo.
   b.   Since she is mildly depressed St. John's Wort could work for her.
   c.   She should see a psychiatrist before choosing treatment for her depression.
   d.   a and b

1.352   The underlying principle of acupuncture in health care includes which of the following?
   a.   Four secrets of enhancing energy refers to movements that improve health
   b.   Stimulation of the appropriate area helps the body correct any imbalance in the flow of energy thereby restoring balance.
   c.   Energy enhances healing by alleviating spiritual blockages
   d.   A therapeutic method that uses pressure to areas or zones that correspond to areas of the body to treat physical disorders.

ANSWER EXPLANATIONS

1.1   **The answer is b.** Cancer pain may be acute, chronic, or intermittent and often has a definable etiology, usually related to tumor recurrence or treatment. In contrast to acute pain, chronic cancer pain is rarely accompanied by signs of sympathetic nervous system arousal. The lack of objective signs may prompt the inexperienced clinician to wrongly conclude the patient is not in pain. Answer **d** is also true, but that is not what the question is asking.

1.2   **The answer is c.** The most common reason for unrelieved pain in American health care systems is the failure of staff to routinely assess pain and pain relief. Many patients silently tolerate unrelieved pain, especially if they are not specifically asked about it.

1.3   **The answer is d.** Changing the dosing regimen or route of the same drug helps to achieve a constant blood level rather than the high peak serum levels that often cause side effects. In general, all strong opioid analgesics have similar side effects, with the exception of fentanyl and oxymorphone, which have little propensity to release histamine, which often causes itching and urticaria. Adding caffeine to counteract sedation or a laxative and nutrition counseling to control constipation or antiemetics for nausea are appropriate to help the patient tolerate the pain medicine.

1.4   **The answer is a.** TCAs, gabapentin, lidocaine patch 5%, and tramadol are effective agents for the treatment of neuropathic pain, diabetic neuropathy, and postherpetic neuralgia. Sedation and orthostatic hypotension are common, which is why TCAs are given at bedtime and may limit the concomitant use of opioid analgesics. The use of low-dose TCAs for neuropathic pain in addition to regular-dose selective serotonin reuptake antidepressants for concurrent depression is common, but Prozac and Paxil block the metabolism of TCAs and may increase their blood levels markedly. This drug interaction is not a problem with citalopram (Celexa) and escitalopram (Lexapro).

1.5   **The answer is d.** When consumed, about 25% of the fentanyl that dissolves in saliva is rapidly absorbed through the oral mucosa; an additional 25% is swallowed and absorbed more slowly through the gastrointestinal tract. Plasma concentrations peak approximately 5–10 minutes after lozenge consumption, which typically takes 15 minutes. Although it may be used off-label, it is indicated only for breakthrough pain in patients with malignancies who already are receiving and who are tolerant to opioid therapy for their underlying cancer pain.

1.6   **The answer is c.** Counterirritant cutaneous stimulation (e.g., massage, heat or cold therapy, transcutaneous electrical nerve stimulation) is thought to help relieve pain by somehow physiologically altering the transmission of nociceptive stimuli referred to in Melzack and Wall's gate control theory of pain. It is also thought that the relief achieved may outlast the actual application of the counterirritant.

1.7   **The answer is a.** Distraction (e.g., conversation, imagery, breathing exercises, watching television) directs attention away from the sensations and emotional reactions produced by pain and blocks awareness of the pain stimulus and its effects. It can be very helpful in reducing pain, but caregivers must remember that simply because a patient is effectively distracted from the pain does not mean that he or she is pain free.

1.8   **The answer is d.** Of the five dimensions of the cancer pain experience described by Ahles et al., the cognitive dimension relates to the manner in which pain influences a person's thought processes, view of self, and the meaning of the pain.

1.9   **The answer is a.** Lorazepam is a sedative. Methylphenidate and dextroamphetamine are the most common treatments for opiate-induced daytime sedation. Donepezil is an oral acetylcholinesterase inhibitor. This class of agents increases central cholinergic activity and therefore reverses cognitive and sedative side effects of opiate treatment.

1.10 **The answer is c.** A great deal of valuable information is available in the field of pain management, but the lack of basic assessment skills, a lack of coordinated and detailed records, and inaccurate knowledge concerning pharmacologic principles all create problems for successfully managing patients' pain. Existing legal statutes and government agencies have contributed to inadequate prescribing by physicians because of fear of regulatory scrutiny.

1

Quality of Life

1.11   **The answer is c.** An assessment of behavioral parameters of pain should include the effect of the pain on activities of daily living, such as eating, mobility, and social interactions, as well as activities/behaviors that increase or decrease the intensity of pain. A behavioral assessment also considers pain behaviors used, including grimacing or other nonverbal communication and the use of medications or other pain control interventions.

1.12   **The answer is b.** Pain cues include changes in overt behaviors (aggressiveness, restlessness, and agitation), sounds (increases or decreases in verbalization or vocalization), or appearances (facial expressions or body language).

1.13   **The answer is c.** Fatigue associated with radiation therapy may be caused by anemia, an accumulation of cell destruction end products, or increased energy requirements to repair damaged epithelial tissue. Fatigue has been reported to affect 65–85% of individuals receiving radiation therapy and has been related to length of treatment, pain, depression, and weight loss. Fatigue has not been found to consistently be influenced by age, stage of disease, time since surgery, weight, or length of time since diagnosis.

1.14   **The answer is d.** In this situation she is not by definition a candidate for erythropoietin because the National Comprehensive Cancer Network guidelines establish a hemoglobin level of 10–11 g/dL as the point for initiating therapy with erythropoietin. Also, fatigue due to anemia does not get better on its own; her fatigue is more likely related to the side effects of her antiemetics. Exercise is an appropriate recommendation, especially with the breast cancer population.

1.15   **The answer is a.** Women who received chemotherapy reported low to moderate fatigue (a year post-treatment) that was significantly related to other symptoms, including poorer sleep quality and more menopausal symptoms.

1.16   **The answer is d.** Although results may be seen in 2 weeks, the time required for erythropoiesis and the red blood cell half-life, an interval of 2–6 weeks may occur between the time of a dose adjustment and significant change in hemoglobin. Patients with uncontrolled hypertension should not be treated with darbepoietin alfa. If blood pressure is difficult to control by pharmacologic or dietary means, the dose of darbepoietin alfa should be reduced or withheld. In patients with a history of congestive heart failure, an increase in the rate of rise of the hemoglobin of more than 1 g/dL in any 2-week period was associated with an increase in cardiac arrest and stroke.

1.17   **The answer is b.** The psychobiological-entropy hypothesis includes propositions that address the importance of achieving a balance between activity and rest.

1.18   **The answer is d.** A pilot study was published in 2002 regarding the efficacy of conservation of energy in the management of fatigue. Although it is somewhat effective in the sense that it is only logical, compared with exercise it is not research based. Rest and sleep are among the most frequently cited self-care strategies but are less effective in relieving fatigue than going to bed early. Motivational strategies to increase self-care beliefs as it applies to fatigue are still theoretically based.

1.19 **The answer is d.** Elderly patients are more susceptible to chemotherapy-induced hematologic toxicity than younger patients. The base number of myeloid cells does not decrease with age, but older patients with cancer are less able to mobilize these cells from the bone marrow into the bloodstream in times of stress. Older patients are chronically anemic as a result of chemotherapy, so drugs that normally bind to circulating red blood cells may reach higher concentrations in the circulation in older patients with depleted numbers of such cells, resulting in greater toxic effects.

1.20 **The answer is c.** The most commonly used definition of fatigue states that it is a sensation of tiredness and is a self-perceived state. The causes of fatigue are multifocal, but most studies address fatigue as a side effect of cancer treatment. This contrasts a national survey of oncologists, who reported that fatigue is a symptom of cancer rather than a side effect of treatment. If fatigue is a symptom, then cancer therapy should decrease the patient's fatigue instead of increasing it.

1.21 **The answer is a.** Biologic response modifiers tend to produce fatigue that is more severe than that associated with surgery, radiation therapy, and the most commonly used chemotherapy regimens.

1.22 **The answer is b.** Fatigue may persist for months after the conclusion of treatment and may in fact worsen for those patients with advanced cancer. Assistive devices may still be necessary and appropriate.

1.23 **The answer is a.** Presenting symptoms for prostate cancer rarely include generalized itching. The other diagnoses are commonly associated with generalized itching, as are vulvar cancer, gastric adenocarcinoma, central nervous system tumors, and Hodgkin's disease and non-Hodgkin's lymphoma.

1.24 **The answer is d.** Itching occurs in approximately 10% of patients receiving epidural opioids and 50% of patients receiving intrathecal opioids. The itching commonly precedes a rash. She could be hypercalcemic, but this is not the best answer. In the absence of other symptoms, itching is not a reason to stop the opioids because itching lessens over time and patients generally tolerate the itching with appropriate pharmacologic management.

1.25 **The answer is d.** Monoamine oxidase inhibitors, opioids, and alcohol can all intensify central nervous system depression in persons taking diphenhydramine HCl and should be avoided if possible. Hydroxyzine is another antihistamine and can be used if diphenhydramine HCl does not work, but it is not given concurrently.

1.26 **The answer is b.** For patients who develop chronic graft-versus-host disease, 80% have skin involvement and complain of itching and burning of the skin.

1.27 **The answer is d.** The most common adverse reactions to isosulfan blue dye during sentinel lymph node mapping for breast cancer is urticaria, a generalized rash, or pruritus.

1.28 **The answer is b.** Pruritus, which frequently accompanies jaundice, is precipitated by irritation of the cutaneous sensory nerve fibers by accumulated bile salts. The use of deodorant soaps should be avoided because they tend to dry skin and intensify pruritus.

1.29 **The answer is d.** Vitamins A, C, D, and B complex can be given to reduce the effect of jaundice, but it is not a treatment for pruritus. Meticulous skin hygiene is needed to cleanse away the accumulated bile salts. Relief is sometimes obtained with oil-based lotions, antihistamines, and cholestyramine.

1.30   **The answer is b.** In patients with Hodgkin's disease, itching is often constant and manifests as a burning sensation in the lower legs. These patients also report pruritus and painful
lymph nodes after alcohol consumption.

1.31   **The answer is d.** Pruritus, or itching, may be localized or generalized and is associated with
many medical conditions. Pruritus may occur in conjunction with thyroid disease, diabetes,
anemia, polycythemia, leukemia, multiple myeloma, adenocarcinoma, Hodgkin's disease,
non-Hodgkin's lymphoma, AIDS, and Kaposi's sarcoma. It may also occur as a consequence
of obstructive biliary disease or treatment side effects, such as dry desquamation following
radiation therapy; as a reaction to opiate analgesics; or an allergic dermatitis following
chemotherapy.

1.32   **The answer is d.** Generalized pruritus may be an early sign of systemic disease as with
Hodgkin's disease and T-cell lymphomas. In central nervous system malignancy, pruritus can
present as a paraneoplastic syndrome.

1.33   **The answer is a.** Constitutional symptoms of fever, malaise, night sweats, weight loss, and
pruritus appear in about 40% of affected patients, and these manifestations, called B symptoms, are more common in patients with advanced disease.

1.34   **The answer is a.** Although some thinning can occur, true alopecia is rare. Severe itching
and pruritus can be intense because of severe skin dryness. Rapid weight gain occurs as a
result of capillary leak syndrome. The most severe nausea, vomiting, and diarrhea occur with
interleukin-2 therapy, particularly high-dose regimens.

1.35   **The answer is a.** Environmental factors include keeping the room humidity at 30–40% and
the room temperature cool.

1.36   **The answer is a.** In both laboratory and natural settings, sleep deprivation after insomnia
has been associated with a decline in cognitive function, inability to engage in work or recre-
ational activities, loss of hedonic capacity, a sharp decline in quality of life, and alterations
to immune and neuroendocrine function.

1.37   **The answer is c.** Lung cancer patients are at least twice as likely to have insomnia compared to others with cancer. In the general population female gender increases the risk of
insomnia twofold, and this is true in the cancer population as well. Sleep disturbance also
increases with age. As with psychiatric disorders, those with a family or personal history of
sleep disturbance are more vulnerable to the onset of sleep difficulties.

1.38   **The answer is b.** Thalidomide, an antiangiogenic, immunomodulatory, and growth factor
inhibitor agent, has been associated with fatigue and somnolence. Opioid toxicity can result
in somnolence associated with hallucinations, nightmares, and confusion. Ketamine, which
is sometimes used with an opioid to increase analgesic effects, has been found to further
increase somnolence. Selective serotonin reuptake inhibitors are associated with disruptions
in sleep architecture, but not somnolence. Most cancer patients taking these medications
report improved subjective sleep quality.

1.39   **The answer is a.** Radiation therapy is commonly associated with increases in daytime
fatigue and somnolence regardless of whether the radiation therapy is for primary brain
tumors or for primary tumors in areas other than the brain. Studies indicate that radiation
results in less sleep efficiency and a higher level of daytime dysfunction and higher levels of
sleep disturbance in patients further along in their radiation treatment protocol. Other medications can disrupt her night-time sleep, causing her to be more fatigued during the day.

1.40   **The answer is d.** Although effective, the benzodiazepines have potential addictive properties, including tolerance. Discontinuation of benzodiazepines is associated with a rebound effect, where insomnia returns to higher than baseline levels. They commonly cause a next-day "hangover" effect, motor slowing, and cognitive difficulties.

1.41   **The answer is a.** The reported incidence of sleep disturbances varies from a low of 29% to a high of 90%, but most estimate that approximately 50% of patients with cancer suffer from insomnia.

1.42   **The answer is a.** Corticosteroids are frequently used in antineoplastic drug regimens and in antiemetic drug protocols and commonly cause sleep disruption, insomnia, restlessness, and increased motor activity.

1.43   **The answer is d.** Anticipatory nausea and vomiting are often brought about by the patient's previous experience with uncontrolled nausea and vomiting. Lorazepam acts as an antianxiety agent but also has some antinausea effects because it works well with other antiemetics. Sleep is an important adjunct to controlling nausea and vomiting with chemotherapy, and lorazepam is sedating.

1.44   **The answer is c.** Herbal agents can be harmful if taken over extended periods of time; kava can cause liver damage. Ginseng is a stimulant used for hypersomnia that should not be taken with monoamine oxidase inhibitors or anticoagulants. There is no evidence that lavender is addicting.

1.45   **The answer is b.** Benzodiazepines have potential addictive properties, including tolerance. They only slightly reduce sleep latency and significantly increase sleep duration. They are associated with a next-day hangover effect, motor slowing, and cognitive difficulties.

1.46   **The answer is a.** It is often difficult to distinguish whether sleep disturbances are a function of the treatment and disease factors or are instead secondary to emotional factors. Affective factors unrelated to the cancer cannot be ignored as etiologic factors in sleep disturbance.

1.47   **The answer is a.** The newer hypnotics are not benzodiazepine derivatives but act similarly without suppressing delta sleep, the stage during which physiologic restoration is thought to be the greatest.

1.48   **The answer is d.** Dyspnea is described as the "invisible" disease because the patient masks it by resting. So unless the patient has lung cancer, they are rarely asked if they are having any difficulty breathing and they are reluctant to report this symptom. Physiologic parameters are rarely present with dyspnea. Dyspnea occurs when an increase (not decrease) in the amount of respiratory muscles is required to maintain adequate breathing, such as in the presence of cachexia, where muscle wasting is occurring. The pain associated with dyspnea can be a presenting symptom of pulmonary effusion and is generally acute rather than chronic.

1.49   **The answer is c.** Continuous pulse oximetry is contraindicated because it provides no useful information and serves only to exacerbate existing fear and anxiety because the family focuses on the monitor rather than on ways to provide comfort. Although antibiotics may help to treat pneumonia, extensive testing will yield information that is immaterial to the outcome. Oxygen therapy is not indicated in the absence of hypoxemia and is not effective in treating the symptom of dyspnea. What is helpful is air therapy—room air directed at the person's face. Opioids are the first-line therapy in relieving dyspnea. Opioids decrease the intensity of dyspnea regardless of the underlying pathophysiology without causing respiratory depression. Low doses of an opioid administered on an as-needed basis are generally very effective in patients with mild to moderate dyspnea who have not previously been taking opioids.

1.50   **The answer is d.** Although it may be appropriate to suppress a dry, persistent, and debilitating cough, this should not be attempted at the expense of removal of secretions. The other strategies suggested promote comfort.

1.51   **The answer is d.** Dyspnea, although a subjective observation, is a general indication of inadequate respiration. Pleuritic chest pain may manifest as rapid shallow breathing. Intercostal retractions on inspiration indicate obstruction of air inflow, and bulging interspaces on expiration are associated with outflow obstruction; either may be an indication of tumor. Stridor is a manifestation of extrathoracic airway obstruction. The use of accessory muscles for breathing, labored prolonged expiration, and wheezing may indicate obstruction of intrathoracic airways.

1.52   **The answer is a.** Agents used for pleurodesis include bleomycin, talc, doxycycline, and minocycline. Tetracycline, formerly the most frequently used sclerosing agent, is no longer available in the injectable form.

1.53   **The answer is d.** Pleural fluid removal through an implanted port and interpleural catheter can be performed by the nurse on an outpatient basis. New technology using small-bore needles may permit management of malignant pleural effusions on an outpatient basis. These radiologically placed small-bore catheters are connected to a plastic bag with a one-way valve system for gravity drainage. In cases of recurrent effusion, a pleuroperitoneal shunt can be inserted to divert fluid from the chest cavity to the abdomen.

1.54   **The answer is d.** Respiratory rate, oxygen saturation, and arterial blood gas levels neither correlate with nor measure dyspnea. For example, patients may be hypoxemic but not dyspneic or may be dyspneic but not hypoxemic. The only reliable indicator of dyspnea in clinical practice is patient self-report.

1.55   **The answer is a.** Agitation is not a side effect of opioids. Lethargy and nausea are common side effects, and patients will become tolerant of these side effects generally within 1–2 weeks. The only side effect that patients do not reach a tolerance for is constipation.

1.56   **The answer is b.** Benzodiazepines, along with oxygen, are useful adjuncts to opioids without fear of respiratory depression, but they are not used alone as first-line therapy for dyspnea. Chlorpromazine, a major tranquilizer, and buspirone, a nonbenzodiazepine anxiolytic, both decrease dyspnea.

1.57   **The answer is d.** Although suctioning visible pooled secretions in the posterior oral cavity may be effective, suctioning is usually ineffective. It may be contraindicated because of the associated discomfort and because the site of the accumulated secretions is generally inaccessible. Anticholinergic medications, including scopolamine or glycopyrrolate, are effective for decreasing oral secretions once the patient is unable to mobilize them himself. Glucocorticoids are ineffective in managing fluid in the oral pharynx, and benzodiazepines only sedate the patient.

1.58   **The answer is a.** The purpose of the bleomycin is to obliterate the pleural space and prevent reaccumulation of fluid.

1.59   **The answer is b.** The cause of dyspnea is thought to be the decrease in cardiac output or the decrease in lung expansion by the pericardium. No adventitious sounds are heard with the disorder because pulmonary congestion is absent.

1.60   **The answer is b.** Most patients who have infection are tachycardic and tachypneic, except when the infection is so severe as to cause acidosis. Bacterial infections produce high spiking fevers with periods of return to normal. Disseminated fungal infections usually produce high spiking fevers without any such return to baseline. Viral infections may be characterized by low continuous fevers.

1.61   **The answer is d.** Intense chills and headache generally occur before fever spike and are predictable within the first 2–4 hours of administering biologics. Ways to minimize the severity of the symptoms is to administer the drug by subcutaneous injection or in the evening so the patient can sleep through the symptoms. Patients should be prepped prophylactically with acetaminophen with or without benzodiazepine to avoid symptoms from becoming so intense they have a negative impact on the patient's quality of life. They should also be informed that these symptoms, including myalgias, arthralgias, and fatigue, are common with flulike syndrome. This syndrome has been identified as one of the most common dose-limiting toxicities associated with therapy with biologics due to its interference with normal activities.

1.62   **The answer is d.** Hypersensitivity reactions are common and are related to the infusion rate. Hypotension, bronchospasm, and angioedema may occur. Stop the infusion if serious cardiac arrhythmias develop. Angina may occur postinfusion, especially in individuals with a prior history.

1.63   **The answer is d.** The nadir for high dose methotrexate is 5–7 days, and diarrhea in the presence of neutropenia requires the patient be tested for *C. difficile*, especially if the patient is also receiving antibiotics. This bacteria causes toxin release and is treated with oral vancomycin or metronidazole.

1.64   **The answer is c.** When the neutrophil count is less than $500/mm^3$, approximately 20% or more of febrile episodes have an associated bacteremia caused principally by aerobic gram-negative bacilli and gram-positive cocci.

1.65   **The answer is b.** In a study of 1130 patients with severe sepsis, only 55% had fevers greater than 38°C, 15% were hypothermic, and 30% were normothermic.

1.66   **The answer is c.** It has been demonstrated that unfiltered platelet concentrates accumulate high levels of cytokines, which can produce the signs and symptoms of a febrile transfusion reaction.

1.67   **The answer is c.** Nonhemolytic transfusion reactions are usually reversible with conservative therapy, and the transfusion may be resumed once the symptoms have subsided. Placing the patient in the Trendelenburg position and administering a fluid bolus are not ideal because of the dyspnea.

1.68   **The answer is c.** Patients who react to the Herceptin usually react the first time with the loading dose but then not again during subsequent dosing. The patients generally do very well once they have the diphenhydramine and can continue their treatment.

1.69   **The answer is b.** Spirituality refers to that dimension of being human that motivates meaning-making and self-transcendence—or intra-, inter-, and transpersonal connectedness. Spirituality prompts individuals to make sense of their universe and to relate harmoniously with self, nature, and others, including any god(s) (as conceptualized by each person). Religion is the representation and expression of spirituality. Ethics involves reflecting systematically about right conduct and how to live as a good person.

1.70   **The answer is c.** Regardless of one's beliefs about religion, prayer (liberally defined) can be a resource to all; conversational and meditative types are usually more directly correlated with spiritual well-being than petitionary and ritualistic approaches to prayer.

1.71   **The answer is b.** The process of deriving meaning in illness has been described as assisting individuals with recognizing positive outcomes from negative experiences, such as seeing the positive changes in life that may result from a cancer diagnosis.

1.72   **The answer is b.** In nursing literature that defines related terms such as spiritual distress, need, or well-being, spirituality is described as an integrating energy, a life principle, an innate human quality. In contrast to spirituality, religiosity often is viewed as a narrower concept.

1.73   **The answer is c.** Gotay found that praying, having faith, and hoping were used more often as coping strategies by women with advanced cancer than by their counterparts with early-stage cancer.

1.74   **The answer is c.** The rationale for nurses who opposed active euthanasia included personal and professional integrity, sanctity of life, and religious beliefs, and the nurses who supported active euthanasia typically cited patient autonomy, families' wishes, severe suffering, and terminal illness as reasons for supporting active euthanasia. It is important to note that private religiosity significantly influences oncology nurses' attitudes about end-of-life options.

1.75   **The answer is c.** Individuals assume that the world is meaningful and that they have worth. Traumatic events such as a cancer diagnosis can shatter these assumptions. When this happens, people work to reconstruct their world view so that it includes assumptions about the event that are wiser and more mature. Cognitive strategies that individuals use for reconstructing the assumptions include making comparisons—for example, "it could be worse." The individuals must construe their own meanings for life's traumas—the nurse cannot do this cognitive work for them.

1.76   **The answer is a.** Spirituality prompts individuals to make sense of their universe and to relate harmoniously with self and others. It motivates meaning-making for one's life.

1.77   **The answer is d.** Because of shifts in health care delivery from inpatient to outpatient due to the increased restrictions of payment, cost-control measures by other insurers, and increased out-of-pocket expenses, patients and their families must assume responsibility for self-care.

1.78   **The answer is d.** Because she works for a small business owner with fewer than 15 employees, she is not protected at the workplace by the ADA and the FMLA. She would not win a suit against her employer given these conditions. She should probably apply for Medicaid, for which she qualifies.

1.79   **The answer is a.** Because cancer is considered a disability under the ADA, employers must make reasonable accommodations. Scheduling changes are considered reasonable, but turning a full-time job into a part-time job is not required. Employers are not required to provide insurance for individuals who are no longer employees, as might be the case if the patient worked for a small business owner who could not afford insurance to cover cancer treatment.

1.80   **The answer is a.** Individuals with low annual incomes are three to seven times more likely to die of cancer than those with high annual incomes.

1.81   **The answer is b.** In the late 1970s the question of the role of poverty in the differences in incidence, mortality, and survival of different ethnic groups was first raised. The disproportionate number of African-Americans in the lower socioeconomic strata accounted for the increased incidence. However, one study concluded that poverty, not race, accounted for the 10–15% lower survival rate from cancer in many ethnic groups.

1.82   **The answer is d.** A primary barrier to cancer care for many ethnic minority populations is access to health care, especially among the socioeconomically disadvantaged. Many programs focus on providing effective cancer screening for ethnic minority populations using culturally sensitive strategies.

1.83   **The answer is b.** Historically in the United States, cancer prevention services have not been reimbursed by payers at all levels. The growth of managed care and capitation and the increasing use of primary health care providers as gatekeepers are driving the coverage of preventive services. Quality control efforts by health plans carefully monitor whether patients receive necessary preventive services. However, funding for preventive services remains inadequate, even in prepaid health systems.

1.84   **The answer is a.** A point of service (POS) plan allows members to access out-of-plan providers but imposes strict utilization strategies.

1.85   **The answer is d.** For middle- and upper-class families with adequate health insurance and relatively secure jobs, out-of-pocket expenditures for deductibles and copayments are not a concern, and with adequate insurance there are no gaps in coverage.

1.86   **The answer is c.** Increasingly, nurses are being called on to justify the resources that are needed to improve patient care. Feasibility studies and cost analysis studies, including cost–benefit analysis and cost-effectiveness analysis, are some techniques at the nurse's disposal. Feasibility studies determine whether a new program should be developed and implemented in a health care agency. Cost–benefit analysis assigns monetary value to all costs and benefits of a potential program or practice, resulting in a cost–benefit ratio. Cost-effectiveness analysis is all the costs, measured in dollars, necessary to achieve a certain benefit, calculated and expressed as cost per unit of effectiveness. This technique is used to compare relative costs of several alternatives.

1.87   **The answer is b.** Approximately 60% of uninsured Americans are in the active workforce but are employed by small companies that do not offer health coverage benefits. This category of worker will continue to increase as the number of small service-oriented companies increases and that of large manufacturing companies declines. The other factors are real but less important.

1.88   **The answer is b.** The evaluation and selection of alternative care arrangements requires individual attention to the needs and goals of the patient. Two important considerations in this selection process are cost and the patient's financial resources, including insurance coverage and benefits, and the quantity and quality of care provided by alternative care settings or agencies.

1.89   **The answer is a.** The stages of the grief process vary and are not typical for all individuals. As awareness increases, the denial decreases. In terms of public expression of grief, some individuals have resources that enable them to cope with the loss experience more efficiently. No behaviors are considered maladaptive or abnormal within a range of acceptable behavior.

1.90   **The answer is c.** Allow the patient/family members the opportunity to express their emotional response to bad news. Allow the patient/family member to cry and wait for them to stop on their own. This may be an appropriate time for silence. It is important to acknowledge their grief, and tears are an appropriate expression of grief. Only if crying is protracted or hysterical should you consider resuming your discussion at a later time.

1.91   **The answer is c.** The success of a coping strategy is determined by its outcome or intended outcome. The behavior of denial is "value neutral," meaning that it is not inherently adaptive or maladaptive. Its adaptiveness is determined by what it can or does achieve. Also, because this patient has "just been diagnosed," we may assume that not enough time has passed for us to determine whether the denial is adaptive or maladaptive.

1.92   **The answer is c.** Age is a sociodemographic factor that is predictive of psychological adjustment to cancer. Younger people report greater adjustment difficulties in comparison to older people.

1.93   **The answer is b.** When psychological boundaries are clear, they touch another boundary but do not get mixed up with the other person's priorities or goals. This is when caring is therapeutic.

1.94   **The answer is d.** A history of comorbidity (whether psychiatric or medical) and the presence of more advanced disease increases the individual's risk for poor psychosocial outcomes after a cancer diagnosis. Social networks have been found to have a protective effect with regard to psychosocial outcomes.

1.95   **The answer is b.** Three different role preferences have been identified among individuals with cancer. Between 12% and 20% of cancer patients expressed a desire to take an active role in making the final selection of treatment. A second group of 32–59% preferred passivity, allowing the physician to make the final decision about treatment. A third group of 28–40% preferred to collaborate with the physician in making decisions.

1.96   **The answer is c.** Although it is possible to achieve complete remission in 93% of children with ALL, the same drug treatment—even with the addition of an anthracycline—produces remission rates of only 70–75% in adults with ALL.

1.97 **The answer is d.** According to stress theory, individuals come to the cancer experience with a history of stress responses. Those who have been unsuccessful in resolving past stress situations, who are dealing with several stressors simultaneously, and who perceive minimal social support in the situations are at higher risk for psychosocial distress.

1.98 **The answer is c.** The primary objective of psychosocial nursing intervention usually is to encourage coping responses by patients. These interventions may be focused on problem-solving choices (**a**, **b**, and **d**) or on emotional expression. Examples of emotion-focused interventions include fostering emotional expression through active listening; creating constructive release of affective responses through play therapy, music, or humor; and providing individual or group testing and counseling to facilitate insight into emotional needs and response patterns.

1.99 **The answer is a.** Denial or minimization may be an effective coping strategy, particularly in the early stages of the disease and at stressful points in the illness trajectory (such as during recurrence). Psychosocial responses cannot be clearly identified as either adaptive or maladaptive; this depends largely on the situation and on the adaptive potential of the particular response in that situation. A perception of uncertainty can result in an appraisal of danger or opportunity, depending on the individual's definition of the situation. Distancing behaviors by health professionals enhance patients' sense of loneliness and fear. Overinvolvement with patients can be countered through supportive collegial relationships.

1.100 **The answer is a.** The idea that depression is to be expected in cancer patients is not supported by empirical data. Cancer patients are no more likely to develop depression than other medical-surgical patients. People with cancer who also suffer from depression are as likely to benefit from its treatment as anyone else. It is a myth that suicide is a logical choice for all cancer patients. With attention to the problems such as depression, unmanaged pain, or other symptoms, suicide is not common.

1.101 **The answer is a.** Fatigue is normal for many months following treatment and often occurs with other symptoms. Depression occurs most commonly when symptoms persist, lending to uncertainty in illness and fear of recurrence. The better the quality of life before diagnosis, the better the patient tolerates treatment and recovery.

1.102 **The answer is c.** Four dimensions that are typically represented in quality of life include physical, functional, psychologic, and social well-being.

1.103 **The answer is a.** The quality of life dimension of social well-being includes social support, family functioning, and intimacy. Psychological well-being refers to emotional state, including both positive and negative moods.

1.104 **The answer is d.** When patients with low and high levels of information about their disease were compared, there was a significant correspondence between patient and spouse perceptions for patient with high information. When the individual with cancer knows little about his or her disease, the couple functions under highly restrictive conditions of denial, fear, isolation, and conjecture.

1.105 **The answer is b.** Social psychologists theorize that significant losses and changes cause individuals to search for meaning as a way of trying to make sense of such a negative experience.

1.106 **The answer is d.** The overwhelming demands and complexity of care for the individual with cancer can result in caregiver burden as well as increased denial, fear and isolation.

1

Quality of Life

1.107   **The answer is c.** A detailed family assessment is important, particularly with regard to the functional abilities of the caregiver, pattern of authority, and support mechanisms available. Families are categorized as supportive, ambivalent, or hostile, and they generally continue to act as they did in previous crises.

1.108   **The answer is d.** Family units can be identified as supportive, hostile, or ambivalent, with their behavior described in terms of cohesion, adaptability, and communication. When crisis occurs or families are faced with the serious and difficult implications of cancer and its treatment, their behavior usually does not change and in some cases can intensify. Therefore if a family was dysfunctional, hostile, or in conflict, it is very likely that their behavior will continue. The home health care nurse's primary concern is to support and care for the patient. The chances are high that the home health care nurse will be unable to change the behavior of the family members in conflict.

1.109   **The answer is c.** Each individual brings to the cancer experience unique personality traits and a personal socialization pattern different from all others. Understanding the uniqueness of the individual is achieved only through study of the commonalities of the personality and social psychological (psychosocial) aspects of illness.

1.110   **The answer is d.** Intensive family therapy may be helpful in selected situations. However, research indicates that most cancer patients and significant others facing care are well adjusted without the need for intensive intervention.

1.111   **The answer is c.** Loss and grief in the care of the cancer patient is concerned with how to help patients die well. To do this they must be aware of their losses first and then embrace the impact of these losses on their life.

1.112   **The answer is d.** Grief is an experience with psychological, behavioral, social, and physical dimensions. It is a reaction to all types of serious loss, not just death. It can change over time, it is a natural reaction, its absence is indicative of pathology, and it is a process dependent on an individual's perception of the loss, independent of society's validation.

1.113   **The answer is a.** Families often believe the information they receive from health care professionals regarding coping is insufficient. The family begins to prepare for the unavoidable pain of loss and the necessary adjustments that must be made (hospice care) if sufficient information is presented to them. Families desire honest communication, despite the use of denial, as well as appropriate referrals. Denial is viewed as a healthy coping mechanism that with appropriate information will help the wife gradually accept the next level of care.

1.114   **The answer is b.** Abnormal grief may manifest itself in exaggerated or excessive expressions of normal grief reactions, such as excessive anger, sadness, or depression. For most hospice programs, therapy for abnormal grief extends beyond the scope of the bereavement care services provided. The hospice program staff should be able to identify and recommend competent referrals for abnormal grief syndromes. It is therapeutic to review a person's life with a loved one. Listening to a family member share stories of their life with the loved one honors the meaning of their relationship and their life together. Funeral planning can be therapeutic and facilitate someone's loss as they do one last thing in a special way for their loved one. Delegating responsibilities that can be overwhelming or too painful might actually be an indicator of the grieving party being aware of their limitations and calling on their resources and support systems.

1.115   **The answer is b.** It is helpful to explore previous losses and coping mechanisms used.

1.116 **The answer is b.** Unresolved grief has been associated with multiple physical and emotional illnesses, including increased risk of suicide.

1.117 **The answer is c.** It is important that the grieving individual adjust only to the environment where the deceased had been living, not unfamiliar environments.

1.118 **The answer is b.** The patient must desire palliative, not curative, treatment. Patients can receive treatments that are aimed at palliation, not cure. Blood is generally not given but can be, for palliative reasons, as can pamidronate.

1.119 **The answer is b.** Loss of a parent during adolescence has been documented as a critical event in the life of a child. Research has shown that during the illness, adolescents describe open information sharing among the family. After the death of the parent, however, adolescents assume the protector role in shielding the remaining parent from discussing distressful feelings. These adolescents frequently found the protector role extremely stressful.

1.120 **The answer is d.** A study of communication patterns between breast cancer patients and children within the family revealed that deteriorated relationships correlate with a poor prognosis for the patient and with poor adjustment scores on the measurement instruments used. The frequency and magnitude of problems with fears related to prognosis, rejection, and refusal to discuss cancer were greatest in mother–daughter relationships.

1.121 **The answer is d.** Anticipatory mourning is considered to be a normal process associated with a chronic disease, whereby a grieving person begins to work through part of his or her grief before the patient dies.

1.122 **The answer is d.** Redeker and colleagues found a cluster of symptoms that were positively correlated in patients with cancer undergoing chemotherapy. Of the symptoms, anxiety and depression had the strongest correlation. The temporal sequence or causal nature of the relationship among the variables remains unclear.

1.123 **The answer is a.** Individual counseling is the most common form of therapy provided to the patient with cancer who is experiencing anxiety. The therapist generally provides short-term psychotherapy based on a crisis intervention model.

1.124 **The answer is c.** SSNRIs target a second neurotransmitter, norepinephrine, that plays a role in triggering the "fight or flight" reaction. These medications work well for those patients who have anxiety with an overlay of depression. Because these medications take up to 2 weeks to work, the short-acting benzodiazepines may be used until they take effect.

1.125 **The answer is a.** The diagnosis of anxiety in healthy persons is made based on somatic symptoms, including anorexia, fatigue, and weight loss, which in cancer are often symptoms of the disease itself and its treatment. The symptoms of worry, distractibility, restlessness, and fearfulness are more important for diagnosing anxiety among cancer patients.

1.126 **The answer is b.** There is a wide range in estimates of prevalence for anxiety in the cancer population. However, when standardized psychiatric interviews and research diagnostic criteria are used, the range is more typically 10–30%.

1.127 **The answer is c.** Anxiety is most likely to occur when an individual experiences a non-specific internal or external stimulus that is perceived as a threat to certain beliefs, values, and conditions essential to a secure existence.

1.128 **The answer is d.** In one study, anxiety levels among the 85 patients studied were above the norms for acutely ill psychiatric patients. In addition to this finding, critical thinking was substantially reduced during hospitalization when compared with 6–8 weeks after discharge.

1.129 **The answer is c.** Loss of self-esteem is more commonly a symptom of depression. In general, nursing interventions that focus on anxiety are based on helping the patient to recognize various manifestations of anxiety, determining whether the patient desires to do anything about the response, and activating coping strategies to control anxiety levels.

1.130 **The answer is a.** Cognitive and behavioral techniques are well suited to the treatment of anxiety because the techniques are often effective not only in symptom control, but also in restoring or enhancing a sense of self-control.

1.131 **The answer is d.** Sexual dysfunction in women is due to a threefold assault on her sexual being: body image, sexual functioning, and fertility.

1.132 **The answer is c.** The most significant independent predictor of erectile dysfunction is age.

1.133 **The answer is d.** TURP commonly causes erectile dysfunction (ED) in 50% of patients. Although radical prostatectomy has been associated with a 90% risk of ED, nerve-sparing radical prostatectomy has been reported to carry a risk of ED as high as 75%, whereas external-beam radiation therapy may be associated with up to a 60% risk.

1.134 **The answer is c.** *Self-concept* is defined as the total self-appraisal of appearance, background and origins, abilities, resources, attitudes, and feelings. Most empirical studies dealing with the relationship of cancer to self-concept have focused on women with gynecologic or breast cancer or on men with testicular or prostate cancer. Additional empirical data are needed on the issues of perception of significant others' responses to the physical and psychological sequelae of cancer and on the interaction of other variables, such as age, depression, and activity status, on the physical as well as psychosocial aspects of sexual health.

1.135 **The answer is d.** In a European multicenter-controlled clinical trial, women receiving goserelin and goserelin plus tamoxifen experienced significantly higher levels of sexual dysfunction at 1- to 2-year follow-up compared with those who received no endocrine treatment. Patients treated with tamoxifen alone did not report significant sexual side effects. In contrast, women treated with chemotherapy had high and frequently increasing levels of dysfunction even after 2 to 3 years independent of treatment.

1.136 **The answer is b.** Beau's lines indicate a reduction in or cessation of nail growth in response to cytotoxic therapy.

1.137 **The answer is a.** The TRAM flap procedure is sometimes known as the "tummy tuck" because the muscle and fat are tunneled from the abdominal muscle to the mastectomy site.

1.138 **The answer is a.** Recent studies have indicated the effectiveness of education and counseling as approaches to treatment of changes in sexual health. One problem with respect to such interventions is that effectiveness is often measured in terms of resumption of sexual intercourse rather than as the effect of the intervention on self-concept or on relationships with others. Another problem is that patients are generally not screened for participation. Screening increases the probability of identifying patients and partners with preexisting problems that may require more intensive therapy.

1.139 **The answer is a.** Among the factors that affect a cancer patient's sexuality are those related to the biologic/physiologic process of cancer, the effects of treatment, the alterations caused by cancer and treatment, and the psychologic issues surrounding the patient and family. Physiologic problems of infertility and sterility, changes in body appearance, and the inability to have intercourse are enhanced by psychologic and psychosexual issues of alteration in body image, fears of abandonment, loss of self-esteem, alterations in sexual identity, and concerns about self. Mutagenicity and psychosexual changes are not closely related.

1.140 **The answer is d.** If more than the anterior third of the vaginal wall is removed, the diameter of the introitus and the vaginal barrel can be severely compromised and intercourse may be restricted. In addition, because of its close proximity to the urethral meatus, the clitoris may be injured or have compromised function because of scarring and fibrosis after surgery.

1.141 **The answer is b.** For women receiving radiation therapy to the vagina, vaginal fibrosis and scarring with a loss of blood supply and elasticity is a major adverse effect. Frequent intercourse can minimize these effects. For patients who are not sexually active, the use of a vaginal dilator with water-soluble lubricants or prescribed estrogen cream starting 2 weeks after treatment are effective prophylactic measures to minimize functional loss.

1.142 **The answer is d.** Researchers found that 50% of patients experience lack of energy and fatigue severe enough to impede normal activities. Most women experience vaginal dryness and dyspareunia after bone marrow transplant and total body irradiation.

1.143 **The answer is d.** Body image includes those elements that refer to the physical self, including how we perceive our bodies, how our bodies actually look and how they function, the impact of sensory inputs (e.g., pain), and what we perceive as an "ideal" body or image.

1.144 **The answer is c.** Grade 0 refers to no change; grade 1 refers to minimal loss; grade 2, moderate patchy loss; grade 3, complete but reversible alopecia; and grade 4, nonreversible complete hair loss. The latter may be due to excessively high-dose long-term chemotherapy (alkylating agents) with or without radiation to the scalp.

1.145 **The answer is a.** Physical exam to document patterns of hair loss include descriptions of patterns of hair loss on the scalp and over entire body; density of remaining hair; shape of the front hairline; length, texture, and curl; color and shine; and condition of the scalp. A history of male pattern baldness may be a factor in predicting hair loss but is not an assessment criteria because it relates to the timing of chemotherapy and hair loss.

1.146 **The answer is a.** Scalp pain is common approximately 3–4 days prior to hair loss. The bulb of the follicle swells as it is about to release the hair. An anti-inflammatory agent, massage, and/or heat can be helpful. Skin metastases to the scalp rarely causes scalp pain.

1.147 **The answer is b.** Research to determine Minoxidil's effect concerning prevention/retardation of hair loss has only been shown to be somewhat effective in the rat model. Researchers found Minoxidil to significantly reduce the period of time required from maximum hair loss to the point of hair regrowth (mean, 50.2 days) in women receiving adjuvant chemotherapy after breast cancer surgery.

1.148 **The answer is a.** In order of decreasing radiosensitivity are scalp, beard, eyebrows, eyelashes, axillary, pubic, and fine hair of the body.

1.149 **The answer is a.** Chemotherapy-induced alopecia occurs rapidly and usually starts 2–3 weeks following a dose of chemotherapy. After discontinuation of the epilating drugs, regrowth is visible in 4–6 weeks, but complete regrowth may take 1–2 years. In situations involving very high doses of alkylating agents, hair may not regrow.

1.150 **The answer is d.** Cyclophosphamide, 5-fluorouracil, and methotrexate commonly cause hair thinning rather than a dramatic loss of hair. The patient may not require a wig over the 6 months of treatment depending on the amount of hair the patient has to begin with.

1.151 **The answer is d.** Recommendations to minimize hair loss include using mild protein-based shampoos with conditioners, avoiding daily shampooing, allowing hair to dry naturally, and grooming hair with a wide-toothed comb. Minoxidil has not been shown to be effective in the prevention of hair loss.

1.152 **The answer is b.** Radiation response is seen mostly in tissues and organs that are within or adjacent to the treatment field (i.e., they are site specific). Thus an individual treated in the abdominal field does not lose scalp hair from radiation.

1.153 **The answer is a.** Chemotherapy agents affect actively growing (anagen) hairs. Because anagen hair is the most rapidly proliferating cell population in the human body, alopecia is a common toxicity.

1.154 **The answer is c.** Chemotherapy agents associated with only mild hair loss include uinorelbine, bleomycin, carmustine, epirubicin, 5-FU, methotrexate, mitoxantrone, and capecitabine.

1.155 **The answer is b.** In southern Thailand cervical cancer accounts for nearly 25% of all cases of cancer in women, and more than half of patients are diagnosed at stage II or higher. The world incidence rates averages about 9%.

1.156 **The answer is d.** African-American women of lower socioeconomic status obtain fewer mammograms, experience premature deaths, and have a lower survival rate.

1.157 **The answer is d.** Among Asian groups, health is a state of harmony in body, mind, and spirit with nature and the universe. A balance between hot (*yang*) and cold (*yin*) is essential for good health. Other explanations for illness include an imbalance of humoral elements, an obstruction of *chi,* a curse, a punishment for immoral behavior, or an imbalance in the body caused by exposure to wind or air.

1.158 **The answer is b.** Cultural sensitivity is having respect for cultures—and the beliefs connected with those cultures—other than your own.

1.159 **The answer is a.** Make linkages with key members of the target community, involving members of the community in the development of educational materials, programs, and community outreach strategies.

1.160 **The answer is a.** Home remedies are first-line treatment in Hispanic cultures. To cure a hot or cold imbalance, the opposite quality of the causative agent is applied.

1.161 **The answer is a.** Among the high-risk behaviors in the Hispanic population are obesity, alcohol consumption, and sexual practices.

1.162 **The answer is c.** In Native American cultures, the singers are healers who treat illnesses and disharmony by laying on of hands, massage, sweat baths, use of herbs and roots, and chanting.

1.163 **The answer is b.** In a culture of poverty, secondary prevention may be absent because of an orientation in which survival needs take precedence over screening and early detection. Delayed tertiary prevention is due to a lack of insurance, inability to pay for service, or limited care access.

1.164 **The answer is a.** The use of professional interpreters, if available, is the optimal choice. Family and/or friends may be used, but the correct or complete message may not be relayed.

1.165 **The answer is a.** The basic unit of society is the family. Cultural values can determine communication with the family, the norm for the family size, and the roles of specific family members.

1.166 **The answer is b.** According to the Common Sense Model, patients process information about their symptoms in two ways. They process cognitively, using knowledge, which assists in their making a plan for addressing the symptom. They also process information emotionally. Emotional processing can impact planning for self-care.

1.167 **The answer is d.** Evidence supports the use of appropriate teaching/learning principles when planning and implementing educational interventions. Key principles include a baseline educational needs assessment, consideration of what barriers and facilitators exist regarding learning, consideration of the roles and needs of the family, and the degree to which symptom distress impacts the individual's ability to learn.

1.168 **The answer is a.** If a patient feels discriminated against it is important to take action sooner rather than later; however, experts advise thinking about legal action only as a last resort. Other steps that should be tried first include documenting the incidents, talking to a supervisor or human resources, speaking to other coworkers who have tread this path before, and citing the law. The individual may be covered by the Americans with Disabilities Act. Also, get help from organizations that regularly help cancer survivors (Cancer Care: 800-813-HOPE).

1.169 **The answer is a.** Education assists the patient in reducing his or her sense of helplessness and inadequacy. The most common means of reducing uncertainty is to provide preparatory information about the specific aspects of the cancer experience faced by the individual. Preparatory information also prevents or alleviates treatment-related symptoms.

1.170 **The answer is a.** Individuals use alternative methods for a variety of stated reasons, such as "I have nothing to lose" or "If it won't hurt me, why not try it?" Often they are confused by conflicting reports of cure rates of standard treatments and frightened by treatment risks and possibly side effects. Many unproven methods promise no side effects and draw on the patient's fantasy of cure involving "the body's natural defenses." By using an unconventional therapy, the patient hopes for an unconventional cure.

1.171 **The answer is c.** In theory, valid data on the efficacy of an alternative method are the best reason for a patient to choose that method, but then the method would no longer be "alternative." The fact remains that none of the various alternative methods discussed in this chapter has stood up to scientific scrutiny, especially the requirement of proven efficacy in human subjects. The reasons stated in the other choices are among the most likely to motivate the cancer patient to seek an alternative therapy.

1.172 **The answer is a.** A living will may be applicable only when it pertains to a terminal illness, but not for a patient whose health is declining for medical reasons other than those that can be classified as terminal or if the patient is in a vegetative state. In general, the power of attorney for health care is more useful than the living will. The living will does not identify another person who can act as the agent for a disabled patient. Verbal instructions are of little value if a family member or anyone else chooses to argue against what has been reportedly communicated verbally. Written instructions are necessary. An order that instructs not to intubate does not address any other interventions that might be suggested.

1.173 **The answer is d.** The purpose of this legislation is to ensure that patients' wishes are carried out in the event they become mentally incapacitated or are incapable of making or communicating their decisions.

1.174 **The answer is d.** In studies of breast self-examination behavior, women who practiced breast self-examination more frequently were those who perceived an internal locus of control. This locus of control is often seen in combination with beliefs in high susceptibility and benefits.

1.175 **The answer is a.** Disruption of family relationships is a key issue for adult children of cancer patients. Behavior problems may become a key issue in the younger child, and assuming the protector role is a documented response of many adolescents to the death of a parent. Other major issues for adult children include involvement in the parent's illness, unresolved relationship problems, and coping with illness demands.

1.176 **The answer is b.** Overall adaptations to illness tends to be poorer in younger persons than in older persons. Advanced stage of disease, relapse or progression, unrelieved symptoms, medications, and body image problems have all been associated with depression. An individual or family history of depression or a history of substance abuse places the person with cancer at greater risk of depression as does disease recurrence, medications, and unrelieved symptoms.

1.177 **The answer is d.** Cancer patients are no more likely to develop depression than other medical-surgical patients. People with cancer who also suffer from depression are as likely to benefit from its treatment as any other individual. Minimal time and psychosocial skill are needed to conduct a brief assessment and make a referral. When correctable problems such as depression, unmanaged pain, or other unrelieved symptoms are dealt with an acceptable quality of life can be attained, making suicide an undesirable choice.

1.178 **The answer is a.** A variety of screening measures for depression is available. The most accurate screening interview consists of a single question: "Are you depressed most of the day nearly every day?" In a study of advanced cancer patients, this single question correctly identified all depressed individuals (100% sensitivity) and all nondepressed individuals (100% specificity). Adding more questions to the one-question screen did not increase the accuracy of the measure.

1.179 **The answer is a.** In addition, the coexistence of signs and symptoms of disease and treatment that are similar to those of depression make the diagnosis of depression difficult.

1.180 **The answer is a.** Choice **b** is an affective response; other affective responses include worthlessness, hopelessness, and sadness. Choices **c** and **d** are cognitive responses; another cognitive response is a decreased ability to concentrate. Other behavioral responses include change in appetite, sleep disturbances, withdrawal, and dependency.

1.181   **The answer is c.** Critical to establishing a diagnosis of reactive (situational) depression in cancer patients is the evaluation of selected defining characteristics commonly attributed to depression among the psychiatrically ill. Some common characteristics of depression, however, may also occur in the cancer patient as a result of the disease, its treatment, or its side effects, or they may have existed in the patient before diagnosis. Therefore the primary criteria for assessment of depression are that the characteristics are a change from previous functioning, are persistent, occur for most of the day and on more days than not, and are present for at least 2 weeks.

1.182   **The answer is b.** The other interventions listed are cognitive or behavioral in approach. Before these interventions are attempted, it is important for the nurse to acknowledge the patient's feelings associated with depression, including hopelessness, despair, anger, and guilt. The nurse can do this in many ways, starting with giving the patient permission to discuss those feelings and then demonstrating acceptance of them by attentive listening and by exploring methods for the patient to deal positively with them.

1.183   **The answer is d.** Hopelessness appears not to pervade the experience of the cancer patient, unlike anxiety and depression. Rather, it waxes and wanes with changes in perceived health, relationships, and spirituality.

1.184   **The answer is a.** Family responses of anxiety, depression, hopelessness, and altered sexual health in response to a diagnosis of cancer have been shown to be similar to those of the patients themselves.

1.185   **The answer is c.** Anxiety and depression can result from the disruption in life-style produced by fatigue. This may occur when fatigue experienced as a side effect of cancer treatment forces the individual to give up usual social roles or makes it impossible to reach desired goals.

1.186   **The answer is d.** For the first time an aromatase inhibitor has shown a survival advantage over tamoxifen in early breast cancer. By replacing tamoxifen with anastrozole, postmenopausal women treated for early breast cancer reduce the likelihood of their disease returning by almost half and, more importantly, reduce their risk of dying by nearly a third.

1.187   **The answer is c.** Colonoscopy is recommended beginning at ages 20–25, repeating every 1–2 years. Transvaginal ultrasound and endometrial aspirate is recommended annually, starting at ages 25–35.

1.188   **The answer is b.** The population of cancer survivors is increasing, with 60% of adults and 77% of children surviving now beyond 5 years after their diagnosis. Fourteen percent of all survivors alive today were diagnosed more than 20 years ago. Of the 24,040 households in the 1992 National Health Interview Survey, 63% of the respondents had a cancer diagnosis more than 5 years and 10% had a cancer diagnosis more than 25 years.

1.189   **The answer is b.** Up to 80% of cancer patients return to work after being diagnosed, and their performance differs little, if any, from others hired for similar assignments. "Job-lock" refers to survivors' fear of losing medical coverage if they changed jobs. Only a few states explicitly protect those with a history of cancer.

1.190   **The answer is d.** Four main considerations affect the adult cancer survivor's ability to achieve optimal physical, social, and psychological function: developmental considerations, disease trajectory considerations, physical function and cosmesis, and socioeconomic considerations.

1

Quality of Life

1.191   **The answer is a.** Advanced disease at diagnosis is the most powerful predictor of cancer survival.

1.192   **The answer is c.** The observation over time of individuals with cancer and the calculation of their probability of dying over several time periods is called survival analysis.

1.193   **The answer is d.** The ability to conceive or father a child after bone marrow transplantation is related to age and treatment with total body irradiation.

1.194   **The answer is b.** A review of the findings from 18 studies that included almost 1600 children born to 1078 mothers or fathers who had previously been treated for cancer indicated no increase in fetal wastage or in congenital defects noted in the offspring when compared to the general population.

1.195   **The answer is a.** The target organs most commonly affected are the thyroid, ovaries, and testes. Late effects can include alterations in metabolism, growth, secondary sexual characteristics, and reproduction.

1.196   **The answer is b.** High doses of radiation to the hypothalamic pituitary axis can damage the hypothalamus and disrupt the production of growth hormone. Growth hormone deficiency with short stature is one of the most common long-term endocrine consequences of radiation to the central nervous system in children.

1.197   **The answer is b.** The largest study of the offspring of long-term survivors involved 5,847 offspring of 14,652 survivors of childhood cancer. These researchers found no increased risk of nonhereditary cancers among offspring, no increased risk of birth defects, and no increased risk of malignancies or anomalies in the offspring.

1.198   **The answer is a.** Radiation exposure during the first trimester represents the greatest risk to the fetus. In the second or third trimester, fetal death is unlikely, but growth retardation, sterility, and cataracts are common. Chemotherapy, particularly when received during the first trimester, has been related to congenital abnormalities, with approximately 10% of fetuses experiencing some type of anomaly.

1.199   **The answer is d.** Chemotherapy in the second and third trimester may cause premature birth or low birth weight, but congenital abnormalities are not increased over the normal pregnancy incidence.

1.200   **The answer is c.** Women over the age of 30 are less likely to regain ovarian function because they have fewer oocytes.

1.201   **The answer is b.** There appears to be no decrease in survival for women who become pregnant after breast cancer treatment. In fact, some researchers believe further pregnancy may actually protect against recurrence.

1.202   **The answer is c.** Therapeutic abortion has not been shown to be beneficial in altering disease progression and should not be considered unless pregnancy will compromise treatment and thus prognosis. Therapeutic abortion is most likely to be recommended when the cancer is diagnosed at an advanced stage during the first trimester of pregnancy and the effects of combination chemotherapy are likely to damage the fetus.

1.203 **The answer is a.** During the first two trimesters, surgery or radiation therapy, without therapeutic abortion, is usually undertaken. Early-stage disease may be treated with radical hysterectomy and pelvic node dissection, whereas radiation therapy is the most common treatment in advanced disease. During the third trimester, fetal viability usually can be awaited and the infant delivered by cesarean section, after which appropriate cancer therapy can be given.

1.204 **The answer is d.** Certain malignancies, notably melanoma, non-Hodgkin's lymphoma, and leukemia, are known to spread from the mother to the fetus. If the mother has any of these cancers, the placenta should be carefully evaluated at delivery and the baby monitored for development of the disease.

1.205 **The answer is c.** Chemotherapy during the first trimester has been associated with fetal wastage, malformations, and low birth weight, although the incidence of fetal malformations is low and may be minimized or avoided with careful selection of agents. Maternal surgery can be safely accomplished with minimal risk to the fetus. Pelvic surgery is more easily accomplished during the second trimester. There is little risk to the fetus from short exposure to anesthetic agents after the first trimester, provided ventilation is adequate and hypotension is prevented. Low doses of radiation associated with diagnostic x-ray studies are not harmful if adequate fetal shielding is provided.

1.206 **The answer is d.** Only a few cancers spread from the mother to the fetus; melanoma, non-Hodgkin's lymphoma, and leukemia are the most common.

1.207 **The answer is c.** Comorbid conditions are often ignored by physicians, and therefore survivors of cancer have significantly poorer health outcomes. Compared with matched control subjects without a cancer history, the cancer survivors were more likely not to receive recommended care for a broad range of chronic medical conditions, such as angina, congestive heart failure, erectile dysfunction, and diabetes. Investigators conclude that survivors are a vulnerable population because their history of cancer may shift attention away from important health problems unrelated to cancer.

1.208 **The answer is b.** Despite using multiple measures of quality of life, sexual dysfunction as determined by Goldberg's clinical interview schedule was the only symptomatic long-term sequela of cancer treatment in cancer cases compared to neighborhood control subjects. The study cites premature menopause as the most commonly reported abnormality in females and performance dysfunctions as the most commonly reported abnormality in males treated for cancer.

1.209 **The answer is d.** Because a direct correlation between attitudes regarding sexuality and practice appears to exist, it is imperative that medical and nursing curricula incorporate teaching that improve knowledge and increase the comfort of health care professionals when discussing alterations in sexual function with patients.

1.210 **The answer is d.** The nerve-sparing procedure is recommended for patients with stage A or B disease who are eligible to undergo radical prostatectomy. Factors identified that promote sexual function after surgery are age less than 50, stage of disease, and the preservation of neurovascular bundles. In patients over 70, only 22% regain potency postoperatively, even if both neurovascular bundles are spared.

1.211   **The answer is b.** Choices **a**, **c**, and **d**, although all associated with sexual dysfunction resulting from gastrointestinal surgery, primarily are psychosexual and not organic issues. For all patients the removal of rectal tissue appears to be the most common denominator to organic sexual dysfunction. If the rectum remains intact, there rarely is an associated sexual dysfunction without direct tumor invasion.

1.212   **The answer is a.** Permanent damage to erectile function with loss of emission and ejaculation may occur with perineal resection or radical prostatectomy. Retrograde ejaculation is common with transurethral and transabdominal resection and erectile dysfunction with transabdominal resection. Bilateral orchiectomy causes sexual dysfunction through gradual diminution of libido, impotence, gynecomastia, and penile atrophy.

1.213   **The answer is c.** Evaluation of sexual dysfunction according to the ALARM model includes
A—Activity or sexual function
L—Libido or desire
A—Arousal and orgasm
R—Resolution or release
M—Medical data

1.214   **The answer is b.** Radiation therapy can cause sexual and reproductive dysfunction through primary organ failure (e.g., ovarian failure and testicular aplasia), through alterations in organ function (e.g., decreased lubrication and impotence), and through the temporary and permanent effects of therapy associated with reproduction (e.g., diarrhea and fatigue). In addition, radiation therapy can cause decreases in sexual enjoyment, ability to reach orgasm, libido, and frequency of intercourse and sexual dreams, as well as vaginal stenosis in women.

1.215   **The answer is d.** Radiation therapy can cause sexual and reproductive dysfunction through primary organ failure, through alterations in organ function, and through the temporary or permanent effects of therapy related to total dose, location, length of treatment, age, and prior fertility status.

1.216   **The answer is c.** Chemotherapy-induced reproductive and sexual dysfunction is related to the type of drug, dose, length of treatment, age, and sex of the individual receiving treatment and to the length of time after treatment, as well as to the use of single rather than multiple agents and drugs to combat side effects of chemotherapy. Combination chemotherapy including alkylating agents such as mechlorethamine have been shown to produce sexual dysfunction and to decrease fertility in both men and women. Androgen therapy affects sexual function in women; estrogen therapy affects sexual function in men. Chemotherapy may deplete the germinal epithelium that lines the seminiferous tubules in men.

1.217   **The answer is c.** Sexual dysfunction is not a normal side effect of chemotherapy. Although it is not uncommon in conjunction with breast cancer and surgery and it is more prevalent among younger women, sexual dysfunction can be treated, usually through therapy or a support group. The rest of these—ovarian failure, hot flashes, night sweats, and irregular menses—are common side effects of chemotherapy.

1.218   **The answer is d.** The traditional bilateral RPLND results in the loss of antegrade ejaculation with resultant infertility from retrograde ejaculation. The ability to experience a normal orgasm is not impaired.

1.219   **The answer is d.** The patient should be allowed to express his fears, concerns, and wishes regarding death; this can provide comfort and emotional healing. When coping with a difficult disease like lung cancer, it is the discovery of meaning in the disease that gives one a sense of mastery. The recurrence of lung cancer can be a greater crisis than the initial diagnosis. Often, the fear of dying is not as profound as the fear of suffering in the process.

1.220   **The answer is b.** Suicide is the intentional taking of one's own life. Euthanasia refers to the act of assisting or enabling a sufferer's death, preferably without pain. Active euthanasia refers to direct intervention causing death, whereas passive euthanasia refers to letting a sufferer die by withholding or withdrawing life-sustaining care.

1.221   **The answer is a.** The most frequently addressed factors contributing to cancer-related suicide or euthanasia are pain and other symptom distress.

1.222   **The answer is c.** Hospice care pivots around the idea of palliative medical management. Palliative management involves a shift in treatment goals from curative toward providing relief from suffering. Euthanasia means active interventions to hasten a person's death, and this is *not* the philosophy of hospice care.

1.223   **The answer is c.** The durable power of attorney is preferable. A living will gives advance directives for the final period of terminal illness, and the durable power of attorney covers any treatment situations at any stage in life. This document names an individual who will speak for the patient if the patient becomes incompetent to make decisions about health care.

1.224   **The answer is c.** This legislation required that all health care institutions receiving Medicare or Medicaid reimbursement ask patients they admit to the hospital whether they have an advance directive. If patients do not, the institution is obligated to provide written information about such directives.

1.225   **The answer is a.** The hospice team's goal is to help the family prepare for their loved one's death. Families need to be prepared for the actual time of the patient's death and what universal signs they can anticipate. Increasing sleep, a gradual decrease in need for food and drink, increased confusion or restlessness, decreasing temperature of extremities, and irregular breathing patterns may occur. Calling the oncologist would be indicating the need for intervention, when in fact the goal of care is purely palliative. The pain relief regimen should not be altered if the patient is comfortable, even if the patient is sleeping more and death is approaching.

1.226   **The answer is b.** Clinical trials are experimental medical trials that are implemented to determine whether there is any disease response to a new antineoplastic regimen. Patients and their families often turn to an experimental procedure when there are limited, if any, options remaining that might halt their disease progress. This choice suggests that the patient has not agreed to palliative care and is still pursuing curative treatment. Further assessment is indicated to make sure this is not the case, because a patient criterion for hospice care is that the patient is agreeable to palliative and not curative care. The remaining three options are actually patient criteria for hospice care: the patient has a primary caregiver, the patient resides in the hospice program's geographic area, and some programs require that the patient have a do-not-resuscitate status before admission to the hospice program.

1.227 **The answer is d.** The federal Patient Self-Determination Act, enacted in December 1991, requires hospices, hospitals, and other health care agencies to provide patients, on admission, with written information about two key areas: (1) their right to accept or refuse treatment under state law, and (2) ways to execute advance directives such as a living will and a durable power of attorney for health care. The purpose is to ensure that patients' wishes are carried out in the event they become mentally incapacitated or are incapable of making or communicating their decisions.

1.228 **The answer is d.** DTCA increases expenditures by patients, health care providers, tax payers, and insurers in terms of more time spent discussing issues as a result of advertising, which increases cost of care. According to the U.S. Food and Drug Administration, DTCA overestimates drug benefits and underestimates their risks. Also, studies indicate that DTCA reinforces gender stereotypes. In a study of 128 advertisements, 46% focused on reproductive or gynecologic issues. When psychiatric products were advertised, two-thirds depicted women only.

1.229 **The answer is c.** In a study of 2,465 first-degree relatives of 316 lung cancer patients who were lifetime never-smokers, researchers found that the first-degree relatives of the lung cancer patients had a 25% excess risk of any type of cancer, including breast, testicular, and lung compared with relatives in a matched control group. The risk of young-onset lung cancer was especially high among relatives of lung cancer patients compared with control subjects. Second-hand smoke exposure is associated with worse survival in early-stage non–small cell lung cancer patients, especially for second-hand smoke exposure at the workplace. These individuals also had the shortest survival.

1.230 **The answer is d.** HIPAA mandates security and privacy regulations for electronic health information.

1.231 **The answer is a.** National, state, and local governments have an impact on cancer control through legislation. Cancer control efforts are affected by the monies specifically appropriated to cancer control in the National Institutes of Health budget. The government can influence advancement in this area by setting national goals for cancer control, such as those in the Healthy People 2000 document.

1.232 **The answer is d.** The Cancer Patient Education Network has developed several resources, such as the Resource Guide to Cancer Patient Education Programs, a complete listing of planned educational programs of the National Cancer Institute–designated centers. An annual conference offers members the opportunity to share information and to explore new developments in patient education.

1.233 **The answer is c.** Hospice care is a medically directed, interdisciplinary, team–managed program of services that focuses on the patient–family as the unit of service. It has been the general experience of those who provide optimal palliative care that their patients do not need or desire euthanasia. Hospice in the United States began as an antimedical establishment and antiphysician movement. This antagonistic bias has unfortunately been a major factor in preventing hospice and palliative care principles from being applied to dying patients on a broader scale.

1.234 **The answer is a.** The American Cancer Society (ACS) and the National Cancer Institute (NCI) are separate organizations. The ACS is a nationwide voluntary health agency dedicated to eliminating cancer as a health problem by preventing cancer, saving lives, and decreasing suffering through research, education, and service. Among its activities are publications, continuing education programs, conferences, scholarships, professorships, and programs for students.

1.235 **The answer is c.** The Food and Drug Act of 1906 called for the truthful labeling of ingredients used in drugs but did not ban false therapeutic claims on drug labels. The Sherley Amendment in 1912 made it a crime to make false or fraudulent claims regarding the therapeutic efficacy of a drug, but proof of intent to defraud the customer was needed. Finally, in 1962 Congress added that drugs must demonstrate efficacy in addition to safety before they can be marketed, and a process was created by which a substance can become approved for prescription use.

1.236 **The answer is b.** Potential hazards associated with the administration of antineoplastic agents have prompted the Occupational Safety and Health Administration to set guidelines for compounding, transporting, administering, and disposing of toxic chemotherapy agents.

1.237 **The answer is a.** Under COBRA, group medical coverage is ensured to those whose circumstances warrant reducing or changing work hours or leaving the job. The employee is eligible for extended benefits for up to 18 months, and spouse and dependents receive these benefits for 36 months.

1.238 **The answer is d.** The Cancer Information Service (CIS) is a toll-free telephone service sponsored by the NCI that answers questions about cancer prevention, control, diagnosis, treatment, and rehabilitation. CIS counselors use the NCI's computerized database, Physician's Data Query, to provide state-of-the-art information to callers. The CIS also functions as a change agent in providing varied techniques to quit smoking, including basic strategies for behavior change.

1.239 **The answer is b.** One of the main reasons for using blood rather than bone marrow–derived cells for autologous transplantation is to avoid tumor contamination from bone marrow. Gene-marking experiments have clearly indicated that relapses can originate from tumor cells contaminating the cryopreserved cells. It is true that there is a shortened nadir with blood-derived cells, but it is not the best answer.

1.240 **The answer is a.** A random donor platelet concentrate may expose the recipient to multiple tissue antigens, leading to platelet refractoriness. A single donor platelet concentrate is taken from one donor or one (human leukocyte antigen) HLA-matched donor; patients are therefore not exposed to multiple antigens. This may be important with patients who are severely immunosuppressed, such as those who have undergone bone marrow transplantation.

1.241 **The answer is a.** These are signs of ABO incompatibility, which is an acute hemolytic transfusion reaction. Choice **b** is a mild allergic reaction, choice **c** is a febrile nonhemolytic reaction, and choice **d** characterizes a delayed hemolytic reaction.

1.242 **The answer is c.** Vitamin K might be administered to a patient experiencing hypocoagulability but not the hypercoagulability caused by DIC. All of the other therapies may provide short-term relief of DIC symptoms. Treatment of the underlying malignancy is vital in treating the patient with DIC, inasmuch as the tumor is the ultimate stimulus.

1.243   **The answer is c.** A serious transfusion complication in patients who are significantly immunosuppressed is the risk of developing graft-versus-host disease. It is generally recommended that all blood products given to the severely immunocompromised host be exposed to pretransfusion irradiation. Blood is irradiated to inhibit proliferation of lymphocytes without impairment of platelets, red cells, or granulocytes.

1.244   **The answer is d.** Leukocytes remaining in donor blood collected for transfusion are responsible for many of the complications related to transfusion therapy, including immunologic effects, nonhemolytic febrile reactions, and transmission of viral infections.

1.245   **The answer is d.** Nonanemic patients can donate up to 6 units of blood before surgery. Blood usually can be donated from 42 days to 72 hours before surgery.

1.246   **The answer is d.** Blood products must be irradiated to destroy T lymphocytes, which can cause graft-versus-host disease in the marrow recipient. Patients whose platelets become refractory to random platelet transfusions can receive (human leukocyte antigen) HLA-matched platelets from family or community donors, and platelets that have undergone plasmapheresis from marrow donors yield optimal increments. Alloimmunization and platelet refractoriness contribute to a 1% case fatality rate from hemorrhage complications.

1.247   **The answer is b.** The causes of anemia frequently seen in patients with cancer include decreased red cell production secondary to myelosuppressive therapy (e.g., chemotherapy and radiation therapy) and the primary disease process.

1.248   **The answer is d.** The most common side effect from erythropoietin is hypertension; therefore the patient's blood pressure should be monitored frequently. Lung cancer commonly metastasizes to the brain and presents as headache. Severe anemia is why Stanley is getting the erythropoietin, which can stop working after a while.

1.249   **The answer is d.** Additional contraindications to enteral nutrition include malabsorptive conditions, intractable vomiting, gastrointestinal fistulas and inflammatory bowel processes, and overall health prognosis not consistent with aggressive nutritional therapy.

1.250   **The answer is d.** Check tube placement, check residuals, and withhold feeding if more than 100 cc remains; keep in Fowler's position; use small-bore tube and place tube distally; and consider drugs to increase motility.

1.251   **The answer is a.** Catheter dislodgement is a common problem with parenteral feeding, and the first symptom of this problem is the patient's complaint of pain with infusion. The fluid should be stopped and the catheter checked for placement. Irrigating the catheter with a small-diameter syringe increases risk for embolism and is contraindicated.

1.252   **The answer is c.** Home care assessment for HPN begins with a visit coincidental with the arrival of equipment. The nurse should review orders for HPN with the supplying agency. The assessment should include the type and status of the venous access device, the patient's and family's knowledge of the management of HPN, and an evaluation of the home for safety factors. Adequate refrigeration should be available in the home for a 2- to 3-week supply of solutions. An electric infusion pump with a battery backup is normally part of the equipment. Choices **a** and eventually **d** are handled by the family; **b** is done by the home infusion therapy company personnel.

1.253   **The answer is a.** Total parenteral nutrition for prolonged periods or home total parenteral nutrition is indicated only in situations in which enteral feeding is not feasible because of advanced disease or severe toxicities of cancer therapies. Patients with enterocutaneous fistulas are not able to use the enteral route for nutrition because oral intake stimulates fistula output and can lead to metabolic and electrolyte disturbances.

1.254   **The answer is c.** Enteral nutrition is much preferred over parenteral nutrition whenever feasible because of the higher incidence of metabolic imbalances and infection with parenteral nutrition. Likewise, enteral nutrition helps to maintain enzymatic and mucosal activity of the gut, which is significantly altered with parenteral nutrition.

1.255   **The answer is d.** Nutritional approaches are the most commonly used questionable treatments and include macrobiotic, metabolic, and megavitamin therapy. Macrobiotic diets can result in protein, vitamins and iron deficiency.

1.256   **The answer is a.** Because Mr. Smith seems to be very healthy otherwise, enteral nutrition is the preferred route, assuming that his gastrointestinal tract is functioning. Total parenteral nutrition (TPN) for brief periods (7–10 days) may be indicated in a severely malnourished patient who cannot be fed via the enteral route. Home TPN or prolonged TPN is indicated only in situations in which enteral feeding is not feasible because of advanced disease or severe toxicities.

1.257   **The answer is a.** Terminally ill patients are not candidates for parenteral nutrition. The largest group of cancer patients receiving home parenteral nutrition are those with severe enteritis following curative radiation treatment. Patients with head and neck cancer generally have enteral nutrition but may also benefit from total parenteral nutrition.

1.258   **The answer is d.** Adding fiber to the formula helps to prevent diarrhea, as does giving the formula at room temperature, diluting it more, and giving it as a continuous infusion.

1.259   **The answer is c.** Enteral feedings, especially in the upper gastrointestinal tract, maintain the normal stimulation of enzymatic and mucosal activity in the gut, an important attribute when oral feeding is resumed.

1.260   **The answer is c.** Oral bisphosphonates are not indicated for the treatment of bone metastasis but prescribed for the prevention and treatment of osteopenia and osteoporosis from hormonal manipulations. Patients are instructed to take oral bisphosphonates on an empty stomach with a sufficient amount of water and to remain upright for 30 minutes afterward.

1.261   **The answer is a.** This is not considered an allergic reaction because it is the result of direct interference with the functions of epidermal growth factor receptor's signaling in the skin and is treated locally with antibiotics. Steroids are discouraged. The drug would only be stopped if the rash covered greater than 60% of the body with symptomatic erythroderma or if vesicular eruption or desquamation occurs.

1.262   **The answer is c.** Research involving women receiving adjuvant chemotherapy for breast cancer indicates that exercise may relieve fatigue. Patients who participated in a supervised aerobic interval training exercise program showed an improvement in fatigue measured as a component of mood, nausea, and functional capacity.

1.263   **The answer is c.** Homeopathy, a medical system developed in the late 18th century, is based on the theory of similars, which holds that a drug that causes symptoms at full strength will cure those symptoms if it is diluted. Energy techniques include reiki, healing touch, and polarity.

1

Quality of Life

1.264 **The answer is d.** Many patients may ultimately use all three speech methods at different times in the rehabilitation period: artificial larynx immediately after surgery; esophageal voice therapy a month or so after surgery; and, after a few months, surgical voice restoration or tracheoesophageal puncture.

1.265 **The answer is c.** Tracheoesophageal puncture enables the patient to divert exhaled pulmonary air through a surgically constructed fistula tract directly into the esophagus.

1.266 **The answer is c.** Liquids are the most difficult thing for the patient to swallow without aspirating.

1.267 **The answer is a.** Because of the absence of thoracic fixation after laryngectomy, the patient's ability to lift heavy objects is compromised.

1.268 **The answer is c.** The success of any cancer survival program depends on the commitment of the health care team to provide ongoing evaluation and planning for change in the lives of survivors. Under such a dynamic program, preventive and restorative goal setting become critical to a long-term survivorship trajectory that is characterized by minimal debilitation and a wellness orientation. Particular attention is also paid to the ongoing and long-range implications of financial burden imposed by cancer.

1.269 **The answer is c.** Rehabilitation refers to the process by which individuals, within their environments, are assisted to achieve optimal functioning within the limits imposed by cancer. The goals are to improve the quality of life for those experiencing cancer and to help the individual regain wholeness.

1.270 **The answer is d.** Severity or duration of disease is the factor most closely related to the cancer patient's rehabilitation needs. The physical needs frequently occurring with a variety of cancers include general weakness, limited activities of daily living, and issues related to limited mobility.

1.271 **The answer is a.** Systemic infections can be thrombus related or caused by intraluminal catheter colonization with a wide variety of infective organisms. Signs and symptoms include fever and chills, especially following vigorous flushing of the catheter. Blood cultures are taken through each lumen of the device (if applicable) as well as peripherally.

1.272 **The answer is a.** During a landmark prospective-randomized study in a surgical intensive care unit, researchers evaluated 10% povidone-iodine, 70% isopropyl alcohol, and 2% aqueous chlorhexidine skin disinfection before central venous catheter insertion and for site maintenance every other day. The chlorhexidine treatment group had a significantly decreased incidence of local catheter-related infection and infusion-related bacteremia.

1.273 **The answer is c.** The peripherally inserted central catheter (PICC) requires daily flushing and central line dressing changes as frequently as every 3–7 days. Although some PICCs have more than one lumen, any lumen can be used for blood withdrawal. The major advantage is that the catheter can be placed by specially trained nurses in the home so the patient can avoid going to the hospital or doctor's office.

1.274 **The answer is d.** In the case of implanted ports, the cause of drug extravasation is usually a misplaced or displaced needle. Another mechanism for drug extravasation from ports involves retrograde subcutaneous leakage from percutaneously inserted catheters obstructed by a fibrin sheath.

1.275 **The answer is d.** Swelling and pain are signs of catheter malfunction or displacement. In the absence of these and a catheter that flushes easily without evidence of occlusion, the lack of blood return is episodic and likely due to either a fibrin sheath or the tip of the catheter impinging on the vessel wall. Tissue plasminogen activator 2 mg instilled into the catheter following catheter flush usually results in a good blood return at the next visit. Approximately 20% of patients with implanted ports experience withdrawal occlusion periodically throughout the use of the catheter.

1.276 **The answer is d.** The Ommaya reservoir is surgically implanted through the cranium. It is placed underneath the skin with the catheter extending from the reservoir to the ventricle. It provides permanent intraventricular access for patients in whom repeated translumbar puncture is impractical. Cerebrospinal fluid is gently aspirated and sent for cytology or laboratory studies. The chemotherapy drug is administered slowly.

1.277 **The answer is a.** PICCs are ideal for short-term access (1 week to several months).

1.278 **The answer is c.** Epidural ports are flushed with 1–2 mL of sterile preservative-free saline after use. Never flush epidural lines with heparin.

1.279 **The answer is c.** Signs and symptoms of a venous thrombosis are related to impaired blood flow and include edema of the neck, face, shoulder, or arm; prominent superficial veins; neck pain; tingling of the neck, shoulder, or arm; and skin color or temperature changes. A venogram with contrast media is used to assess for a venous thrombosis.

1.280 **The answer is d.** When giving a vesicant, it is always better to have a blood return throughout the injection, so a smaller gauge needle is not preferable in that situation. For patients with small veins, choose an angiocatheter that is thin walled with an over-the-needle cannula.

1.281 **The answer is d.** A patient undergoing BCT requires a catheter that is stiffer than the traditional central venous catheter used for ABMT because of the need for high volume and pressure during pheresis.

1.282 **The answer is c.** Serious refractory infections occur in patients with cancer with complex polymicrobial infections, infections lasting more than 21 days, infectious lesions larger than 5 cm, hematologic malignancy, shock associated with infection, and low albumin at the onset of symptoms of sepsis.

1.283 **The answer is d.** Contraindications to ambulatory oral antimicrobial therapy for treatment of fever in neutropenic patients include hematologic malignancy, blood and marrow transplantation, suspected pneumonia, history of invasive fungal infection, active malignant disease, serious comorbid health conditions, and hospital-acquired infections.

1.284 **The answer is c.** Aggressive antiviral therapy with intravenous acyclovir is the standard therapy.

1.285 **The answer is c.** Patients with HIV and neutropenia, who have had prolonged treatment with corticosteroids, or who have had prolonged immunosuppression should be assessed for the development of *Pneumocystis carinii*. Because symptoms are insidious, a prolonged fever that is unresponsive to antibiotics and associated with a nonproductive cough and dyspnea on exertion may indicate infection.

1

Quality of Life

1.286   **The answer is d.** Because ribavirin is potentially mutagenic, tumor promoting, and gonadal toxic, health care workers must take precautions to reduce exposure during administration.

1.287   **The answer is d.** Anecdotal reports and clinical observations suggest that use of masks and garment covers is declining. Cost–benefit analysis does not ensure that such methods eliminate or reduce infection. Hand washing, scrupulous hygiene, and protective isolation may be the most cost-effective and meaningful conventions for infection control.

1.288   **The answer is b.** Immunosuppressive medications are aimed at removing or inactivating T lymphocytes that attack target organs. Cyclosporine and methotrexate inhibit T lymphocytes that are believed to be responsible for acute graft-versus-host disease and are the first-line therapy.

1.289   **The answer is c.** Venoocclusive disease (VOD) is almost exclusive to bone marrow transplantation (BMT) and is the most common nonrelapse life-threatening complication of preparative regimen–related toxicity for BMT. Patients at risk for developing VOD include those with hepatitis and infections before BMT and those who receive repeated doses of chemotherapy before transplant in addition to high-dose irradiation in pretransplant conditioning regimens. An additional risk factor is the use of antimicrobial therapy with acyclovir, amphotericin, or vancomycin and mismatched or unrelated allogeneic marrow grafts.

1.290   **The answer is b.** Side effects of trimethoprim include rash, nausea, vomiting, hepatotoxicity, and myelosuppression.

1.291   **The answer is c.** Amphotericin B is the drug of choice for treatment of systemic fungal infections. However, it is associated with significant side effects and toxicity, including fever, chills, rigors, nausea, vomiting, hypotension, bronchospasms, and occasionally seizures.

1.292   **The answer is a.** Premedication with acetaminophen and the addition of hydrocortisone sodium succinate to the intravenous solution generally reduces the reactions associated with the amphotericin. Intravenous meperidine can be used to ameliorate fever and chills that frequently accompany the initial administration of amphotericin.

1.293   **The answer is a.** Arthralgias and myalgias with the taxanes is thought to be due to an inflammatory process. Corticosteroids are effective because of their ability to reduce the symptoms of inflammation and inhibit a variety of proinflammatory genes. Although arthralgias and myalgias are not associated with muscle inflammation per se, corticosteroids are effective in relieving the aches and pains associated with these symptoms.

1.294   **The answer is b.** Corticosteroids are usually avoided with biotherapy because they may block the effects of these drugs on the immune system. Corticosteroids inhibit prostaglandin synthesis.

1.295   **The answer is d.** NSAIDs interfere with the enzyme prostaglandin synthetase, which blocks the conversion of arachidonic acid to prostaglandins. Prostaglandins are known to sensitize tissues to the effects of inflammatory mediators such as bradykinin. Inhibition of prostaglandin synthesis leads to relief of inflammation and pain. These agents are also antipyretic.

1.296   **The answer is d.** Adverse effects of corticosteroids and NSAIDs together include hypertension, hyperglycemia, immunosuppression, and psychiatric reactions. Although corticosteroids were previously believed to cause peptic ulcers, this effect probably occurs more with the concomitant use of NSAIDs.

1.297 **The answer is c.** Treatment strategies for graft-versus-host disease include systemic immunosuppressive therapy; topical steroids, which may or may not be beneficial; and fluoride therapy for patients at risk for caries secondary to xerostomia.

1.298 **The answer is d.** Aspirin has been demonstrated to increase the risk of bleeding. The clinical risk for bleeding associated with nonsteroidal anti-inflammatory drugs is much less than that for aspirin; however, they should be used cautiously in patients with already low platelet counts.

1.299 **The answer is c.** Because shorter infusion times and higher doses of bisphosphonates correlate with a higher incidence of renal adverse events, doses of zoledronic acid higher than 4 mg and infusion times less than 15 minutes are not recommended.

1.300 **The answer is c.** Medications such as phenothiazines, tricyclic antidepressants, heparin, cimetidine, thiazide diuretics, and estrogen may suppress platelet activity, but aspirin is the medication most commonly associated with platelet dysfunction.

1.301 **The answer is c.** Aspirin and other NSAIDs inhibit the platelet secretory process, diminish collagen-induced aggregation and epinephrine-induced aggregation, and inhibit platelet function.

1.302 **The answer is c.** An example of how chemoprevention may potentially be applied to high-risk populations is the use of nonsteroidal anti-inflammatory drugs for the prevention of colorectal cancer.

1.303 **The answer is d.** The NSAIDs inhibit cyclooxygenase in peripheral tissues, which prevents arachidonic acid from converting to prostaglandin. The loss of the cytoprotective effect of prostaglandin on the GI epithelium causes the occurrence of the GI side effects.

1.304 **The answer is b.** Substance P is the neurotransmitter that acts at neurokinin-1 receptors centrally in the brain and in the peripheral nervous system. Substance P has been shown clinically to play a role in both acute and delayed nausea and vomiting after highly emetic chemotherapy. Aprepitant effectively blocks these receptors, thereby preventing substance P from binding to the neurokinin-1 receptor sites in the medulla, resulting in inhibition of emesis.

1.305 **The answer is d.** Delayed nausea and/or vomiting occurs more than 24 hours after chemotherapy administration. It often peaks 48–72 hours after chemotherapy and can last 6–7 days. Serotonin receptor antagonists are effective on days 1–3, but after that serotonin levels drop and substance P, the neurotransmitter that acts at neurokinin-1 receptors, becomes the dominant mediator of nausea and vomiting. Benzodiazepine may or may not be given with other antiemetics because of sedating effects that are therapeutic for preventing nausea.

1.306 **The answer is b.** Successful antiemetic regimens interrupt the stimulation of the vomiting center. Combination regimens must be individualized and developed according to the emetic potential of the chemotherapy regimen, expected duration of the nausea and vomiting, and current pattern of symptoms. The addition of the serotonin inhibitors has improved the management of chemotherapy-induced nausea and vomiting. The serotonin antagonists have a different mechanism of action (compared to the dopamine antagonists such as prochlorperazine) so they are ideal to use in combination antiemetic therapy.

1

Quality of Life

1.307   **The answer is b.** The mechanism of nausea and vomiting is unclear, but prostaglandin synthesis appears to play a role. Dexamethasone appears to inhibit prostaglandin synthesis and therefore helps to prevent nausea and vomiting.

1.308   **The answer is c.** Despite effective antiemetic regimens, 93% of patients receiving a high dose of cisplatin experience delayed nausea and vomiting up to 6–7 days.

1.309   **The answer is c.** The combinations of dopamine antagonists with steroids have been found to provide complete control of nausea and vomiting in up to 100% of patients undergoing high-dose cisplatin-base regimens. The combination of ondansetron and dexamethasone has been found to be more efficacious than ondansetron alone in controlling emesis.

1.310   **The answer is c.** Serotonin antagonists and dopamine antagonists have different side effects, which make them ideal for combination therapy to prevent nausea and vomiting. One of the primary side effects of dopamine antagonists is extrapyramidal reactions.

1.311   **The answer is c.** The vomiting center lies close to the respiratory center on the floor of the fourth ventricle and is directly activated by the visceral and vagal afferent pathways from the gastrointestinal tract, chemoreceptor trigger zone, vestibular apparatus, and cerebral cortex.

1.312   **The answer is a.** Serotonin is released from the enterochromaffin cells in the small intestine. Serotonin activates 5-HT$_3$ receptors on visceral and vagal afferents, sending a message to the chemotherapy trigger zone and the vomiting center.

1.313   **The answer is a.** Aprepitant is an example of a new class of agents called substance P/neurokinin-1 receptor antagonists, which are used in combination with other antiemetics to prevent acute and delayed chemotherapy-induced nausea and vomiting.

1.314   **The answer is b.** Anticipatory nausea and vomiting occur in 25% of patients as a result of classic operant conditioning from stimuli associated with chemotherapy, usually 12 hours before administration. Nausea commonly occurs in patients receiving oral cyclophosphamide.

1.315   **The answer is d.** Meperidine (Demerol) is not recommended for the treatment of chronic cancer pain. Even though its use has declined considerably, some clinicians are not aware of its risk for producing serious toxic side effects such as agitation, tremors, myoclonus, and seizures. Proproxyphene, the active opioid in Darvocet, is structurally similar to methadone but is a very weak opioid with significant toxicity, especially in the elderly.

1.316   **The answer is b.** Bisphosphonates such as pamidronate and zoledronic acid effectively palliate pain in patients who have metastatic disease, especially in situations where NSAIDs and steroids are no longer effective. Zoledronic acid has been found to be more effective than pamidronate.

1.317   **The answer is b.** Fentanyl is 75–100 times more potent than morphine.

1.318   **The answer is d.** Naloxone is the drug of choice in the treatment of respiratory depression related to opioid overdosing. The amount of naloxone a patient receives should be titrated to changes in respiratory rate. Rapid injections of naloxone should be avoided in opioid-tolerant patients, so as not to precipitate an abstinence syndrome that may include intense pain.

1.319   **The answer is c.** All these are common side effects, except increased motility; opioids commonly decrease motility.

1.320 **The answer is a.** Antidepressants (e.g., amitriptyline, desipramine, imipramine) control pain by inhibiting the uptake of neurotransmitters into nerve terminals. They are used in the treatment of many types of nonmalignant pain, such as migraine headaches, but are also believed to be useful in neuropathic pain that is due to tumor infiltration of nerves, often described as having a continuous burning quality.

1.321 **The answer is d.** Psychostimulants may be indicated when the dose of the opioid causes extreme sedation, produces no other side effects, and the dose cannot be lowered.

1.322 **The answer is b.** Steroids are extremely efficacious for managing the pain caused by epidural cord compression. Some side effects of steroid use, such as mood elevation and increased appetite, may also be desirable in some patients. However, the use of these drugs as adjuvant analgesics early in the course of a patient's pain problem is not recommended.

1.323 **The answer is a.** Except in a few circumstances, oral pain medication should be on a fixed-interval basis. Although the evidence is not conclusive, most caregivers agree that round-the-clock scheduling is most effective in treating pain.

1.324 **The answer is c.** Drug-induced toxicities such as urinary retention, pruritus, nausea, vomiting, and respiratory depression can occur with intraspinal therapy. Cardiac toxicity is not generally reported.

1.325 **The answer is c.** Avinza is the brand name for a morphine sulfate extended-release capsule. It is composed of two components: immediate release and extended release. When ingested, approximately 10% of the morphine is available immediately for absorption and the remaining 90% is released continuously during a 24-hour period. The capsule beads are not to be chewed, crushed, or dissolved because of the risk of rapid release of the morphine from the beads, which may result in absorption of a potentially fatal dose of morphine.

1.326 **The answer is b.** Psychostimulants are useful in counteracting the sedation that accompanies opioid analgesics and may potentiate opioid analgesia. Unpleasant side effects of psychostimulants include confusion, agitation, dysphoria, and apprehension. Recent research indicates that psychostimulants like methylphenidate significantly counteract fatigue.

1.327 **The answer is c.** The opioid dose should be changed all together or reduced by at least 50%. This toxicity is usually due to neuroexcitatory metabolites of the opioids. Naloxone is not effective in reversing this toxicity. Benzodiazepines, including diazepam and midazolam, are recommended and available in parenteral forms.

1.328 **The answer is d.** Cannabinoids have significant side effects, including dysphoria, disorientation, and impaired concentration, especially in the elderly.

1.329 **The answer is a.** Psychopharmacologic agents exert their clinical effects primarily through the increased availability or reduced degradation of neurotransmitters integral to the regulation of mood states. The clinical efficacy of antidepressants in abating depressive symptoms is primarily due to their effects on the 5-HT neurotransmission system with secondary effects on the norepinephrine and dopamine neurotransmitter systems that influence mood states.

1.330 **The answer is d.** Antidepressants are useful for patients with a neuropathic component to their pain. These drugs act by inhibiting the uptake of neurotransmitters into nerve terminals.

1

Quality of Life

1.331   **The answer is d.** Liver failure or dysfunction is a common problem secondary to cancer or its treatments and inhibits the individual's ability to properly metabolize antidepressants. Most antidepressants are metabolized by enzymes located in the liver. Metabolism by P-450 enzymes inactivates most antidepressants, as does alcohol use and isoniazid therapy.

1.332   **The answer is a.** The highest risk for suicide occurs in patients with unmanaged symptoms (including depression), hopelessness, preexisting psychopathology, suicide history, and inadequate social support.

1.333   **The answer is d.**

1.334   **The answer is b.** There have been reports of serious, sometimes fatal, reactions in patients receiving Prozac in combination with a monoamine oxidase inhibitor (MAOI) and in patients who have recently discontinued Prozac and then started on an MAOI. Some patients present with extreme agitation and progress to delirium and coma. Because Prozac and its major metabolite have a very long half-life, at least 5 weeks should be allowed before starting an MAOI.

1.335   **The answer is c.** Methylphenidate counteracts the sedation that accompanies opioid analgesics.

1.336   **The answer is d.** Haloperidol can be used to treat opioid-induced acute confusional states (e.g., hallucinations, agitation from delirium).

1.337   **The answer is d.** Colony-stimulating factors mediate all these steps.

1.338   **The answer is b.** Granulocyte and granulocyte-macrophage colony-stimulating factors decrease myelosuppression, febrile episodes, and number of hospital days when given in conjunction with chemotherapy. Both mucositis and anorexia are complications of chemotherapy and have no relationship to biotherapy.

1.339   **The answer is d.** High levels of epidermal growth factor receptors (EGFRs) on cells from cancers of the breast and bladder indicate a worse prognosis. High levels of EGFRs are noted on many epithelial carcinomas, and mutant EGFRs have been found on high-grade glioblastomas.

1.340   **The answer is c.** HGFs activate the production and maturation of distinctive cell lineages, thereby enhancing the activity of mature neutrophils–phagocytosis, oxidative burst, antibody-dependent cytotoxicity, and chemotaxis. These actions allow the neutrophils to be more aggressive and effective in destroying pathogens. HGFs lessen the duration and severity of neutropenia, but they do not speed the onset.

1.341   **The answer is d.** Colony-stimulating factors are appropriate when febrile neutropenia is expected in more than 40% of patients, such as results from high-dose chemotherapy. It is not appropriate as routine prevention of neutropenia.

1.342   **The answer is b.** Tissue hypoxia is the single most potent factor in erythropoietin production. In the presence of hypoxia, the kidneys increase production and secretion of endogenous erythropoietin. This in turn stimulates red blood cell production by the bone marrow, thereby correcting hypoxia.

1.343   **The answer is c.** Procrit is contraindicated in patients with uncontrolled hypertension. Hypertension, associated with rapid increases in hematocrit, rarely has been noted in cancer patients treated with Procrit. Nevertheless, blood pressure should be monitored carefully, particularly in patients with an underlying history of hypertension or cardiovascular disease.

1.344   **The answer is d.** Granulocyte colony-stimulating factor has been shown to decrease the duration of neutropenia, the number of episodes of neutropenic fever, and the number of hospital days in patients receiving chemotherapy.

1.345   **The answer is c.** Hematopoietic growth factors are used as supportive therapy for patients receiving myelosuppressive therapy or undergoing a bone marrow transplant.

1.346   **The answer is b.** FDA-approved hematopoietic growth factors include granulocyte-macrophage colony-stimulating factors, granuloctye colony-stimulating factors, erythropoietin alfa, and interleukin-11, which prevents thrombocytopenia.

1.347   **The answer is a.** Stimulating the bone marrow to produce white blood cells when chemotherapy is given would enhance cell kill of the white blood cells and potentially cause mutations of myeloid cells and even leukemia. After 24 hours the chemotherapy is generally excreted and administration of HGFs is deemed to be safe.

1.348   **The answer is a.** There is an inverse correlation between epidermal growth factor receptors and ER status, with ER-negative tumors tending to have a higher level of epidermal growth factor receptor than ER-positive tumors.

1.349   **The answer is c.** When patients were asked to disclose their use of complementary and alternative medicine therapies the majority selected prayer. Megavitamins, special diets, massage, herbs and relaxation were cited about one third as often as prayer.

1.350   **The answer is d.** Patients' attitudes regarding symptoms (patients' belief in their ability to manage symptoms or their knowledge of which factors are causing specific symptoms) will affect their ability to manage symptoms. Cognitive Behavioral Therapy is based on the idea that the manner in which patients perceive a situation affects their behavior and beliefs regarding their ability to control it. Patients can change the way they perceive a situation (cognitive reframing), and their ability to control a situation effectively can be improved by changing their perspective.

1.351   **The answer is d.** Little is known about many complementary therapies that the patient may wish to use. One of the few exceptions was a randomized, controlled trial evaluating St. John's Wort versus placebo in individuals with severe depressive illness. Unfortunately, St. John's Wort was not proven to be superior to placebo in this setting. It is still possible, however, that this supplement could be effective in less severe forms of depression, which is how it is commonly used in Europe and more recently in the United States.

1.352   **The answer is b.** The underlying principle of acupuncture is that *qi* (pronounced 'chee' and translated as meaning "energy" is present at birth and maintained throughout life. Health is a balance of yin and yang. Disease is a result of imbalance. Acupuncture results in correcting any imbalance in the flow of energy, thus restoring balance. The four secrets of qi gong means energy cultivation and refers to movement that are believed to improve health, longevity, and harmony. Reiki refers to the creation of energy that alleviates physical, emotional, and spiritual blockages. Reflexology is a therapeutic method that uses manual pressure applied to certain areas of the feet, hands or ears that are believed to correspond to areas of the body, in order to relieve stress and prevent and/or treat physical disorders.

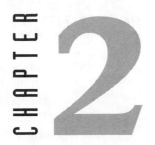

CHAPTER 2

Protective Mechanisms

ALTERATIONS IN MOBILITY

2.1   Assessment of cerebellar function focuses on the ability to
    a.   Coordinate movement
    b.   Maintain normal muscle tone
    c.   Maintain equilibrium
    d.   All of the above

2.2   Which of the following is *not* a typical complication of allograft bone reconstruction?
    a.   Rejection
    b.   Infection
    c.   Fracture
    d.   Nonunion

2.3   Mr. Pen has metastatic prostate cancer to the bone and is receiving leuprolide acetate, a lutenizing hormone-releasing hormone (LH-RH) agonist, as his primary therapy. One and one-half weeks into his treatment, he calls complaining of worsening bone pain and difficulty in walking. He is concerned that the leuprolide acetate is not working. Your *most* appropriate response would be which of the following?
    a.   He is probably correct. The increase in pain may be because the leuprolide acetate is not working and he may need to talk to his doctor about switching therapy.
    b.   The pain is probably caused by release of calcium from lytic lesions in the bone.
    c.   The leuprolide acetate causes an initial increase in testosterone levels and a "flare" in symptoms.
    d.   There is a rapid decrease in testosterone levels that causes intense pain in the area of the tumor.

2.4 Mrs. Wu has metastatic breast cancer that has spread to her bones and has recently begun pamidronate in conjunction with paclitaxel therapy. She does not fully understand why she is being offered bisphosphonate therapy. Your teaching would *not include* which of the following?
   a. Bisphosphonate therapy should help to make the paclitaxel work better because they are synergistic.
   b. Bisphosphonate therapy helps to manage her bone pain.
   c. Bisphosphonate therapy reduces her hypercalcemia and risk for fractures.
   d. Bisphosphonate therapy may help to inhibit the development of bone metastases.

2.5 A patient's physical performance classification is established before treatment and is intended to accomplish *all but* which of the following?
   a. Determine whether or not the individual is a candidate for a research study
   b. Influence the type of treatment planned
   c. Establish the individual's quality of life using numeric values
   d. Provide prognostic information

2.6 Mrs. Geoffry has lung cancer metastatic to her bones. She has recently completed 3 weeks of radiation to her thoracic spine. She phones you with complaints of recent onset of repeatedly dropping things and radicular pain. Which of the following *best* describes the etiology of her symptoms and appropriate nursing action?
   a. Her symptoms are most likely due to delayed effects of radiation; she should be cautioned against dropping items and instructed to take an analgesic for pain.
   b. Her symptoms are related to her cancer in her bones and will get better in a few weeks because that is when the radiation has its peak effect.
   c. Her symptoms are new and are most likely indicative of spinal cord compression at the level of her thoracic spine. She should see her physician immediately for evaluation.
   d. Her symptoms are probably related to metastatic disease in her brain, and she should be evaluated immediately.

2.7 Tumor spreads from the primary site to bone by which of the following mechanisms?
   a. Direct extension to adjacent bone
   b. Arterial embolization
   c. Direct venous spread
   d. All of the above

2.8 Mrs. George has multiple myeloma and has been confined to bed because of a pathological fracture. Her daughter calls the nurse because her mother is sleeping more and is becoming difficult to arouse. The patient's symptoms are *most likely* due to which of the following?
   a. Hyperviscosity syndrome due to multiple myeloma
   b. Hypocalcemia due to multiple myeloma
   c. Steroid psychosis
   d. All of the above

2.9 Which of the following would *not* be an appropriate therapeutic intervention for chronic phantom limb pain after an above-the-knee amputation?
   a. Relaxation to minimize emotional/psychological stress
   b. Morphine sulfate with immediate-release morphine as needed
   c. Muscle relaxants and tranquilizers
   d. Stump shrinker to exert pressure, alternating with heat compresses

2.10   Which of the following chemotherapy agents is *not* commonly associated with palmar-plantar erythrodysesthesia (hand and foot) syndrome?
    a.   Topotecan
    b.   Doxorubicin hydrochloride liposomal
    c.   Capecitabine
    d.   Cytarabine

2.11   Which of the following would *not* be considered treatment for osteoporosis?
    a.   Thyroid hormone replacement therapy
    b.   Vitamin D
    c.   Calcitonin
    d.   Oral calcium

2.12   The risk for osteoporosis is increased in men with prostate cancer being treated with androgen-ablative therapy because
    a.   Osteoblastic bone formation is decreased
    b.   Osteoclastic activity is decreased
    c.   Estrogen therapy increases osteoblasts
    d.   a and c

2.13   Which of the following *best* describes the therapeutic action of bisphosphonates?
    a.   Bisphosphonates act as inhibitors of osteoclasts.
    b.   Bisphosphonates bind to bone to stabilize the bone mineral and inhibit breakdown.
    c.   Bisphosponates are natural inhibitors of bone mineralization.
    d.   a and b

2.14   All of the following are goals in the treatment of primary malignant bone cancer *except*
    a.   Preservation of maximum function
    b.   Early intervention in children believed to be at high risk
    c.   Eradication of tumor
    d.   Avoidance of amputation

2.15   All of the following are considered to be indications for limb-salvage surgery *except*
    a.   A locally aggressive chondrosarcoma
    b.   The absence of soft tissue invasion
    c.   A child older than 10 years
    d.   All of the above

2.16   After amputation, Mr. Riley reports pain in the missing lower leg. The nurse should be aware that this phantom limb pain
    a.   Generally decreases substantially during the first year
    b.   Is likely to worsen with aging
    c.   Indicates a patient's inability to cope with loss
    d.   Usually occurs immediately after surgery

2.17   The rationale for the use of preoperative chemotherapy in patients with osteosarcoma includes *all but* which of the following aspects?
    a.   It treats micrometastases.
    b.   It decreases the size of the primary tumor, possibly facilitating limb-salvage surgery.
    c.   It enhances the effect of postoperative radiation.
    d.   It demonstrates the effectiveness of the chemotherapy.

2.18 The most common sites of occurrence for chondrosarcoma are the
   a. Femur, tibia, patella, and metatarsal
   b. Vertebrae and shoulder girdle
   c. Shoulder girdle, hip girdle, and trunk
   d. Mandible and maxilla

2.19 Treatment of metastases to the bone may include surgery, chemotherapy, and/or radiotherapy. When radiation therapy is used, the primary goal often is to
   a. Eliminate the need for surgical intervention
   b. Palliate pain
   c. Decrease the likelihood of further metastases
   d. Treat the primary cancer

NEUTROPENIA

2.20 Infection in the neutropenic patient is a serious complication of chemotherapy and can be fatal in what percentage of patients?
   a. 15%
   b. 30%
   c. 60%
   d. 75%

2.21 Kate is being treated with chemotherapy for Hodgkin's disease and is monitored weekly for myelosuppression. This is appropriate because neutropenia
   a. Is the most common dose-limiting side effect of chemotherapy
   b. Is potentially the most lethal side effect of chemotherapy
   c. Is most severe with antimetabolites and vinca alkaloids
   d. a and b

2.22 Mr. Mendez, who is receiving high-dose chemotherapy, has developed neutropenia. The usual symptoms of infection will likely be absent or muted in this patient because
   a. Most infections are due to organisms that are part of the body's normal flora
   b. The white blood cells drop rapidly and recovery time is slow
   c. Neutrophils are necessary to produce an inflammatory response
   d. The immunoglobulins are reduced

2.23 How many days after chemotherapy does neutropenia typically develop, and what is the usual time for recovery?
   a. Develops 4–6 days after chemotherapy with recovery in 2 weeks
   b. Develops 16–20 days after chemotherapy with recovery in 6 weeks
   c. Develops 8–12 days after chemotherapy with recovery in 3–4 weeks
   d. Develops 4 weeks after chemotherapy with recovery in 6 weeks

2.24 The most common site of infection in the granulocytopenic patient is which of the following?
   a. Perineal region
   b. Respiratory tract
   c. Urinary tract
   d. Gastrointestinal tract

2.25 Which of the following *best* describes the difference between sepsis and septic shock?
   a. Septic shock involves hypotension that is unresponsive to fluid resuscitation.
   b. Sepsis involves elevated heart rate and temperature with or without evidence of infection.
   c. Septic shock involves organ dysfunction.
   d. a and c

2.26 Which of the following is considered to be the *most important* risk factor for sepsis in individuals with cancer?
   a. Systemic candidiasis
   b. Granulocytopenia
   c. Bone marrow infiltration by tumor cells
   d. Cytotoxic chemotherapy

2.27 Which of the following risk factors increases the degree and duration of cytopenia?
   a. Tumor cells in the bone marrow
   b. Prior treatment with chemotherapy or radiation
   c. A high negative nitrogen balance
   d. All of the above

2.28 Colony-stimulating factors (CSFs) are indicated as adjuvant therapy in *all but* which of the following circumstances?
   a. Patients with cancer undergoing chemotherapy with greater than 10% risk of febrile neutropenia
   b. Patients with cancer undergoing chemotherapy with greater than 20% risk of febrile neutropenia
   c. Patients receiving dose-dense high-dose chemotherapy
   d. Patients with cancer undergoing chemotherapy with greater than 30% risk of febrile neutropenia

2.29 Oral candidiasis can be a serious complication of cancer chemotherapy. Under which of the following circumstances would prophylactic antifungal therapy be indicated?
   a. All neutropenic patients receiving chemotherapy
   b. Patients with acute leukemia and those undergoing hematopoietic stem cell transplantation
   c. Afebrile patients with an absolute neutrophil count less than 1000/mm^3 for more than one week
   d. b and c

2.30 Your patient is scheduled for chemotherapy and has a white blood cell count of 2100 cells/mm^3 with 28% polymorphonuclear neutrophils (PMNs), 18% bands, and 42% lymphocytes. He is informed that his treatment will be delayed. The reason for this is *most likely* which of the following?
   a. His white count is too low.
   b. His absolute neutrophil count (ANC) is less than 1000/mm^3.
   c. His ANC is less than 500/mm^3.
   d. None of the above; his ANC is adequate for treatment.

2.31 Alfred is a patient with colon cancer who is scheduled to have a vascular access port placed before beginning continuous infusion of 5-fluorouracil. He has recently experienced diarrhea and fever of unknown origin. His hemogram reveals a hemoglobin of 11.0 g/100 mL, a white blood cell count of 2000/mm³ with an absolute neutrophil count of 750/mm³, and platelets of 92,000/mm³. His surgeon has delayed his port placement for another week. The likely cause of this delay is which of the following?
   a. Diarrhea is a common cause of fever of unknown origin.
   b. Platelets less than 100,000/mm³ are associated with bleeding during surgery.
   c. Neutropenia is the primary risk factor for infection with vascular access catheters.
   d. Anemia is associated with postoperative complications.

2.32 The administration of colony-stimulating factors as prophylaxis following highly myelosuppressive chemotherapy is intended to accomplish primarily which of the following?
   a. Maintain white blood cell count above 10,000 cells/mm³
   b. Prevent pancytopenia
   c. Minimize infection and stomatitis
   d. Decrease the number of days that the white blood cell count is at its nadir

2.33 What percentage of cancer patients develop sepsis?
   a. 10%
   b. 20%
   c. 45%
   d. 70%

2.34 Five days after chemotherapy for lung cancer your 72-year-old patient calls with fever and chills. Blood counts reveal an absolute neutrophil count of 429/mm³. Which of the following constitutes appropriate management of this patient?
   a. Begin oral antibiotics and monitor fever.
   b. Administer antibiotics immediately and arrange for admission to the hospital.
   c. He is at the nadir of the white blood cell count and will gradually improve on his own.
   d. He needs a chest x-ray to rule out pneumonia.

2.35 The most common and lethal side effect of chemotherapy is
   a. Respiratory distress
   b. Electrolyte imbalance from nausea, vomiting, and diarrhea
   c. Myelosuppression
   d. Increased liver function tests

THROMBOCYTOPENIA

2.36 Thrombopoietin
   a. Reduces the duration of the thrombocytopenia
   b. Stimulates multipotential progenitor cells that later result in increased numbers of platelets
   c. Stimulates the differentiation and proliferation of megakaryocytes into platelets
   d. a and c

2.37   Thrombocytopenia in cancer patients can be caused by any of the following factors *except*
    a.   An abnormal distribution of platelets that results in increased platelet sequestration
    b.   Rapid platelet destruction characterized by a shortened platelet life span
    c.   Overstimulation of normal coagulation causing rapid platelet thrombosis
    d.   Decreased production of platelets in the bone marrow due to tumor involvement

2.38   The anemia associated with multiple myeloma is believed to be caused by
    a.   The effects of radiation
    b.   A normochromic iron deficiency
    c.   The replacement of erythrocyte precursors with plasma cells
    d.   Erythrocyte destruction by white blood cells

2.39   Ms. Drake has myelodysplastic syndrome (MDS). She reports being asymptomatic for a prolonged time and asks you why she still has to endure ongoing monitoring. The best explanation you can offer is that
    a.   T-cell abnormalities increase the risk of opportunistic infections.
    b.   Compliance with the prescribed treatment delays or prevents the onset of symptoms.
    c.   All patients with MDS eventually develop anemia, thrombocytopenia, and/or neutropenia.
    d.   All patients with MDS eventually develop acute leukemia.

2.40   A cumulative and delayed thrombocytopenia has been associated with *all but* which of the following chemotherapeutic agents?
    a.   Methotrexate
    b.   Mitomycin
    c.   Lomustine
    d.   Streptozocin

2.41   Mr. Jones has a malignant brain tumor and has been receiving 5-fluorouracil and carmustine every 6 weeks. His blood counts today reveal a white blood cell count of 3000 cells/mm^3, hemoglobin of 10 g/100 mL, and platelet count of 50,000 cells/mm^3. His treatment is delayed today. The best explanation for delaying his treatment is which of the following?
    a.   He is moderately to severely immunosuppressed.
    b.   He is moderately anemic.
    c.   He is at moderate risk for bleeding due to thrombocytopenia.
    d.   He is at severe risk for bleeding due to thrombocytopenia.

2.42   When platelets decrease to 10,000 cells/mm^3, the patient is most at risk for which of the following?
    a.   Spontaneous central nervous system bleeding
    b.   Gastrointestinal bleeding with black tarry stools
    c.   Respiratory tract hemorrhage
    d.   All of the above

2.43   During the physical exam of a new patient you notice that he has small red eruptions on his upper and lower extremities. He appears pale and states that he is exhausted most of the time. His physical exam is suspicious for which of the following?
    a.   Severe anemia and bleeding
    b.   Disseminated intravascular coagulopathy
    c.   Thrombocytopenia
    d.   Leukemia

2.44   Allen has prostate cancer with metastasis to the bone. He has had chemotherapy and radiation therapy to control his disease. He comes to the clinic for further chemotherapy. His blood counts are as follows: white blood cell count, 2700 cells/mm³; hemoglobin, 8.7 g/100 mL; and platelets, 88,000 cells/mm³. His thrombocytopenia is most likely due to which of the following?
  a. Tumor invasion of the bone marrow
  b. Acute or delayed effects of chemotherapy
  c. Delayed effects of radiation therapy
  d. All of the above

2.45   The most common cause of thrombocytopenia in patients with cancer is
  a. Infection
  b. Hypersplenism
  c. Decreased megakaryocytopoiesis
  d. Immune-mediated thrombocytopenia

2.46   Jenny has chronic lymphocytic leukemia. She has immature platelets in the bone marrow and a platelet count of 45,000 cells/mm³. She has evidence of petechiae, purpura, and ecchymosis. Her condition is *most likely* associated with which of the following platelet disorders?
  a. Thrombocytopenia
  b. Idiopathic thrombocytopenic purpura
  c. Thrombocytosis
  d. Hypocoagulopathy

2.47   The use of interleukin-11 is specifically aimed at which of the following blood components?
  a. Granulocytes
  b. Erythrocytes
  c. Platelets
  d. All of the above

2.48   Which of the following is *not* a side effect of interleukin-11?
  a. Fluid retention
  b. Dyspnea
  c. Conjunctival redness and blurring
  d. Hyperthermia

2.49   Your patient just started a new regimen of chemotherapy including vincristine and methotrexate 1 week ago. He is elderly and has historically had some problems with constipation. Other significant problems include a platelet count of 20,000 cells/mm³ and stomatitis. Nursing action would include which of the following?
  a. Stool softener and a laxative each day as needed
  b. Rectal exam to rule out impaction
  c. Rectal suppository followed by a tap water enema
  d. All of the above

2.50   Which of the following chemotherapeutic agents is *not* considered to be platelet sparing?
  a. Ifosfamide
  b. Mitoxantrone
  c. Mitomycin
  d. Vincristine

2.51   Mr. Czar has an enlarged spleen and has been started on corticosteroid therapy. The primary purpose of this therapy is which of the following?
    a.   Steroids have a capillary-stabilizing effect.
    b.   Steroids help to control platelet sequestration.
    c.   Steroids help to minimize bleeding potential.
    d.   All of the above

2.52   Your patient with leukemia has developed sepsis and is suffering from severe thrombocytopenia. Despite several platelet transfusions his platelet count is only 20,000 cells/mm^3. Which of the following is the most logical explanation for why multiple platelet transfusions are less effective in some situations?
    a.   The patient must be bleeding somewhere.
    b.   The platelets must not have been stored properly.
    c.   Fever and infection destroy platelets.
    d.   The leukemia cells destroy platelets.

2.53   Your patient has received multiple transfusions of random-donor platelets and is experiencing no increase in his platelet count. What is this process called?
    a.   Refraction
    b.   Alloimmunization
    c.   Hyperimmunization
    d.   Autoimmunization

ALTERATIONS IN SKIN INTEGRITY

2.54   After the administration of doxorubicin, you notice that swelling has occurred at the injection site. The patient complains of some burning. You determine that there is a lack of blood return. These clues alert you that the patient may be experiencing
    a.   Venous flare
    b.   Erythema
    c.   Extravasation
    d.   All of the above

2.55   Rosa is about to receive radiation therapy for the first time. She says, "I have such sensitive skin. I'm worried about the effect radiation could have on my skin." You tell Rosa that acute radiation effects
    a.   Result from the depletion of actively proliferating cells
    b.   Are characterized by dilation, local edema, and inflammation
    c.   Are usually temporary and manageable
    d.   All of the above

2.56   Which of the following is *not* true regarding radiation-induced skin reactions?
    a.   Higher doses given over shorter periods of time to larger volumes result in more severe acute skin reactions.
    b.   Electrons produce greater skin reactions than photons.
    c.   Placing tissue-equivalent material on the skin creates a skin-sparing effect during radiation therapy, minimizing dose at the level of the skin.
    d.   When treatment is targeted at areas of skin apposition, increased reaction secondary to warmth and moisture can be expected.

2.57   Following radiation therapy to the chest, your patient plans a trip to Bermuda. You instruct her to use a sunscreen with an SPF of 30 or more because radiation has undoubtedly affected her skin via
a.   Skin-sparing effect during radiation therapy
b.   Slower rate of melanin production in new epidermal cells in the radiation field
c.   Faster rate of melanin production in new epidermal cells in the radiation field
d.   Destruction of lymphocytes in the irradiated epidermis

2.58   The signs and symptoms of an extravasation from chemotherapy can be subtle. Which of the following might be considered a definite sign of infiltration of a vesicant agent?
a.   A bleb formation at the injection site
b.   Swelling that occurs in more deeply accessed veins
c.   Loss of a blood return
d.   a and b

2.59   A 60-year-old woman reports a flesh-colored, raised, firm papule on the top of her nose. It is examined and found to be a squamous cell carcinoma (SCC). How do SCCs differ from most basal cell carcinomas (BCCs)?
a.   They tend to be less aggressive than BCCs, even though they have faster growth rates.
b.   Their margins are well demarcated, as compared with those of the BCCs.
c.   They tend to have greater metastatic potential.
d.   a and c

2.60   In the days *immediately* after a major open-field abdominal surgery,
a.   One should not be surprised to see a temporary suppression of wound healing; healing becomes more proliferative after 21 days.
b.   Chemotherapy agents can be used to best advantage.
c.   Granulation tissue is usually formed in the first 3–25 days after surgery, providing the characteristic strength of the wound.
d.   b and c

2.61   A graft or flap is most often used in the surgical treatment of a nonmelanoma cancer when
a.   The lesion is large or located in an area with insufficient tissue for closure
b.   Risks of bleeding are high and vasculature must be maintained
c.   The extent of the tumor must be accurately assessed and margins are relatively unclear
d.   The lesion is small, superficial, or recurrent

2.62   Side effects of radiation to the skin are least likely to include
a.   Mild erythema and moist desquamation
b.   Fibrosclerotic changes that make skin smooth, taut, and shiny
c.   Permanent tanning
d.   Complete or patchy alopecia

2.63   Three months after sentinel lymph node biopsy (SLNB) your patient complains of tenderness and soreness at the site. The most appropriate response to her complaint would include which of the following?
a.   She should call her doctor to report these symptoms because they are unusual.
b.   She probably bumped herself and should not be concerned.
c.   These sensations are common for up to 6 months after SLNB, and she should not worry.
d.   Tenderness this long after the procedure could mean hematoma formation, and hot packs could help.

2.64   One week after doxorubicin hydrochloride liposomal therapy, Mrs. Allen, a 58-year-old woman with ovarian cancer, complains of swelling, pain, and erythema on her hands and feet. Your advice to her would include which of the following?
    a.   She should stop her chemotherapy, as this reaction could progress to ulcerations on her hands and feet.
    b.   She is probably protein deficient and anemic, which often present as swelling and erythema of the feet.
    c.   This reaction is common, will resolve in 1–2 weeks, and will not interfere with her scheduled therapy.
    d.   Ascites occurs commonly with ovarian cancer, and these symptoms are caused by this condition.

2.65   Monique is experiencing hyperpigmentation. You explain to her that this may be a reaction to
    a.   Asparaginase
    b.   Bleomycin
    c.   Paclitaxel
    d.   Cisplatin

2.66   High-risk factors for cutaneous melanoma (CM) include all of the following *except*
    a.   Skin pigmentation
    b.   A persistently changed or changing mole
    c.   The presence of a precursor lesion such as dysplastic nevi
    d.   Oral contraceptives

2.67   Following her third course of capecitabine oral therapy your patient presents with grade 3 diarrhea, stomatitis, and pronounced hand–foot syndrome. She states she did not report her side effects because she did not want to have to stop the medicine. Your teaching would include which of the following true statement(s)?
    a.   Dose interruption or reduction does not affect efficacy.
    b.   Untreated toxicity can negatively affect treatment outcomes.
    c.   She made the right choice because larger doses of capecitabine are generally better if the side effects can be tolerated.
    d.   a and b

2.68   Alicia has metastatic cancer with a grade 2 performance status. She returns today for her second course of doxorubicin hydrochloride. Her chief complaint is not being able to eat, fatigue, and a rash that has newly formed on her scalp, and spread to her temple just below her left eye. Appropriate nursing action would include which of the following?
    a.   Continue with chemotherapy as ordered because her disease has obviously spread to her scalp.
    b.   Hold her therapy and notify the physician immediately.
    c.   Prevent contact with persons who may be immunocompromised.
    d.   b and c

2.69   Which of the following statements about dysplastic nevi (DN) is *not* correct?
    a.   DN may be familial or nonfamilial.
    b.   Most persons affected by DN have about 25–75 abnormal nevi.
    c.   DN develop from precursor lesions of cutaneous melanoma.
    d.   A distinctive feature of DN is a "fried egg" appearance with a deeply pigmented papular area surrounded by an area of lighter pigmentation.

2.70   The phase of cutaneous melanoma tumor growth that is characterized by invasion into and through the dermis is the
   a.   Radial phase
   b.   Vertical growth phase
   c.   Nodular phase
   d.   Acral lentiginous phase

2.71   Which of the following statements about primary prevention of skin cancers is *false*?
   a.   Ultraviolet radiation is strongest during the mid-part of the day.
   b.   For most people sunscreen is not required on overcast days.
   c.   Certain medications (e.g., oral contraceptives) can make individuals photosensitive.
   d.   Surfaces such as sand and water can reflect more than one-half of the ultraviolet radiation onto the skin.

2.72   Which of the following is effective in preventing neurotoxicities associated with cisplatin, paclitaxel, and carboplatin?
   a.   Pyroxidine (vitamin B_6)
   b.   Amifostine
   c.   Nortriptyline
   d.   Carbamazepine

NEUROPATHIES

2.73   Davis is taking vincristine. You are able to discern from his conversation that although he is familiar with some of vincristine's adverse effects, he seems unfamiliar with its neurotoxic effects. Thus, you tell him that vincristine is well known for potential
   a.   Encephalopathy
   b.   Peripheral neuropathy
   c.   Acute cerebellar dysfunction
   d.   Leukoencephalopathy

2.74   Which of the following chemotherapy agents is *not* associated with peripheral neuropathies?
   a.   Cytarabine
   b.   Cisplatin
   c.   Methotrexate
   d.   Carboplatin

2.75   A patient receiving paclitaxel has recently complained that she has some trouble walking without stumbling. After examining the patient, the physician changes her chemotherapy. What is the most logical explanation for switching her chemotherapy?
   a.   She probably has a brain tumor, and the chemotherapy is not working.
   b.   The paclitaxel is causing a cerebellar dysfunction.
   c.   The paclitaxel could be causing progressive peripheral neuropathy.
   d.   The cancer could be impinging on the spinal nerves.

2.76   Which of the following chemotherapy drugs is *not* associated with arthralgias and myalgias?
   a.   Paclitaxel
   b.   Docetaxel
   c.   Ifosfamide
   d.   Vinorelbine

2.77 Which of the following is *not* considered a risk factor for ifosfamide-induced encephalopathy?
a. Hepatic insufficiency
b. Previous taxane therapy
c. Low serum albumin
d. High serum creatinine

2.78 Mr. Rogers has a metastatic cancer of unknown origin. He originally went to his doctor because of ataxia and lower extremity weakness. His doctor described his symptoms as being related to a paraneoplastic syndrome. Which of the following statements best describes the cause of the patient's weakness?
a. Cerebellar function is impaired because of the effect of the tumor.
b. The cancer is in the brain and is pressing on the cerebellum.
c. Chemotherapy is the most likely cause of the weakness.
d. Muscle wasting is common in metastatic cancer.

2.79 Your patient has a possible brain tumor involving the frontal lobe. He is unable to coordinate skilled movements but is not paralyzed. This clinical manifestation is called
a. Dysphasia
b. Apraxia
c. Aphasia
d. Dysreflexia

2.80 Which of the following symptoms may accompany peripheral neuropathy associated with chemotherapy?
a. Ataxia
b. Diminished temperature sense
c. Diminished touch sense
d. All of the above

2.81 You are beginning treatment of a patient who is receiving oxaliplatin and 5-fluorouracil. Before the oxaliplatin you administer calcium gluconate (1 g) and magnesium sulfate 50% (1 g) over 15 minutes. The purpose of this is to prevent which of the following side effect of oxaliplatin?
a. Renal toxicity
b. Neurotoxicity
c. Ototoxicity
d. Allergic/anaphylactic reactions

2.82 The cause of peripheral neuropathy caused by chemotherapy is best described by which of the following?
a. Sensory and motor axons are injured.
b. Demyelination reduces nerve conduction velocity.
c. Deep tendon reflexes are lost.
d. Nerve cells are damaged by the cytotoxic effects of the drugs.

2.83   Jonas has finished his last course of chemotherapy including carboplatin and etoposide. He comes for an office visit complaining of colicky abdominal pain, constipation, urinary retention, and impotence. You are concerned because you know that his symptoms are *most likely* due to which of the following?
a.   Tumor recurrence
b.   A paraneoplastic syndrome
c.   The effect of chemotherapy on autonomic fibers
d.   Opstipation from chemotherapy

2.84   Which of the following is *not* considered to increase the risk of vincristine-induced peripheral neuropathy?
a.   Vincristine 2 mg intravenous twice a month
b.   Age greater than 60
c.   Hepatic dysfunction
d.   Concomitant etoposide therapy

2.85   Which of the following statements regarding the effect of cisplatin on hearing loss is *not* true?
a.   The drug causes loss of the hairs in the inner ear.
b.   Hearing loss begins with asymptomatic loss of high-frequency tones.
c.   Tinnitus is the first symptom to appear.
d.   Loss of medium-frequency sounds is always permanent.

2.86   Annie has just completed her 10 treatments of weekly paclitaxel. Over the last few weeks she has complained of difficulty buttoning her clothes and asks how soon it will get better. Your *most* appropriate response would be which of the following?
a.   Her symptoms will probably get worse before they get better.
b.   This means she cannot receive more paclitaxel.
c.   Most symptoms will improve 2–3 weeks after treatment ends.
d.   Her symptoms will improve but may never completely resolve.

2.87   The risk of ototoxicity from cisplatin therapy is increased by *all but* which of the following?
a.   Continuous infusion therapy
b.   Aminoglycoside therapy
c.   Dehydration
d.   Rapid drug delivery

2.88   Metabolic encephalopathy manifested as blurred vision, seizures, motor system dysfunction, and irreversible coma has been reported in up to 30% of patients receiving which drug?
a.   High-dose cisplatin
b.   Etoposide continuous infusion
c.   Ifosfamide
d.   Cytarabine

2.89   Mr. Jones is an elderly gentleman who has been receiving 5-fluorouracil and leucovorin weekly as treatment for his colon cancer. His wife phones you to say that he is unsteady on his feet and complains of intermittent double vision. You encourage her to bring him in right away because you suspect which of the following?
a.   Acute cerebellar dysfunction due to the 5-fluorouracil
b.   Leukoencephalopathy from the cumulative effect of the drugs
c.   Dehydration due to severe diarrhea from the 5-fluorouracil
d.   Metastatic disease to the brain causing ataxia and diplopia

ALTERATIONS IN MENTAL STATUS

2.90 When a patient at the end of life complains of dyspnea, the nurse should *most* appropriately focus on which of the following?
  a. Determine degree of dyspnea by assessing arterial blood gases and pulmonary function tests
  b. Monitor pulse oximetry to determine need for oxygen
  c. Administer opioids to lessen the sensation of breathlessness
  d. Administer bronchodilators as needed

2.91 Delirium is common in the final days of life. Which of the following nursing interventions would be counterproductive in the management of delirium?
  a. Concentrate on orienting the individual to what is real and what is not.
  b. Administer low-dose haloperidol to decrease anxiety.
  c. Discontinue benzodiazepines because they can worsen delirium.
  d. Encourage the individual to speak about a loved one that has died.

2.92 As your patient nears death, his daughter is distressed and believes he is suffering because he is unable to drink fluids. She insists you give him intravenous fluids. In an attempt to help her understand her father's condition and provide optimal end-of-life care, which of the following is the *most* appropriate response?
  a. She is right; dying of thirst is painful and you will call the doctor for intravenous hydration.
  b. Assure her that he is not suffering or experiencing any discomfort from dehydration.
  c. Suggest they insert a small nasogastric tube to administer fluids to prevent dehydration.
  d. Suggest that she try to encourage her father to drink fluids in small amounts.

2.93 The single most important adjunctive treatment to combat the effects of vasogenic cerebral edema is the use of glucocorticoids. Which of the following is *not* a therapeutic mechanism of action of glucocorticoids?
  a. Inhibition of the capillary permeability factor produced by tumor cells
  b. Increase in cerebral blood flow
  c. Suppression of antidiuretic hormone
  d. Reduction in the rate of cerebral fluid formation

2.94 After his emergency treatment for carotid hemorrhage, Mr. Jessup begins to experience tingling in his extremities on the ipsilateral side as well as progressive motor loss and changes in the level of consciousness. You suspect, therefore, that he might have
  a. Cushing's syndrome, in response to progressive tumor
  b. Intermittent pulmonary failure with cardiac episodes secondary to carotid artery ligation
  c. Cerebral ischemia secondary to carotid artery ligation
  d. None of the above

2.95 A patient who is receiving high-dose cytosine arabinoside for acute myelogenous leukemia (AML) begins to experience slight difficulty with articulation of words. She smiles apologetically and says, "I guess I didn't get enough sleep. My mouth is pretty dry too." Your response is to
  a. Do an oral examination, offer mouth care, and continue chemotherapy
  b. Withhold her chemotherapy dose and do a neurological evaluation
  c. Withhold her medication and check her renal function tests
  d. Interview the patient to identify factors contributing to sleeplessness, which is also contributing to dry mouth

2.96   Mrs. Ely has breast cancer and is receiving treatment for metastatic disease to bone, liver, and skin. She feels markedly fatigued, is not eating well, is losing weight, is slightly constipated, and at times is confused. Her symptoms are likely due to which of the following?
   a.   Brain metastasis
   b.   Liver failure
   c.   Chemotherapy
   d.   Hypercalcemia

2.97   Which of the following signs and symptoms could be associated with hypercalcemia?
   a.   Difficulty concentrating
   b.   Diarrhea
   c.   Ataxia
   d.   All of the above

2.98   In severe hypercalcemia a patient exhibits which of the following symptoms?
   a.   Hypotension, dysrhythmias, severe diarrhea, and stupor
   b.   Atrioventricular block and asystole, hypertension, and coma
   c.   Extreme agitation, hypertension, and constipation
   d.   Diarrhea, hypotension, and coma

2.99   A patient with breast cancer has meningeal carcinomatosis that commonly manifests as
   a.   Headache
   b.   Cranial nerve palsies
   c.   Radiculopathies
   d.   All of the above

2.100   Which of the following is considered to be a classic sign of increased intracranial pressure?
   a.   Headache at the base of the brain
   b.   Change in level of consciousness
   c.   Agitation
   d.   Forgetfulness

2.101   Which of the following statements regarding primary central nervous system lymphoma (PCNSL) is correct?
   a.   PCNSL is often associated with acquired or congenital immunosuppression.
   b.   PCNSL is generally disseminated within the central nervous system at diagnosis.
   c.   Patients with PCNSL show no evidence of a systemic lymphoma.
   d.   All of the above

2.102   Your patient has lung cancer metastatic to the brain. He is admitted because he has lost his balance and complains of severe nausea and vomiting. After three doses of whole brain radiation his wife states he is getting worse. Which of the following statements would *most* appropriately explain why her observations might be true?
   a.   Hospitalization is a frequent cause of disorientation in patients with central nervous system malignancies.
   b.   The radiation treatments take weeks to be effective.
   c.   Depending on the dose, radiation can lead to increased intracranial pressure due to cerebral edema.
   d.   His symptoms are probably due to abrupt cessation of his steroids.

2.103 About 1 month after whole brain radiation your patient's wife calls, stating that her husband is more sleepy, lethargic, and complaining of fatigue and lack of appetite. The physician states that the patient's tumor has decreased in size as expected. Therefore your response would include which of the following nursing interventions?
   a. Reassure the family that these symptoms are expected and will gradually improve.
   b. Encourage proper nutrition and ambulation as tolerated.
   c. Explain that these symptoms could mean the cancer has returned, and they should make an appointment to see the doctor.
   d. a and b

2.104 Allison has been on tapering doses of steroids over the past week after the completion of radiation therapy to her brain for metastatic breast cancer. She is now sleeping more and seems confused. The cause of changes in her mental status is *most likely* due to
   a. Tapering of steroids
   b. Recurrence of her cancer
   c. Hypercalcemia
   d. Steroid psychosis

2.105 Which of the following is *not* considered to be a side effect of dronabinol?
   a. Excessive salivation
   b. Euphoria
   c. Dysphoria
   d. Orthostatic hypotension

2.106 A common manifestation of central nervous system lymphoma is
   a. A change in personality
   b. Syndrome of inappropriate antidiuretic hormone (SIADH)
   c. Frontal headache
   d. Spinal cord compression

2.107 The most common acute-onset sign of malignant cerebral edema is
   a. Headache
   b. Nausea/vomiting
   c. Seizure
   d. Disorientation

2.108 In most instances, the earliest and most sensitive indicator of a central nervous system tumor is a change in
   a. Level of consciousness
   b. Cognitive ability
   c. Motor and sensory function
   d. All of the above

INFECTION

2.109 The consequence of infection with gram-negative organisms that can quickly lead to death is
   a. Dehydration
   b. Gastrointestinal bleeding
   c. Endotoxic shock
   d. Anaphylaxis

2.110   *Pneumocystis carinii* is potentially fatal and requires treatment with
   a.   Foscarnet
   b.   Ganciclovir
   c.   Trimethoprim-sulfamethoxazole
   d.   An aminoglycoside

2.111   Risk factors for development of refractory infection and sepsis in patients with cancer include *all but* which of the following?
   a.   Hematologic malignancy
   b.   Infections lasting less than 7 days
   c.   Infectious lesions larger than 5 cm
   d.   Low albumin at the onset of symptoms of sepsis

2.112   In septic shock, fever is defined as which of the following?
   a.   A single oral temperature of 38.3°C or higher
   b.   A temperature of 38.0°C for longer than an hour
   c.   Chills without fever in the elderly
   d.   All of the above

2.113   When treating the patient with sepsis it is important to consider combinations of antimicrobials. Which of the following is the primary benefit of combination therapy?
   a.   Drugs are potentially synergistic.
   b.   Doses of drug may be markedly reduced, thereby minimizing toxicity.
   c.   Drugs used in combination decrease incidence of development of drug-resistant strains.
   d.   a and c

2.114   Numerous acute hepatic complications can arise following hematopoietic cell transplantation (HCT). Which of the following is *not* diagnostic for venoocclusive disease?
   a.   Fluid retention
   b.   Hyperbilirubinemia
   c.   Hypernatremia
   d.   Right upper quadrant pain

2.115   Correctly identify the sequence of events in the pathophysiology of venoocclusive disease:
   1.   Cytokine and tumor necrosis factor activation
   2.   Injury of the endothelial lining of hepatic venules and sinusoids
   3.   Hypercoagulation and thrombosis
   4.   Impaired blood flow
   5.   Renal insufficiency
   a.   2, 1, 3, 4, 5
   b.   5, 2, 1, 3, 4
   c.   2, 4, 1, 5, 3
   d.   4, 1, 2, 3, 5

2.116   Which of the following is *not* considered to be a classification of Kaposi's sarcoma (KS)?
   a.   Non–HIV-related KS, occurring primarily in men of Mediterranean descent
   b.   Endemic KS, occurring in men, women, and children in certain areas of Africa
   c.   Epidemic or HIV-related KS
   d.   Malignant KS with a genetic component

2.117 Which of the following is considered to be the cardinal symptom of infection?
a. Pus formation
b. Inflammation
c. Fever
d. Elevated white blood cell count

2.118 The primary cause of infection in cancer patients continues to be
a. Gram-positive organisms
b. Gram-negative organisms
c. Fungal infections
d. Mycobacterial infections

2.119 Melanie is about to undergo treatment with cyclophosphamide and doxorubicin. She is at risk for developing hemorrhagic cystitis. What preventive measures can be taken?
a. Protection of the bladder focuses on reduced hydration.
b. Intravenous acrolein may produce sulfhydryl complexes and subsequent detoxification.
c. She is instructed to drink 8–10 glasses of fluid a day and void frequently.
d. She should receive amifostine therapy daily.

2.120 The body's first line of defense against bacteria, which is commonly altered by cancer therapies, is
a. Granulocytes
b. The skin
c. Macrophages
d. The acid pH of fluid

2.121 The specific white blood cell that constitutes 55–70% of circulating white blood cells and responds quickly to bacterial invasion is the
a. Polymorphonuclear neutrophil
b. Monocyte
c. Macrophage
d. Lymphocyte

2.122 What is the name given to the microbes that normally live in the body and lead to over 80% of infections in cancer patients?
a. Exogenous organisms
b. Intracellular organisms
c. Extracellular organisms
d. Endogenous organisms

2.123 Meticulous skin care is required when caring for the patient with reactivated varicella zoster virus to
a. Minimize spread to other areas of the body
b. Prevent a secondary bacterial infection
c. Promote drainage of the vesicles
d. Provide the primary source of pain relief

2.124 The single most important measure to prevent infection when caring for the patient with granulocytopenia is
a. Promptly instituting empiric antibiotics
b. Washing the hands meticulously
c. Providing optimal nutrition
d. Restricting the presence of live flowers and plants

2.125   Ms. Daniels has developed profound immunosuppression that has resulted in neutropenia, along with a denuding of the mucosa in the gastrointestinal tract. This combination puts her at particular risk for
a.   Gram-negative bacteremia
b.   *Aspergillus* infection
c.   Epstein-Barr virus infection
d.   *Pneumocystis carinii* pneumonia

2.126   The leading cause of liver cancer throughout the world is
a.   Chronic hepatitis B virus
b.   Chronic hepatitis C virus
c.   Chronic cirrhosis
d.   Chronic hepatitis A virus

2.127   The occurrence of non-Hodgkin's lymphoma (NHL) in persons infected with HIV appears to be related to
a.   The destruction of helper T cells as a result of infection by cytomegalovirus
b.   Decreased levels of serum protein/albumin as a result of internal coalesced lesions
c.   Opportunistic infections of the central nervous system related to toxoplasmosis
d.   The proliferation of B lymphocytes as a result of Epstein-Barr virus (EBV) and HIV infection

HEMORRHAGE

2.128   The most important measure in the early detection of bleeding is
a.   Accurate screening, beginning with a platelet count
b.   Observation for subtle diagnostic signals, such as skin petechiae
c.   A family history, focusing on possible congenital bleeding disorders
d.   Diagnostic testing of the complete cardiovascular system

2.129   Ms. Edwards, a cancer patient, is being assessed for abnormal bleeding. She is to receive a prothrombin time test. This test is a measure of
a.   Coagulation pathway deficiencies
b.   The concentration of functional factors in plasma
c.   Platelet plug formation
d.   Diminished or absent coagulation factors

2.130   The typical response of the body to a reduction in the platelet count, such as that caused by bleeding, is
a.   An increase in the fibrinolytic activity of remaining platelets
b.   A release of adenosine diphosphate (ADP) into the bloodstream, which increases the oxygen-carrying capacity of available platelets
c.   Sequestering of red blood cells in the spleen
d.   Increased production of megakaryocytes in the bone marrow

2.131   Circulating platelets perform several vital functions, including all of the following *except*
a.   Fibrinolysis, or the lysis of fibrin clots and vessel repair
b.   The release of plasminogen activators required for clot formation
c.   Furnishing a phospholipid surface for the biochemical phase of hemostasis
d.   The formation of a mechanical hemostatic plug at the site of vessel injury

2.132 Bleeding with cancer is most often due either to the mechanical pressure of tumors on organs or to
a. Interference with vasculature
b. Damage to the spleen
c. Hypocoagulability of the blood
d. Infection

2.133 Acute bleeding that occurs as a result of tumor-induced structural damage to vasculature is best managed by
a. Radiotherapy
b. Oral or parenteral iron supplements to reduce anemia
c. Mechanical pressure (e.g., nasal packing during epistaxis)
d. Chemotherapy

2.134 The single most significant measure for predicting bleeding in an individual with cancer is
a. Tumor site
b. Platelet count
c. Abnormal platelet function
d. An imbalance in coagulation factors

2.135 Mr. Jessup, who has a tracheostomy, is having a carotid hemorrhage. Besides controlling the bleeding, what should you do first to prevent aspiration of the blood?
a. Suction his throat and oral cavity
b. Deflate the cuff and remove the tracheostomy tube to clear the airway
c. Inflate the tracheostomy cuff
d. Transport him immediately to the operating room for ligation of the carotid artery

2.136 You are monitoring Liza to ensure that she does not develop complications associated with leukostasis. The most common and most lethal complication is
a. Intracerebral hemorrhage
b. Cerebellar toxicity
c. Blast crisis
d. Disseminated intravascular coagulation

2.137 The individual who has recently had an ultrasound-guided percutaneous needle biopsy of the liver must be monitored closely for symptoms of
a. Spinal cord compression
b. Hematemesis
c. Headache
d. Hemorrhage

2.138 Patients with liver cancer are more at risk for bleeding due to
a. A decrease in vitamin K absorption
b. Varices from portal hypertension
c. Increase in prothrombin time and activated partial thromboplastin time
d. All of the above

2.139 A patient with a brain tumor is suspected of having possible hemorrhage. The test most likely needed to determine this is
a. Noncontrast computed tomography (CT)
b. CT with contrast
c. Magnetic resonance imaging
d. Cerebral angiography

2.140 Postoperative care of an individual who has undergone palliative surgery for pancreatic cancer includes all of the following *except*
    a. Administration of pancreatic enzyme supplements
    b. Providing a diet that is low in fat, is high in protein, and includes a glass of red wine with lunch and dinner
    c. Observing for hemorrhage, hypovolemia, and hypotension
    d. Examining stools for steatorrhea

2.141 One of the common sequelae of liver cancer is
    a. Esophageal varices
    b. Visual disturbances
    c. Fat intolerance
    d. Urinary retention

2.142 The risk of carotid artery rupture after radical neck dissection is associated with all of the following *except*
    a. Coverage of the artery with a skin flap
    b. Infection of the surrounding area
    c. A small trickle of blood from the area
    d. Persistent tumor in the area

2.143 An example of a postoperative situation requiring immediate nursing intervention is
    a. A smooth suture line with no sign of swelling
    b. Hematoma formation beneath a skin flap
    c. Bleeding on a dressing the size of a quarter
    d. Clearing of airway secretions by coughing

2.144 Patients with cancers may at times have bleeding, despite normal platelet counts and coagulation factors. An example is bleeding caused by
    a. Platelet sequestration
    b. Disseminated intravascular coagulation
    c. Decreased platelet adhesiveness
    d. Hypocoagulability

2.145 There are numerous steps in the cascade of events leading to blood clot production. Which of the following substances results from both the intrinsic and the extrinsic pathway and is necessary for conversion of prothrombin to thrombin?
    a. Factor XII
    b. Factor VII
    c. Thromboplastin
    d. Fibrinogen

ANSWER EXPLANATIONS

2.1 **The answer is d.** Assessment of cerebellar function focuses on the ability to coordinate movement and to maintain normal muscle tone and equilibrium.

2.2 **The answer is a.** The bone is freeze-dried and irradiated, which decreases the bacteria of the graft. Bone allograft recipients do not require immunosuppressive agents.

2

PROTECTIVE
MECHANISMS

2.3   **The answer is c.** LH-RH agonists initially increase testosterone levels, but after 3–4 weeks of therapy testosterone levels fall to castration level. The surge of testosterone production after initiation of an LH-RH agonist is called a "flare." During a flare, patients need to be aware that symptoms can worsen and require prompt medical intervention.

2.4   **The answer is a.** Pamidronate treatment in women with breast cancer and bone metastases led to reductions in the occurrence of hypercalcemia, severe bone pain, and skeletal complications from bone metastases. Pamidronate has been found to inhibit bone metastases.

2.5   **The answer is c.** Performance scales that measure a person's functional status are used frequently in the eligibility criteria for cooperative group clinical trials and also periodically to evaluate the effects of treatment and disease. It may be helpful to interpret a person's quality of life, but it is not a primary objective of performance status.

2.6   **The answer is c.** Individuals with spinal metastasis may have radicular pain, paresthesias, heaviness of limbs, leg buckling, and episodes of dropping items. Compression of the spinal cord is likely and needs immediate treatment to prevent progressive neurological injury.

2.7   **The answer is d.** The three mechanisms by which a tumor spreads from the primary site to bone are (1) direct extension to adjacent bones, (2) arterial embolization, and (3) direct venous spread through the pelvic and vertebral veins.

2.8   **The answer is a.** Mental status changes can be an initial sign of hypercalcemia, hyperviscosity syndrome, or drug toxicity.

2.9   **The answer is b.** Phantom limb pain is caused by the nerve pathways that have been transected during surgery. This transection results in the transmission of abnormal impulses. Patients may feel pain, burning, itching, cramping, and throbbing sensations in the limb. These sensations can be exacerbated by stress, fatigue, and emotional stressors. Medications include muscle relaxants and tranquilizers. Simple measures like the use of a stump shrinker that exerts pressure, heat packs, or distraction may reduce the problem. Although narcotics have been used, they are not the best treatment option.

2.10   **The answer is a.** The hand–foot syndrome is characterized by an often painful rash and swelling of the palms of the hands and soles of the feet. Patients can have difficulty walking, especially if the cause is capecitabine. Topotecan has similar effects as capecitabine but less dermatologic toxicity.

2.11   **The answer is a.** Treatment of osteoporosis involves intake of oral calcium, vitamin D, calcitonin, and bisphosphonates. Thyroid hormone replacement therapy increases the risk for osteoporosis.

2.12   **The answer is a.** When patients with prostate cancer receive androgen therapy, osteoblastic bone formation activity is decreased and osteoclastic activity is increased, creating an opportunity for osteoporosis to occur.

2.13   **The answer is d.** Because bisphosphonates inhibit osteoclast activity in bone (causes bone breakdown), they are ideal in the treatment of patients with bone metastases. When bisphosphonates bind to bone, they help to stabilize the bone mineral and inhibit calcium release and further breakdown.

2.14 **The answer is b.** Avoidance of amputation, preservation of maximum function, and eradication of tumor are all goals in the treatment of primary malignant bone cancer. Although there is evidence of a familial tendency for some of the bone cancers, early intervention in these cases is not common practice.

2.15 **The answer is d.** The scenarios in which limb salvage is not a treatment option are (1) when the surgeon is unable to attain adequate surgical margin, (2) when the neurovascular bundle is involved, and (3) when the patient is younger than 10 years. In the latter case limb salvage is contraindicated because of the resultant limb length discrepancy, although recent advances in expandable prostheses make it possible for more children afflicted with bone cancer to retain their limbs during surgery.

2.16 **The answer is a.** Although phantom limb sensations (i.e., itching, pressure, tingling) are often experienced shortly after surgery, phantom limb pain (i.e., cramping, throbbing, burning) usually occurs within 1–4 weeks after surgery. For most individuals, phantom limb pain resolves in a few months; however, some may be troubled for years. This worsening may be a sign of a neuroma or of locally recurrent cancer in the stump.

2.17 **The answer is c.** Currently, chemotherapy is given preoperatively. The rationale for preoperative chemotherapy is to treat micrometastasis, decrease the size of the primary tumor (thereby increasing the likelihood of limb-salvage surgery), and assess the effectiveness of the chemotherapeutic agents for 2–3 months before postoperative chemotherapy is given.

2.18 **The answer is c.** Chondrosarcoma is a tumor arising from either the interior medullary cavity of the cartilage (central chondrosarcoma) or from the bone through malignant changes in benign cartilage tumors (peripheral chondrosarcoma). The most frequent sites for this cancer are the shoulder girdle, hip girdle, and trunk. Less common sites include the bones of the hands and feet.

2.19 **The answer is b.** Radiation to the involved sites is used primarily to relieve pain, improve bone strength, and improve neurological deficits.

2.20 **The answer is b.** Infection in the neutropenic patient is always considered a potentially life-threatening emergency. Mortality rates in individuals with cancer who are neutropenic exceed 30%.

2.21 **The answer is d.** Myelosuppression is not only the most common dose-limiting side effect of chemotherapy, it is also potentially the most lethal. Antimetabolites, vinca alkaloids, and antitumor antibiotics are most damaging to cells that are in a specific phase of the cell cycle; thus myelosuppression is less severe with these agents.

2.22 **The answer is c.** The patient with neutropenia is unable to mount an inflammatory response. Fever is usually the first sign of infection. Choices **a**, **b**, and **d** are all true, but they explain why the neutropenic patient is at greater risk for infection rather than why the usual signs and symptoms of infection are often absent.

2.23 **The answer is c.** Neutropenia typically develops in 8–12 days after chemotherapy, with recovery in 3–4 weeks.

2.24 **The answer is b.** The respiratory tract is the most common site of infection in neutropenic patients. A high incidence of pneumonia in immunocompromised patients warrants thorough assessment of the respiratory tract. The mouth and oropharynx are also high incidence sites for infection.

2.25   **The answer is d.** Sepsis is the presence of systemic inflammatory response syndrome with evidence of infection. Septic shock occurs with hypotension that is unresponsive to fluid resuscitation plus organ dysfunction or perfusion abnormalities.

2.26   **The answer is b.** A decrease in the number of functional granulocytes is termed granulocytopenia. Granulocytopenia can occur as a result of leukemia, bone marrow infiltration by tumor cells in solid tumors, total body irradiation, and cytotoxic chemotherapy. It is the single most important risk factor for sepsis in individuals with cancer.

2.27   **The answer is d.** Risk factors such as tumor cells in the bone marrow, prior treatment with chemotherapy or radiation, and a high negative nitrogen balance all compromise the marrow and increase the degree and duration of cytopenia.

2.28   **The answer is a.** Patients with cancer undergoing chemotherapy would receive CSFs if they were at a 20% risk or greater of febrile neutropenia. Patients receive CSFs when they receive dose-dense chemotherapy to facilitate treatment in the time frame indicated.

2.29   **The answer is d.** In general, antifungal prophylaxis is not recommended for all neutropenic patients receiving chemotherapy. It is recommended for high-risk patients such as those with acute leukemia or those undergoing hematopoietic stem cell transplantation. Antifungal prophylaxis is indicated for severely neutropenic afebrile patients with an absolute neutrophil count less than 1000/mm^3 for more than 1 week.

2.30   **The answer is b.** The ANC is determined by multiplying the percentage of PMNs and bands by the total number of white blood cells. The individual in this example is considered neutropenic because the ANC is less than 1000/mm^3.

2.31   **The answer is c.** The incidence of catheter-related bacteremia is influenced by specific therapy, degree of catheter use, patient population, catheter insertion technique, and care and maintenance procedures. However, neutropenia remains the primary risk factor for patients with an infection who have a vascular access catheter

2.32   **The answer is d.** Infections, due to invasion and overgrowth of pathogenic microbes, increase in frequency and severity as the absolute neutrophil count decreases. Risk for severe infections increases when the nadir persists for more than 7–10 days. The purpose of colony-stimulating factors is to reduce the number of days that the nadir is below 500 cells/mm^3.

2.33   **The answer is c.** Approximately 45% of individuals with cancer develop sepsis.

2.34   **The answer is b.** In the setting of neutropenia, the general standard of care is a time frame of 2 hours from fever to administration of the first antimicrobial agent. Chest x-rays are usually ordered, but the yield is relatively low, and this step is considered a lower priority than starting antimicrobial therapy, especially in an elderly patient.

2.35   **The answer is c.** Myelosuppression is the most common and lethal side effect of chemotherapy. Because hematopoietic cells divide rapidly, they are vulnerable to chemotherapy, potentially resulting in dangerously low levels of red blood cells, white blood cells, and platelets. When this occurs, patients are at risk for bleeding, infection, and circulatory compromise.

2.36   **The answer is d.** Thrombopoietin is the factor that stimulates the differentiation and proliferation of megakaryocytes into platelets. It has been shown to reduce the duration of thrombocytopenia.

2.37   **The answer is c.** The other choices all result in lowered platelet count. Choice **a** is often associated with splenomegaly, an enlarged spleen; **b** is frequently due to an autoimmune response in which antibodies are formed against the person's own platelets; **d** may also be the consequence of cancer therapy on bone marrow. A fourth cause of thrombocytopenia is platelet dilution, often caused by the use of stored platelet-poor blood.

2.38   **The answer is c.** A multifactorial model for multiple myeloma-associated anemia has been postulated, including the replacement of erythrocyte precursors with plasma cells.

2.39   **The answer is c.** All patients with MDS eventually develop life-threatening anemia, thrombocytopenia, and/or neutropenia. Regular evaluation of patients with MDS is important to monitor the need for supportive therapy with red blood cells, platelets, or antibiotics. MDS can transform to acute leukemia; however, this does not occur in all patients with MDS.

2.40   **The answer is a.** A cumulative and delayed onset of thrombocytopenia has been observed with carmustine, fludarabine, lomustine, mitomycin C, streptozocin, and thiotepa.

2.41   **The answer is c.** When platelets are lower than 50,000 cells/mm^3, there is a moderate risk of bleeding. As the platelets continue to decrease below 10,000 cells/mm^3, a severe risk exists for fatal bleeding.

2.42   **The answer is d.** As the platelets continue to decrease below 10,000 cells/mm^3, a severe risk exists for fatal gastrointestinal, central nervous system, and respiratory tract hemorrhage.

2.43   **The answer is c.** Manifestations of thrombocytopenia are easy bruising; bleeding from gums, nose, or other orifices; and petechiae on the upper and lower extremities.

2.44   **The answer is d.** A decreased production of platelets may be due to tumor invasion of the bone marrow or to acute or delayed effects of chemotherapy or radiation. Pancytopenia is usually present.

2.45   **The answer is c.** The most common cause of thrombocytopenia in patients with cancer is a disorder involving decreased megakaryocytopoiesis (i.e., platelet production in the bone marrow).

2.46   **The answer is b.** Idiopathic thrombocytopenic purpura occurs most frequently in individuals with lymphoproliferative disorders such as chronic lymphocytic leukemia. It rarely is associated with solid tumors.

2.47   **The answer is c.** Interleukin-11 is used for the prevention of chemotherapy-induced thrombocytopenia. It also shortens the duration of thrombocytopenia.

2.48   **The answer is d.** The side effects of interleukin-11 treatment are dyspnea, fluid retention, and conjunctival redness and blurring.

2.49   **The answer is a.** Rectal manipulation may place the thrombocytopenic patient at risk for bleeding. The use of suppositories or enemas is contraindicated. Stool softener and a laxative are important for preventing constipation in the patient who is receiving vincristine.

2.50   **The answer is c.** Mitomycin causes cumulative and often delayed thrombocytopenia.

2.51   **The answer is d.** Transient control of platelet sequestration has been achieved with corticosteroid therapy. Steroids have a capillary-stabilizing effect that is important in minimizing the bleeding potential of thrombocytopenia.

2.52 **The answer is c.** Fever and infection enhance the consumption of platelets and can increase the occurrence of hemorrhage. Patients with fever or sepsis may require more frequent platelet transfusions to maintain adequate platelet counts.

2.53 **The answer is b.** Platelet survival is greatly decreased when alloimmunization to the platelet transfusion develops. Alloimmunization results when repeated transfusions of random-donor platelets fail to provide a therapeutic increment in the platelet count.

2.54 **The answer is c.** Symptoms that could indicate extravasation include swelling; stinging, burning, or pain at the injection site (not always present); redness (not often seen initially); and lack of blood return. Lack of blood return alone is not always indicative of an extravasation. An extravasation can occur even if a blood return is present. This patient is presenting the classic signs of extravasation, and the possibility of a flare reaction is inappropriate.

2.55 **The answer is d.** Acute radiation effects result from the depletion of actively proliferating parenchymal or stromal cells and is characterized by vascular dilation, local edema, and inflammation. They are usually temporary and occur after higher doses are given over shorter periods of time to larger volumes of tissue.

2.56 **The answer is c.** Factors that determine the degree, onset, and duration of radiation-induced skin reactions include the following, among others: Higher doses given over shorter periods of time to larger volumes result in more severe acute skin reactions; electrons produce greater skin reactions than do photons; and placing tissue-equivalent material on the skin reduces the skin-sparing effect of radiation therapy, allowing for maximum dose at the level of the skin. Finally, when treatment is targeted at areas of skin apposition, increased reaction secondary to warmth and moisture can be expected.

2.57 **The answer is b.** Following radiation therapy the skin's ability to protect itself from ultraviolet rays is decreased as a result of destruction of melanocytes in the irradiated epidermis and the slower rate of melanin production in new epidermal cells in the radiation field.

2.58 **The answer is d.** The obvious sign of drug infiltration is a bleb formation at the injection site or swelling that occurs in more deeply accessed veins. The absence of a blood return does not confirm an extravasation. The needle bevel or cannula tip may be positioned against the vein wall, preventing appropriate and obvious blood return.

2.59 **The answer is c.** SCC is more aggressive than BCC because it has a faster growth rate, less well-demarcated margins, and a greater metastatic potential. SCC appears as a flesh-colored or erythematous raised firm papule. It is usually confined to areas exposed to ultraviolet radiation.

2.60 **The answer is c.** During the proliferative phase of wound healing, which lasts from 3 to 25 days after surgery, granulation tissue is formed and provides the characteristic strength of a wound. Most chemotherapy agents act by interfering with protein synthesis. Thus wound healing could be disrupted by the administration of most chemotherapeutic agents in the early phases of wound healing.

2.61 **The answer is a.** A graft or flap is indicated when a lesion is large or located in an area in which insufficient tissue for primary closure would result in deformity, for example, after excision of large carcinomas of the eyelid and lip. Function is preserved in this manner. A skin flap consists of skin and subcutaneous tissue that are transferred from one area of the body to another. A flap contains its own blood supply, whereas a graft is avascular and depends on the blood supply of the recipient site for its survival.

2

PROTECTIVE
MECHANISMS

2.62 **The answer is d.** Except in cases of whole body irradiation or irradiation to the head, alopecia should not occur.

2.63 **The answer is c.** Tenderness and soreness remain highly prevalent after SLNB at 3 and 6 months after the procedure. Tenderness, soreness, tightness, and numbness are among the most severe and distressing symptoms associated with both SLNB and axillary lymph node dissection.

2.64 **The answer is c.** In ovarian cancer patients, 37.4% of patients experience palmar-plantar erythrodysesthesia (PPE) characterized by swelling, pain, erythema, and, for some patients, desquamation of the skin on the hands and the feet. PPE is generally seen after two or three cycles of treatment but may occur earlier. In most patients the reaction is mild and resolves in 1–2 weeks, so prolonged delay of therapy need not occur.

2.65 **The answer is b.** Hyperpigmentation occurs with bleomycin. Other drugs inducing this reaction include cyclophosphamide, busulfan, carmustine, nitrogen mustard, 5-FU, and etoposide. The other drugs listed as choices in this question have in common hypersensitivity reactions.

2.66 **The answer is d.** Multiple etiologic and risk factors are associated with skin cancers. High-risk factors for CM include a persistent changed or changing mole and the presence of irregular pigmented precursor lesions, including dysplastic nevi, congenital nevi, and lentigo maligna. Other possible risk factors for CM include ultraviolet (UV) radiation, age, hormonal factors, immunosuppression, and a previous history of melanoma. There is no conclusive evidence regarding the use of oral contraceptives and the increased risk of CM.

2.67 **The answer is d.** It is important early on to discuss the dose-modification schedule for capecitabine to decrease anxiety concerning the possibility of dose reductions and what that might mean. Although initial doses should be reduced in certain circumstances (e.g., for grade 2 or higher toxicity and moderate kidney dysfunction), dose interruption or reduction does not affect efficacy. Timely management of capecitabine-related side effects generally allows patients to continue therapy, whereas toxicity can worsen quickly if left untreated, resulting in a cascade of problems that may affect treatment outcomes negatively.

2.68 **The answer is d.** Persons who are immunocompromised are at high risk for activation of varicella zoster virus which once activated spreads down the sensory nerve to skin level. Therapy is generally held until the extent of the spread is known and treatment is underway. The physician should be notified immediately if the eye is in close proximity because ocular dissemination can result in systemic spread and loss of vision.

2.69 **The answer is c.** DN may develop throughout life. They may be familial or nonfamilial. The age-adjusted incidence of melanoma is approximately 15 times higher among persons with DN as compared to the general population. DN are often larger than 5 mm and can number from 1 to 100. They appear typically on sun-exposed areas, especially on the back, but also may be seen on the scalp, breasts, and buttocks. Pigmentation is irregular, with mixtures of tan, brown, and black or red and pink. A distinctive feature is a "fried egg" appearance.

2.70 **The answer is b.** Melanoma has two growth phases. In the radial phase tumor growth is parallel to the skin surface, risk of metastasis is slight, and surgical excision is usually curative. The vertical growth phase is marked by deep penetration into the dermis and subcutaneous tissue. Penetration occurs rapidly, increasing the risk of metastasis.

2.71   **The answer is b.** Sunscreen should always be applied on overcast days because 70–80% of ultraviolet radiation can penetrate cloud cover.

2.72   **The answer is b.** Amifostine is used to prevent neurotoxicities associated with cisplatin, paclitaxel, and carboplatin. Patients must be pretreated with an antiemetic, dexamethasone, and intravenous hydration. Nortriptyline and carbamazepine are used to manage symptoms rather than to prevent them.

2.73   **The answer is b.** Vincristine is well known for potential peripheral neuropathy.

2.74   **The answer is c.** Methotrexate is associated with cerebellar dysfunction, such as unsteady gait and seizures, but not with peripheral neuropathies. Cytarabine, cisplatin, and carboplatin are all associated with peripheral neuropathies, particularly at higher doses.

2.75   **The answer is c.** Paclitaxel can produce profound peripheral neuropathy. Symptoms are progressive and include paresthesia, numbness, loss of sensory qualities, and a decrease in deep-tendon reflexes.

2.76   **The answer is c.** Ifosfamide can cause cerebellar and cranial dysfunction but not myalgia or arthralgia.

2.77   **The answer is b.** Risk factors associated with ifosfamide encephalopathy include duration of administration, hepatic insufficiency, previous cisplatin use, presence of bulky disease, low serum albumin, and high serum creatinine.

2.78   **The answer is a.** Subacute cerebellar degeneration is a group of paraneoplastic neurologic disorders caused by antibodies that attack nerve cells, such as Purkinje cells, resulting in this neurologic syndrome.

2.79   **The answer is b.** Apraxia is the condition in which an individual cannot coordinate skilled movements but is not paralyzed.

2.80   **The answer is d.** Patients who develop peripheral neuropathy as a side effect of chemotherapy may develop sensory abnormalities such as diminished temperature and touch sense in addition to the numbness and tingling commonly experienced. Proprioceptive losses in the lower extremities can lead to ataxia.

2.81   **The answer is b.** Persistent neurotoxicity is a dose-limiting toxicity of oxaliplatin, occurring with increasing frequency after approximately 10–12 cycles and manifesting as a peripheral neuropathy with dysesthesia in a stocking–glove distribution. Calcium gluconate and magnesium sulfate prevent this complication to some degree.

2.82   **The answer is d.** The sensory and motor axons are injured. Demyelination reduces nerve conduction velocity, leading to loss of deep-tendon reflexes, but the cause is the effect of the drug on the microtubules in the axon transport system, which results in axonal degeneration.

2.83   **The answer is c.** Damage to the autonomic fibers can occur from chemotherapy and cause dizziness, constipation, abdominal colicky pain, ileus, impotence, urinary retention, and syndrome of inappropriate antidiuretic hormone secretion (SIADH).

2.84   **The answer is a.** Factors that increase the risk of neurotoxicity with vincristine are frequent drug administration (such as weekly); dose greater than 2 mg; age greater than 60 years; concomitant isoniazid, teniposide, or etoposide therapy; and severe liver dysfunction as the drug undergoes hepatic metabolism and clearance.

2.85   **The answer is d.** With continued drug use, symptomatic loss of medium-frequency sound occurs and may be permanent.

2.86   **The answer is d.** Although mild symptoms may appear 1–3 days after high-dose paclitaxel of 250 mg/m^2 or greater, resolving 3–6 months after drug discontinuance, more severe symptoms, such as loss of fine motor movements, may resolve only partially.

2.87   **The answer is a.** Rapid drug delivery, simultaneous administration of aminoglycosides, and dehydration seem to increase the potential for ototoxicity.

2.88   **The answer is c.** Neurotoxicity characterized by metabolic encephalopathy manifested as blurred vision, seizures, motor system dysfunction, urinary incontinence, cranial nerve dysfunction, or irreversible coma has been reported in 5–30% of patients treated with ifosfamide.

2.89   **The answer is a.** 5-Fluorouracil may cause an acute cerebellar dysfunction, which is usually more common in the elderly. It is characterized by rapid onset of gait ataxia, limb incoordination, dysarthria, nystagmus, and diplopia.

2.90   **The answer is c.** Although continuous pulse oximetry is used widely, patients and family members often focus on the monitor, which can increase anxiety and fear. Opioids are the first-line therapy in relieving dyspnea, without causing respiratory depression. Bronchodilators can relieve bronchospasm but can also increase anxiety.

2.91   **The answer is a.** Reality orientation is not considered beneficial in actively hallucinating patients. In fact, correcting the patient's perceptions may only increase anxiety and agitation. Be open to comments by dying patients about "going home" or seeing loved ones who have previously died. These are common behaviors seen during the dying process.

2.92   **The answer is b.** Research demonstrates that patients do not suffer or experience discomfort due to dehydration. Tube feedings may actually contribute to decreased survival due to aspiration and abdominal distention. Family members may inadvertently try to force patients to eat or drink, leading to aspiration or simply to discomfort for the patient.

2.93   **The answer is c.** Glucocorticoids rapidly reduce the rate of edema fluid formation by the tumor by inhibiting the capillary permeability factor produced by tumor cells. The aim of steroid therapy is to reduce intracranial pressure and increase cerebral blood flow.

2.94   **The answer is c.** Numbness or tingling of the extremities on the ipsilateral side, diplopia, blindness, progressive motor loss, and changes in the level of consciousness alert the nurse to possible cerebral ischemia secondary to carotid artery ligation.

2.95   **The answer is b.** The cytosine arabinoside should be withheld because dysarthria is a symptom of cerebellar toxicity from the drug. High-dose cytosine arabinoside can cause cerebellar toxicities that may be irreversible. A full neurological examination should be done before each dose, even in the absence of symptoms.

2.96   **The answer is d.** Symptoms of hypercalcemia in order of reported frequency are fatigue, anorexia, weight loss, bone pain, constipation, polydipsia, muscle weakness, nausea and vomiting, mental changes, and polyuria.

2.97   **The answer is a.** Initial central nervous system dysfunction can present as personality changes, impaired concentration, mild confusion, drowsiness, and lethargy. Personality changes occur subtly and often are unnoticed by the family or individual. Extreme restlessness, irritability, overt confusion, and progressive deterioration in cognitive function may develop.

2.98   **The answer is b.** Atrioventricular block leading to complete heart block and asystole may occur when the serum calcium level reaches 16 mg/dL or more. Hypertension may occur due to the direct effect of hypercalcemia on arterial smooth muscle.

2.99   **The answer is d.** Clinical manifestations of meningeal carcinomatosis are headache, mental status changes, gait disturbances, hydrocephalus, cranial nerve palsies, back pain, radiculopathies, weakness, and paresthesias.

2.100   **The answer is b.** Change in the level of consciousness is a classic sign of elevated intracranial pressure.

2.101   **The answer is d.** The incidence of PCNSL has increased dramatically in recent years, primarily due to the AIDS epidemic. Of patients diagnosed with PCNSL, about 95% have a brain lesion, and 50% of these lesions are multifocal. These lymphomas are primarily of B-cell origin confined to a single extranodal site.

2.102   **The answer is c.** Increased intracranial pressure, secondary to cerebral edema, is often present at diagnosis. The incidence of radiation-induced elevated intracranial pressure increases with the dose of the initial fraction(s) (i.e., fractions of 200 cGy or more per day). Symptoms include exacerbation of patient's presenting neurologic symptoms.

2.103   **The answer is d.** Somnolence syndrome is a cluster of symptoms consisting of excessive sleepiness and drowsiness, lethargy, and fatigue with anorexia. The cause is related to transient demyelination secondary to radiation. Symptoms occur 4–12 weeks after radiation and can last for 2–8 weeks. Patients need reassurance as the syndrome runs its course.

2.104   **The answer is a.** The purpose of the steroids is to minimize swelling of the brain tissue caused initially by the tumor and the radiation. When steroids are tapered or stopped, the swelling may resume and the patient can become more somnolent.

2.105   **The answer is a.** Side effects from dronabinol that are particularly bothersome in middle-aged and older adults include dry mouth, sedation, orthostatic hypotension, ataxia, dizziness, and euphoria or dysphoria.

2.106   **The answer is a.** Central nervous system lymphoma commonly causes neurologic dysfunction, apathy, confusion, and/or personality changes. It does not typically cause the headaches that are common to brain tumors, spinal cord compression, or SIADH.

2.107   **The answer is c.** Malignant cerebral edema produces diffuse signs and symptoms reflecting its more global effects on brain functioning, as opposed to the focal signs and symptoms caused by direct destruction of tissue by tumor. Subtle early changes in the patient's status are vague and usually are observed only by someone who knows the patient well. Seizure is the most common acute-onset sign. Headache, another common early symptom, is due to distortion and traction of pain-sensitive structures by the edema.

2.108   **The answer is a.** In most instances the first, earliest, and most sensitive indicator of dysfunction is a change in the level of consciousness. Mental status and cognitive ability, as well as motor and sensory function and cranial nerve function, are also assessed.

2 PROTECTIVE MECHANISMS

2.109　**The answer is c.** The most significant consequence of gram-negative infection is the potential for endotoxic or systemic shock. The release of endotoxins initiates a cascade of events that, unless interrupted, rapidly lead to death for the neutropenic patient.

2.110　**The answer is c.** *P. carinii* is a protozoan that causes infection in children with primary immunodeficiency disorders, persons with AIDS, and those with cancer who are undergoing immunosuppressive therapy. Untreated, *P. carinii* is fatal, and even with therapy mortality is high. The treatment of choice is trimethoprim-sulfamethoxazole.

2.111　**The answer is b.** Risk factors for development of refractory infection and sepsis include complex polymicrobial infections, infections lasting more than 21 days, infectious lesions larger than 5 cm, hematologic malignancy, shock associated with infection, and low albumin at the onset of symptoms of sepsis.

2.112　**The answer is d.** Signs and symptoms of sepsis are often subtle or absent. Fever may be absent, especially in the elderly.

2.113　**The answer is d.** The primary advantages of combination therapy are potential synergistic effects of the drugs against some gram-negative bacilli and decreased development of drug-resistant strains during treatment.

2.114　**The answer is c.** The diagnosis of venoocclusive disease is based on clinical findings in the first 21 days after HCT. Diagnostic criteria include two or more of the following symptoms: hyperbilirubinemia, hepatomegaly, right upper quadrant pain, and fluid retention.

2.115　**The answer is a.** The pathophysiology of the syndrome begins with injury of the endothelial lining of hepatic venules and sinusoids. This endothelial injury leads to cytokine and tumor necrosis factor activation, which stimulates coagulation and thrombosis. The resulting impairment of blood flow produces the syndrome of hepatic venoocclusive disease, which leads to renal insufficiency and, ultimately, to multiorgan failure and death.

2.116　**The answer is d.** There are four separate classifications of KS: (1) classic or non–HIV-related KS, usually in men of Mediterranean descent; (2) endemic KS, occurring in men, women, and children in certain areas of Africa; (3) KS associated with iatrogenic immunosuppression, sometimes referred to as renal transplant KS; and (4) epidemic or HIV-related KS, which occurs primarily in men who have sex with men. The genetic reference refers to the fact that there appears to be a genetic predisposition related to the HIV virus (the *tat* gene). However, this is not related to the classification system.

2.117　**The answer is c.** Fever is the cardinal symptom of infection. The neutropenic condition of marrow recipients masks the classic infection-related symptoms of inflammation, pus formation, and elevated white blood cell counts.

2.118　**The answer is a.** Gram-positive organisms are responsible for approximately 75% of all infections.

2.119　**The answer is c.** To help prevent hemorrhagic cystitis during therapy with cyclophosphamide, patients are encouraged to drink 8–10 glasses of fluid a day and to void frequently.

2.120　**The answer is b.** The skin is the first line of defense against invading bacteria and subsequent infection. When a break in the skin occurs, environmental microbes and those that normally inhabit hair follicles and sebaceous glands can enter the body and cause infection.

2.121   **The answer is a.** Polymorphonuclear neutrophils (PMNs) comprise 55–70% of white blood cells and are the first to respond to invading bacteria. The primary function of PMNs is the destruction and elimination of microorganisms through phagocytosis, the process of engulfing and ingesting foreign matter.

2.122   **The answer is d.** Undisturbed endogenous microbial flora exist as a carefully balanced synergistic microenvironment within the host. Alterations in normal flora predispose persons with cancer to serious opportunistic or nosocomial infection. More than 80% of infections developing in cancer patients arise from endogenous organisms, nearly half of which are acquired during hospitalization.

2.123   **The answer is b.** Diagnosis of varicella zoster virus infection is based on a history of chickenpox, characteristic dermatomal distribution of vesicular lesions, and positive culture results. Because skin lesions (vesicles) can become confluent, meticulous skin care is required to prevent secondary bacterial infection.

2.124   **The answer is b.** Meticulous hand washing, by every person who enters the room or comes in contact with the individual at risk, is the single most important preventive measure against infection in the patient with granulocytopenia. Neutropenic individuals are advised of their risk and are encouraged to remind family, visitors, and staff about hand-washing precautions.

2.125   **The answer is a.** Profound immunosuppression with resulting neutropenia concomitant with denuding of the mucosa in the gastrointestinal tract places patients at risk for gram-negative bacteremia.

2.126   **The answer is a.** Chronic hepatitis B virus infection is the leading cause of hepatocellular carcinoma throughout the world.

2.127   **The answer is d.** AIDS-associated NHLs are typically intermediate- to high-grade B-cell malignancies. They appear to be associated with a rise in polygonal B-cell lymphoproliferation that results from EBV and HIV infection. AIDS-NHL has been associated with persistent generalized lymphadenopathy, suggesting polyclonal B-cell activation. One possibility is that once HIV infection occurs, EBV may trigger lymphocyte proliferation that remains unchecked as a result of HIV-induced immune dysfunction. This proliferation, in turn, may allow the expression of two oncogenes, resulting in a polygonal or monoclonal NHL.

2.128   **The answer is b.** Because diagnostic signals may be subtle (e.g., skin petechiae that may be noticed while bathing the person, traces of blood during brushing of teeth), it is important for the nurse to be keenly observant. A family history and various screening tests may be valuable in assessment, but they do not substitute for observation.

2.129   **The answer is d.** This screening test is called prothrombin time. Choice **a** is the activated partial prothromboplastin test, **b** is the specific factor assays test, and **c** is the bleeding time test.

2.130   **The answer is d.** Megakaryocytes mature in the bone marrow and fragment to form platelets, which are then released into the bloodstream. Under normal circumstances any reduction in platelet count—from bleeding, malignancy, chemotherapy or radiotherapy, or other causes—produces an increase in the production of megakaryocytes and platelets in the bone marrow. This activity is controlled by a regulatory hormone called thrombopoietin.

2.131   **The answer is b.** Plasminogen activators are enzymes that are present in most body fluids and tissues. They are responsible for the conversion of plasminogen to plasmin in the presence of thrombin. It is plasmin that is responsible for the lysis (and not the formation) of fibrin clots.

2.132   **The answer is a.** All the other choices can be factors in bleeding, but erosion and rupture of vessels precipitated by tumor invasion or pressure is the other major cause of bleeding in persons with cancer. Any tumor involvement of vasculature tissue or any tumor lying in close proximity to major vessels is seen as a threat of bleeding. Bleeding may also be the result of radiotherapy, surgery, or various platelet and coagulation abnormalities.

2.133   **The answer is c.** If acute bleeding does occur, direct methods to halt the hemorrhage should be instituted immediately. Choices **a**, **b** and **d** are preventive methods. Another example of the use of mechanical pressure to stop acute bleeding is the insertion of an occlusion balloon catheter into the bronchus.

2.134   **The answer is b.** Although all the other choices are factors in bleeding as well, platelet count is the single most important factor in predicting bleeding in the individual with cancer. Patients with platelet counts below 20,000 cells/mm^3 have a high risk of bleeding. Low platelet count (thrombocytopenia) is also the most frequent platelet abnormality associated with cancer.

2.135   **The answer is c.** The nursing actions during a carotid hemorrhage focus on maintenance of the airway and control of bleeding. If the patient has a tracheostomy, the cuff should be inflated to prevent aspiration. Firm pressure should be applied to the neck using a towel or dressing material. If an internal carotid bleed is suspected, a vaginal pack or fluff dressing should be used to tightly pack the oral cavity and oropharynx. The patient is then transported to the operating room for ligation of the carotid artery.

2.136   **The answer is a.** Leukostasis occurs as the leukemic blast cells accumulate and invade vessel walls, causing rupture and bleeding. Patients with extremely high numbers of circulating blasts (white blood cell count > 50,000/mm^3) are at increased risk for leukostasis. Intracerebral hemorrhage is the most common and most lethal manifestation of this complication.

2.137   **The answer is d.** Because most liver tumors are highly vascular, the person having an ultrasound-guided percutaneous needle biopsy of the liver must be monitored closely for intraabdominal hemorrhage. In general, this procedure is rapid, safe, and commonly used; however, some clinicians strongly believe that needle biopsies should be avoided at all costs if there is any potential for curative resection, because of the potential for seeding and spreading the cancer during the procedure.

2.138   **The answer is d.** Patients with liver cancer are more at risk for bleeding because of a decrease in vitamin K absorption, an increase in prothrombin time and partial thromboplastin time, and varices from portal hypertension.

2.139   **The answer is a.** Noncontrast CT can be performed rapidly and is the technique of choice for evaluating acute hemorrhage. Contrast is then administered to delineate the margins and extent of blood–brain barrier disruption. Magnetic resonance imaging is the more definitive and preferred imaging study for the individual with a central nervous system tumor. Cerebral angiography may be used to confirm that the lesion in question is a vascular malformation or an aneurysm rather than a neoplasm.

2.140 **The answer is b.** Hemorrhage, hypovolemia, and hypotension pose the greatest threats to an individual who has just undergone surgery for cancer of the pancreas. As soon as possible after pancreatectomy, small feedings are started with a diet that is usually bland, low in fat, and high in carbohydrates and protein. Restrictions include caffeine, alcohol, and overindulgence. The stool should be examined daily for the characteristic signs of steatorrhea: frothy foul-smelling stool with fat particles floating in the water.

2.141 **The answer is a.** As liver cancer advances, serious complications arise, usually involving many body systems. Portal vein obstruction may lead to necrosis, rupture, and hemorrhage. Esophageal varices and unrelenting ascites are also common sequelae of either primary or secondary liver cancer.

2.142 **The answer is a.** Skin flaps are usually made to cover and protect the carotid artery. However, skin flap necrosis would leave the artery unprotected, and infection and persistent tumor raise the risk of rupture. Carotid artery rupture usually is preceded by a small trickle of blood from the area.

2.143 **The answer is b.** Hematoma formation can adversely affect the adherence of skin flaps, resulting in flap necrosis. Excessive bleeding may require a return to the operating room for ligation of the bleeding vessel. Choices **a** and **d** are positive surgical outcomes; as for choice **c**, bleeding is expected postoperatively. The area is observed and noted but requires no immediate action.

2.144 **The answer is c.** Choices **b** and **d** are coagulation abnormalities; choice **a** is a quantitative abnormality. Qualitative abnormalities such as choice **c** refer principally to alterations in platelet function, which may include a decreased procoagulant activity of platelets, decreased platelet adhesiveness and decreased aggregation in response to adenosine diphosphate (ADP), thrombocytosis associated with myeloproliferative disorders, and the coating of platelets by fibrin degradation products as a result of the increased activation of coagulation factors.

2.145 **The answer is c.** Thromboplastin is needed for conversion of prothrombin to thrombin, and its formation results from both pathways of the clotting cascade—the intrinsic and the extrinsic pathways.

CHAPTER 3

Gastrointestinal and Urinary Function

ALTERATIONS IN NUTRITION

Dysphagia

3.1   What is the best treatment approach for radiation esophagitis?
   a.   Symptom relief and supportive care
   b.   Dietary manipulation
   c.   Topical anesthesia and systemic analgesia, when needed
   d.   All of the above

3.2   Your patient has completed 2 weeks of radiation therapy and concomitant chemotherapy for carcinoma of the pyriform sinus. He complains of dysphagia, odynophagia, and intermittent epigastric pain. He is most likely suffering from which of the following?
   a.   Mucositis
   b.   Bronchitis
   c.   Esophagitis
   d.   Cholangitis

3.3   Pain in the throat and difficulty swallowing following radiation to that area are common. Sucralfate suspension is often recommended and is intended to accomplish which of the following?
   a.   Promote comfort and possibly healing by binding to exposed mucosa
   b.   Promote comfort by numbing exposed nerve endings
   c.   Promote healing by reducing infection
   d.   Pain control only

3.4   Which of the following chemotherapy agents is likely to potentiate the problem of esophagitis in patients also receiving radiation therapy to the esophagus?
   a.   Cyclophosphamide
   b.   5-Fluorouracil
   c.   Paclitaxel
   d.   Procarbazine

3.5 Complications and side effects of radiotherapy for esophageal cancer include all of the following *except*
  a. Esophageal stricture
  b. Radiation pneumonitis
  c. Skin reaction
  d. Diarrhea

3.6 An elderly woman presents with a thyroid mass and symptoms of dyspnea and dysphagia. Assessment indicates carcinoma of the thyroid with metastases to the lung. Her symptoms of dyspnea and dysphagia are *most likely* to be the result of which of the following?
  a. Involvement of the parathyroid gland and associated hypercalcemia
  b. Compressive effects of the tumor on the larynx and esophagus
  c. Infection caused by irritation of the oral mucosa
  d. A high concentration of iodine in the follicular cells of the thyroid

3.7 Dysphagia is the most common presenting symptom of persons with which of the following?
  a. Tracheal cancer
  b. Esophageal cancer
  c. Epiglottal cancer
  d. Laryngeal cancer

3.8 A patient has aspiration pneumonia from a tracheoesophageal fistula. He is terminal and in hospice care. The physician has ordered scopolamine (0.6 mg intramuscularly) three to four times a day as needed. You explain to the patient and family that the purpose of the scopolamine is which of the following?
  a. To decrease the amount of secretions
  b. To manage his pain
  c. To decrease anxiety
  d. To help manage dyspnea

3.9 A patient has difficulty swallowing without aspirating following a hemilaryngectomy for a supraglottic carcinoma. You consult a swallowing specialist, who recommends which of the following to help the patient relearn swallowing without aspiration?
  a. Try liquids first and then semisolids
  b. Try crackers or toast followed by a sip of liquid
  c. Try semisolids first and then solids followed by liquids
  d. None of the above until he can manage his own secretions

Anorexia

3.10 The primary difference between primary and secondary cachexia in cancer is which of the following?
  a. Primary cachexia is where the individual is underweight before cancer.
  b. Secondary cachexia results from voluntary starvation.
  c. Primary cachexia results from tumor-produced metabolic abnormalities.
  d. Secondary cachexia results from chemical toxins and liver failure.

3.11   While teaching your patient with prostate cancer about treatment, his wife mentions he takes nutritional supplements, including saw palmetto because it is purported to promote prostate health. Your most appropriate response to this family would include which of the following?
    a.   Nutritional supplements are encouraged and will help him maintain his weight.
    b.   It is acceptable to continue on what he is currently taking, but he should not take mega-doses of any medication, including vitamins.
    c.   He should be instructed to stop taking saw palmetto because it could interfere with the effectiveness of hormonal drug treatment for prostate cancer.
    d.   He should continue the saw palmetto because it reduces prostate size, but he should stop all other supplements.

3.12   Anorexia or loss of appetite is a common problem in individuals with cancer. Which of the following is *most likely* to contribute to anorexia?
    a.   Cytokines
    b.   Circulating amino acids and lactic acid
    c.   Serotonin or tryptophan
    d.   All of the above

3.13   Patients with metastatic cancer often have difficulty maintaining their weight because of a lack of appetite. Your patient has just received a prescription for megestrol acetate, 800 mg per day. While discussing her new medication, you are sure to include *all but* which of the following?
    a.   Weight gain is likely to occur due to increase in body fat.
    b.   The purpose of the medication is to treat the cancer.
    c.   She may experience edema, hyperglycemia, and risk of embolism.
    d.   The medication will increase her feeling of well-being.

3.14   Vinny has started radiation therapy to his left leg for a sarcoma. He complains of anorexia and slight nausea following his radiation treatment. Your explanation would include which of the following?
    a.   Because the radiation port does not include his stomach, it is not likely that his symptoms are related to the radiation.
    b.   His feeling of nausea and anorexia are probably more psychological than real.
    c.   The waste products of tissue destruction are likely the cause of his symptoms.
    d.   The Cori cycle is producing excess urea.

3.15   Anorexia is characterized by which of the following?
    a.   Abnormalities of carbohydrate, protein, and fat metabolism
    b.   Visceral and lean body mass depletion
    c.   Early satiety
    d.   All of the above

3.16   Which of the following is *not* considered to be a reflection of immune status in an individual suffering from anorexia?
    a.   Hypoalbuminemia
    b.   Decreased macrophage mobilization
    c.   Depressed lymphocyte function
    d.   Impaired phagocytosis

3.17 Which of the following places an individual with cancer at significant high risk for protein-calorie malnutrition?
   a. Loss of 10% body weight within the previous 6 months
   b. An unintentional weight loss of more than 1 kilogram a week
   c. A macrobiotic diet
   d. All of the above

3.18 A newly diagnosed unresectable lung cancer patient complains that he has not had an appetite for many weeks and is concerned because he is losing weight. What is the *most likely* cause of his weight loss?
   a. Anorexia and cachexia are common manifestations of lung cancer.
   b. He is probably depressed over his situation and should improve with treatment.
   c. The chemotherapy and radiation cause weight loss.
   d. Liver disease is most likely causing his loss of appetite.

3.19 Mr. Dillon is dying from lung cancer and has had no appetite for some time. His living will asks for no life-saving measures; however, his family states they are uncomfortable with their loved one starving to death and want him to be force fed. Which of the following is *not* an appropriate rationale for intervention?
   a. If the family wants the patient to have enteral or parenteral nutrition, this is a therapeutic option.
   b. Artificial nutrition can lead to congestive heart failure, nausea, vomiting, and diarrhea.
   c. Anorexia is an adaptive protective mechanism that leads to a gentler death.
   d. Dehydration commonly accompanies other signs of impending death as the organs begin to fail.

3.20 The etiology of anorexia-cachexia syndrome is best explained by which of the following?
   a. Reduced food intake due to tumor byproducts
   b. Multiple metabolic and physiologic abnormalities
   c. Loss of appetite due to changes in taste and smell
   d. All of the above

Mucositis

3.21 Following a course of high-dose chemotherapy your patient complains of mouth soreness. Upon physical inspection you notice the lining of her mouth to be ulcerated with red patches. Your care recommendations are based on which of the following facts regarding oral care?
   a. She should increase the frequency of her oral care because her symptoms are worse.
   b. She should decrease the frequency of her oral care because the lining of her oral cavity is becoming irritated.
   c. She should rinse with a sodium bicarbonate solution because bacteria thrive in an acid environment.
   d. a and c

3.22 Mucositis is observed more often when
   a. 5-FU is combined with other mucositis-producing drugs, such as methotrexate and doxorubicin
   b. 5-FU is given alone
   c. Bleomycin is used to abruptly replace 5-FU
   d. None of the above

3.23   Which of the following is considered an effective measure to minimize oral stomatitis?
 a.   Oral cryotherapy during chemotherapy treatment
 b.   Sucralfate oral suspension
 c.   Frequent oral hygiene
 d.   All of the above

3.24   Which of the following factors is considered a risk factor for stomatitis with cancer treatment?
 a.   Dehydration
 b.   Preexisting dental problems
 c.   Malnutrition
 d.   All of the above

3.25   A patient who has been treated with radiation to the mouth and oropharynx has developed mucositis. Effective management of this side effect incorporates all of the following *except*
 a.   Encouraging the patient to avoid alcohol and cigarettes
 b.   Administering an appropriate systemic analgesic such as morphine
 c.   Removing the plaque-like tissue that forms with mucositis
 d.   Administering Maalox to coat and soothe the mucosa

3.26   Which of the following increases the risk of mucositis to a patient receiving radiation to the base of the tongue?
 a.   Metal tooth fillings
 b.   Tobacco usage
 c.   Alcohol consumption
 d.   All of the above

3.27   The dose-limiting toxicity of 5-fluorouracil when given as a continuous infusion is
 a.   Myelosuppression
 b.   Mucositis
 c.   Nausea and vomiting
 d.   Cerebellar ataxia

3.28   A bone marrow transplant patient has an oral herpetic lesion and asks you how she could have gotten it. Which of the following statements is *not* accurate concerning oral herpes simplex virus (HSV) infections?
 a.   Most oral infections are due to reactivation of latent infections.
 b.   HSV infections in this population present as soft-tissue ulcerations rather than vesicles.
 c.   The incidence of HSV infection in this population is about 50%.
 d.   This population is more at risk for disseminated HSV infection than other immunocompromised patients.

3.29   Patients with acute myelocytic leukemia frequently have gingival hypertrophy with swelling, necrosis, and infection of the gums. All of the following treatments are appropriate. Which one is *most* effective in relieving the problem?
 a.   Oral care with a solution of one quart water with one teaspoon each of salt and sodium bicarbonate
 b.   Antifungal mouth rinses
 c.   Local or systemic analgesics as needed
 d.   Initiating chemotherapy

Xerostomia

3.30   Which of the following would be considered an example of direct stomatotoxicity?
a. The cytotoxic action of drugs on the cells of the oral basal epithelium causes a decrease in the rate of cell renewal.
b. Bleeding from the gums following flossing in the patient with low platelets.
c. Cellular breakdown is due to high alcohol content in mouthwashes.
d. Pancytopenia and gingivitis occur.

3.31   The radioprotectant amifostine has been shown to be effective in reducing which of the following complications of radiation to the head and neck region?
a. Mucositis
b. Acute and chronic xerostomia
c. Dysphagia
d. All of the above

3.32   Your patient is receiving chemotherapy and complains of a dry mouth and thick ropy saliva. The condition interferes with his appetite and speech. Which of the following is *not* part of your patient education plan regarding this reaction?
a. This reaction is permanent, and, although not life-threatening, it can eventually lead to oral caries and candidal infections.
b. Xerostomia is a dysfunction of the salivary gland that occurs following chemotherapy.
c. Xerostomia is a decrease in the quality and quantity of saliva.
d. Saliva substitutes, frequent rinses with ice water, and sugarless gum may provide relief.

3.33   Which is *not* part of your treatment plan for the patient experiencing xerostomia?
a. Oral care before meals helps to freshen the mouth and stimulate appetite.
b. Increasing fluid intake during meals and snacks helps to lubricate food and ease swallowing.
c. Lemon glycerin is an excellent substitute for the more irritating commercial mouthwashes.
d. Butter or cooking oil placed in the mouth may be a cost-effective alternative for artificial lubrication.

3.34   What can be used to dissolve and thin thick saliva?
a. Sugar-free lemon candy and sugar-free gum
b. Papain (found in papaya) and amylase (found in pineapple)
c. Sialagogues
d. Pilocarpine

3.35   After radiation treatment, Michelle complains of a dry mouth and within 3 weeks develops a thick ropy saliva. What is the side effect Michelle is experiencing?
a. Xerostomia
b. Mucositis
c. Trismus
d. Desquamation

3.36   Four weeks after radiation therapy ends, Mr. Allen complains that the xerostomia is not improving. The physician prescribes oral pilocarpine. Your teaching includes which of the following points?
a. The pilocarpine is used to suppress the exocrine gland production.
b. Side effects include diaphoresis, lacrimation, and increased gastric secretion.
c. Photosensitivity worsens over time.
d. All of the above

3.37   Xerostomia, a decrease in saliva secretion, is a side effect of
    a. Oral surgery
    b. Bone marrow transplantation
    c. Cisplatin administration
    d. Head and neck irradiation

3.38   Besides a dry mouth, the primary problem with xerostomia is
    a. Lack of pH balance in the mouth
    b. Enamel decalcification
    c. Heightened taste sensation for sweet and sour foods
    d. Increased tracheal and esophageal irritation

Nausea and Vomiting

3.39   Mr. Zahir is receiving cisplatin therapy for testicular cancer and requires a 5-HT$_3$ receptor antagonist and a corticosteroid daily during his treatment. The rationale for this combination is based on which of the following?
    a. Cisplatin is often associated with cumulative and delayed nausea.
    b. The corticosteroid is used to boost the immune system.
    c. The corticosteroid enhances the antiemetic effect of the serotonin antagonist.
    d. a and c

3.40   According to evidence-based practice, which of the following is likely to be effective in managing nausea and vomiting from chemotherapy?
    a. Guided imagery
    b. Acupuncture and acupressure
    c. Progressive muscle relaxation
    d. All of the above

3.41   Which of the following antineoplastic agents is commonly associated with delayed nausea?
    a. Doxorubicin
    b. Cisplatin
    c. Cyclophosphamide
    d. All of the above

3.42   Anticipatory nausea and vomiting during the 12-hour period before chemotherapy occurs in approximately what percentage of patients?
    a. 15%
    b. 20%
    c. 25%
    d. 30%

3.43   Degree and severity of chemotherapy-induced nausea and vomiting vary based on many factors. Which of the following is *not* considered to be a factor in predicting the degree and severity of chemotherapy-induced nausea and vomiting?
    a. History of nausea due to radiation therapy
    b. Rate of chemotherapy infusion
    c. Drug sequencing
    d. Age

3.44   Which of the following chemotherapy agents is *not* associated with a moderate to high incidence of emesis?
   a.   Vincristine
   b.   Methotrexate
   c.   Doxorubicin
   d.   Topotecan

3.45   5-HT$_3$ antagonists represent a class of drugs used to prevent and manage chemotherapy-induced nausea and vomiting. Which of the following best describes the characteristics of these agents compared to the dopamine antagonists?
   a.   Unlike the phenothiazines, 5-HT$_3$ antagonists are not associated with extrapyramidal reactions.
   b.   5-HT$_3$ antagonists work both centrally and peripherally, whereas the dopamine antagonists work only centrally.
   c.   5-HT$_3$ antagonists have toxicities that can be cumulative.
   d.   a and b

3.46   Protracted nausea and vomiting is common following chemotherapy and total body irradiation, but which of the following could also be *responsible* for the protracted nature of this problem?
   a.   Graft-versus-host disease (GVHD)
   b.   Cytomegalovirus (CMV) esophagitis
   c.   Gastrointestinal infections
   d.   All of the above

3.47   Your patient is receiving high-dose chemotherapy and received prophylactic antiemetics, including ondansetron 16 mg orally on day 1 and daily for 2–4 days with dexamethasone 12 mg orally on day 1 with 8 mg orally on days 2–4. She states she started vomiting on day 2 and continued with nausea and vomiting for 3 days. According to current recommendations, which of the following is an appropriate approach to manage her symptoms for the next course?
   a.   Administer her antiemetic drugs intravenously because they are more effective that way.
   b.   Double the dose of her antiemetics and extend them out to 5 days posttreatment.
   c.   Admit her for intravenous fluids and antiemetics.
   d.   Administer aprepitant tri-pak and consider a different oral serotonin antagonist.

3.48   Emesis is a complex physiologic response to the toxic effects of chemotherapy. Which of the following is *not* considered to be a part of the chemotherapy-induced nausea–vomiting response mechanism?
   a.   Stimulation of cells that line the duodenum
   b.   Serotonin stimulation of the vagal nerve
   c.   Physical injury to cancer cells
   d.   Vagal stimulation of the medulla oblongata

3.49   John has a lung tumor with a single brain lesion for which he has received a full course of radiation therapy. He has been doing well on paclitaxel and carboplatin, until he experiences vomiting that seemed to come on without warning. Select the *most appropriate* advice to give this patient.
   a.   His vomiting is most likely due to the chemotherapy, and he should take an antiemetic and call back if he does not feel better.
   b.   He is probably experiencing delayed nausea and vomiting from the combination of the radiation and the chemotherapy. An antiemetic is appropriate.
   c.   His symptoms could be related to increased intracranial pressure, and he should come to the emergency room as soon as possible.
   d.   His symptoms could be due to chemotherapy or to increased intracranial pressure, and he should be advised to take dexamethasone, which is appropriate in either case.

3.50   Your 28-year-old patient is receiving doxorubicin and cyclophosphamide for her breast can-
        cer. She complains of feeling jittery and nervous following her chemotherapy. She is taking
        ondansetron 24 mg plus dexamethasone 10 mg and prochlorperazine 15 mg according to
        her schedule. Which of the following interventions is *most appropriate* and why?
        a.   Eliminate the dexamethasone from her protocol because it is making her jittery.
        b.   Discontinue the prochlorperazine because she is allergic to it.
        c.   Administer diphenhydramine 25 mg with the prochlorperazine because she is young and
             likely to be sensitive to it.
        d.   Discontinue both the dexamethasone and the prochlorperazine because either one can
             cause jitteriness and a hypersensitivity reaction.

Taste Alterations

3.51   Your patient is beginning radiation therapy to the mandible and is concerned about how this
        will affect his ability to taste and smell. Your teaching would include *all but* which of the fol-
        lowing?
        a.   If xerostomia occurs, loss of taste is more likely.
        b.   Loss of taste is usually permanent.
        c.   Acidic foods may increase glossodynia.
        d.   Taste acuity is usually restored within 4 months.

3.52   You decide to do some research to find out how and why chemotherapy causes an effect on
        nutrition. In your reading, you learn *all but* which of the following?
        a.   Chemotherapy can indirectly cause food aversions.
        b.   Chemotherapy can alter the intestinal absorptive surface.
        c.   Chemotherapy does not interfere with specific metabolic reactions.
        d.   Chemotherapy may cause excitation of the true vomiting center.

3.53   Which of the following medical terms is used to describe taste abnormalities in cancer
        patients?
        a.   Hypogeusia
        b.   Dysgeusia
        c.   Hyposmia
        d.   All of the above

3.54   Which of the following is *not* considered to be a cause of altered taste and smell in individ-
        uals with cancer?
        a.   Deficiencies in zinc, copper, nickel, and niacin
        b.   Direct tumor invasion
        c.   Hypercalcemia
        d.   Tumor-associated circulating factors

3.55   Jim complains that food does not taste the same and that everything tastes like cardboard.
        He especially dislikes the taste of red meat. This is best explained by the fact that persons
        with cancer commonly experience which of the following?
        a.   An increased threshold for sweet, sour, and salt and a decreased threshold for bitter foods
        b.   A decreased threshold for sweet, sour, and salt and an increased threshold for bitter foods
        c.   Difficulty digesting their food
        d.   Intolerance to bland foods

3.56   Lason is receiving radiation to his posterior hypopharynx. Your teaching would include which of the following points regarding the effects of radiation on taste?
a.   He can expect to experience alterations of taste about 2–3 weeks into treatment.
b.   The most severely affected taste qualities are salt and bitter.
c.   Sweet taste is generally least affected.
d.   All of the above

3.57   Common symptoms of carcinoma of the nasal cavity and paranasal sinuses include all of the following *except*
a.   Diplopia
b.   Hyperesthesia of the cheek
c.   Taste changes
d.   Headache pain

3.58   Because of the changed configuration of the aerodigestive tract, the person who has undergone a laryngectomy can expect change in all of the following functions *except*
a.   Speaking
b.   Eating
c.   Taste
d.   Smell

3.59   An example of a chemotherapeutic agent that may cause a metallic taste during administration, leading to taste changes, is
a.   Etoposide
b.   Cyclophosphamide
c.   Doxorubicin
d.   Dacarbazine

Electrolyte Imbalances

3.60   Janie has ovarian cancer and is beginning her cancer treatment with enthusiasm. In addition to chemotherapy, she wants to begin a macrobiotic diet and take dietary supplements. You want to encourage her and guide her in the right direction. Which of the following is *not* appropriate advice to give this patient?
a.   Alternative therapies have not been proved to be effective, and she should not take any vitamins or dietary supplements.
b.   Macrobiotic diets tend to be deficient in protein, calories, iron, and vitamin B_{12}.
c.   Megadose vitamin supplements tend to be excessively high in the B complex, C, A, D, and E vitamins.
d.   Megadose vitamins can cause liver damage, kidney stones, and coagulation abnormalities.

3.61   Mr. Johns is undergoing chemotherapy for high-grade testicular cancer. He complains of being jittery, and his lab tests reveal low magnesium, albumin, and calcium. He is *most likely* experiencing which of the following complications of chemotherapy?
a.   Anorexia and weakness due to chemotherapy
b.   Low magnesium due to cisplatin therapy
c.   Low calcium due to uremia syndrome
d.   A paraneoplastic syndrome

3.62   Rita has lung cancer and wants to try alternative approaches to nutrition to help improve her immune system. She is leaning toward a macrobiotic diet and asks if there are any adverse effects associated with this type of diet. The major problem with a macrobiotic diet is which of the following?
    a. Colitis and electrolyte imbalance
    b. Deficiencies in vitamin B_{12}
    c. Protein deficiencies
    d. All of the above

3.63   Health food stores are replete with vitamin supplements to treat everything from fatigue to terminal cancer. Your patient wants to be as healthy as she can be and wants you to teach her about megavitamin supplementation as an adjunct to her cancer treatment. Trying to give accurate, objective, and scientific information, which of the following would you include as potential hazards of vitamin therapies?
    a. Vitamin therapy usually includes high doses of B complex, C, A, D, and E vitamins
    b. Cardiac abnormalities and liver damage
    c. Kidney stones and coagulation abnormalities
    d. All of the above

3.64   Paracentesis is a procedure commonly used to manage peritoneal ascites. While caring for patients and teaching them about the procedure, it is important to remember which of the following?
    a. The procedure is therapeutic.
    b. The procedure can lead to severe protein depletion and electrolyte imbalance.
    c. Patients can experience postural hypotension.
    d. b and c

3.65   Which of the following metabolic disorders is common in patients who receive cisplatin therapy?
    a. Hypokalemia
    b. Hypomagnesemia
    c. Hypophosphatemia
    d. Hypocalcemia

3.66   Individuals with cancer may experience fluid and electrolyte imbalances related to hyperuricemia. In this condition
    a. A sudden decrease in levels of serum uric acid causes renal failure.
    b. Tumor lysis releases calcium deposits in the renal tubules, which leads to renal failure.
    c. Tumor lysis causes the syndrome of inappropriate antidiuretic hormone secretion.
    d. Urate crystals may be deposited in the kidneys, causing renal failure.

3.67   Which of the following is *not* considered to be a reliable test of protein stores?
    a. Mid-arm muscle circumference
    b. Skinfold thickness measurement
    c. Serum albumin
    d. Serum transtyretin

3.68   An analysis of biochemical data often yields information regarding nutritional status. Decreased levels of urinary creatinine may be an indicator of
    a. Decreased mortality
    b. Fat depletion
    c. Increased gastrointestinal absorption
    d. Decreased lean body mass

Weight Changes

3.69   Betty will be having a mastectomy. In planning ahead and helping her to get ready for the surgery, you tell her that
   a.   Because of the bed rest required in recovery, surgery will decrease her energy requirements
   b.   Nutritional problems resulting from her surgery will probably extend well past the immediate perioperative period
   c.   Surgery on her breast cancer should not have any direct implication for her nutritional needs
   d.   Surgery can increase her energy requirements to 1.5 times what she normally needs

3.70   The three classic signs of a pancreatic tumor located in the head of the pancreas are progressive jaundice, pain, and
   a.   Profound weight loss
   b.   Projectile vomiting
   c.   Confusion
   d.   Hyperkalemia

3.71   Mrs. Allen is beginning adjuvant cyclophosphamide, methotrexate, and 5-fluorouracil (CMF) as treatment for her breast cancer. She is concerned about her weight during chemotherapy. Which of the following most accurately depicts the appropriate nursing response?
   a.   She should be referred to a nutritionist to avoid weight gain.
   b.   She should take nutritional supplements to promote adequate nutrition.
   c.   Weight change during chemotherapy is minimal, and she should not worry.
   d.   It is of no concern because weight loss or gain has no impact on survival or response to treatment.

3.72   Your patient Sean has been participating in professional athletics for several years. At 170 pounds he weighs far more than he should for his height of 5 feet 6 inches, but he does not appear to be overweight. In trying to determine whether you should counsel Sean to reduce his caloric and fat intake, you decide to use _____ to determine his percentage of body fat.
   a.   A body mass index
   b.   A resting metabolic nomogram
   c.   A skinfold measure
   d.   Resting energy expenditure

3.73   Weight loss is predictive of negative outcomes in cancer therapy. Which of the following is considered significant weight loss and diagnostic of cancer-associated cachexia?
   a.   Involuntary weight loss equal to or greater than 10% of usual body weight over a 6-month period
   b.   Involuntary weight loss equal to or greater than 5% of usual body weight over a 1-month period
   c.   Voluntary weight loss of 15% of usual body weight over a 6-month period
   d.   a and b

3.74 You are attempting to choose an instrument to gain a more complete diet history from Carlos. He has already told you that he doesn't pay much attention to what he eats, and he has a hard time remembering what he had for lunch (or if he had lunch) yesterday. Carlos is very upset about his recent diagnosis, and this has changed his eating habits considerably. However, he is willing to cooperate with you, and he understands the importance of being honest in the things he tells you. Keeping in mind that Carlos is in the hospital now but he will not be for most of his treatment, you choose
   a. A calorie count
   b. A 24-hour dietary recall
   c. A food frequency record
   d. A diet diary

3.75 Postoperative care of an individual who has undergone palliative surgery for pancreatic cancer includes all of the following *except*
   a. Administration of pancreatic enzyme supplements
   b. Providing a diet that is low in fat, is high in protein, and includes a glass of red wine with lunch and dinner
   c. Observing for hemorrhage, hypovolemia, and hypotension
   d. Examining stool for steatorrhea

3.76 Of women who receive adjuvant chemotherapy for breast cancer, many will gain weight and even become obese. What percentage of women on adjuvant chemotherapy for breast cancer gain weight?
   a. 15–25%
   b. 30–40%
   c. 40–70%
   d. 60–90%

Cachexia

3.77 William asks you for an appetite stimulant. Keeping in mind that he is on an extensive chemotherapy regimen, is diabetic, and has not had problems with nausea or vomiting, which of the following drugs is the *best possible* intervention for him?
   a. Corticosteroids
   b. Megestrol acetate
   c. Metoclopramide
   d. Tetrahydrocannabinol (THC)

3.78 Cancer-associated nutritional problems, rather than treatment-related nutritional problems, are best reversed by
   a. Extensive verbal counseling
   b. Self-care actions
   c. Medications
   d. Successful treatment of the tumor

3.79 Tumor-related cytokines are known to play a role in the etiology of metabolic and neuroendocrine syndromes associated with cachexia. Which of the following best describes how cytokines contribute to cachexia?
   a. Cytokines such as tumor necrosis factor promote protein loss.
   b. Cytokines dull the brain's perception of hunger and suppress appetite.
   c. Cytokines alter gastric emptying and small bowel motility.
   d. All of the above

3.80 Charles is one of your patients with lung cancer. Because he is diabetic and already well under his ideal weight, one of your major concerns is to provide Charles with adequate nutrition and prevent cachexia. You are dismayed to learn that he "lost his appetite" when he recently received his diagnosis and almost entirely stopped eating. Which of the following is probably *not* a factor that would have contributed to the loss of appetite?
   a. Circulating cytokines
   b. Cancer-induced sepsis
   c. Psychological distress
   d. Bombesin

3.81 When you give Ravi a complete assessment, you find he is suffering from anorexia, skeletal muscle atrophy, and asthenia. His hepatic glucose production is at normal levels, perhaps even a bit higher. What is your diagnosis?
   a. Primary cachexia
   b. Secondary cachexia
   c. Starvation
   d. Marasmus

3.82 The incidence of cachexia is in the range of which of the following?
   a. 15–40% at the initial diagnosis of cancer
   b. 24% at the early diagnosis of advanced cancer
   c. 80% at the terminal stages of cancer
   d. All of the above

3.83 Which of the following statements regarding cachexia is *true*?
   a. Cachexia is the same as anorexia.
   b. Cachexia is due to the tumor consuming the body's nutrients.
   c. Cachexia is not reversible with appropriate feeding.
   d. Cachexia is the same as starvation.

3.84 Mr. Thomas has been steadily losing weight and progressively deteriorating from his pancreatic cancer. He is experiencing severe muscle wasting and energy loss. The appropriate term for this condition is
   a. Cancer cachexia
   b. Malnutrition
   c. Inanition
   d. Undernutrition

3.85 Mr. Thomas has pancreatic cancer and feels as if he cannot get out of bed at times and that if he tried he would probably be up for only a few minutes due to an overwhelming loss of strength. This loss of strength is referred to as which of the following?
   a. Asthenia
   b. Marasmus
   c. Protein-calorie malnutrition
   d. Anorexia-cachexia syndrome

Ascites

3.86 The cancer *most often* associated with malignant ascites is
   a. Ovarian cancer
   b. Pancreatic cancer
   c. Breast cancer
   d. Esophageal cancer

3.87 Beth has slowly progressing ascites due to liver failure associated with metastatic ovarian carcinoma. She is uncomfortable from the pressure and asks what can be done. Which of the following supportive measures is *most appropriate* to manage her discomfort?
   a. Fluid and sodium restriction
   b. Diuretic therapy
   c. Paracentesis
   d. All of the above

3.88 Ascites is a presenting symptom in what percentage of women with ovarian cancer?
   a. 10%
   b. 30%
   c. 50%
   d. 70%

3.89 Approximately what percentage of women with ovarian carcinoma eventually develop ascites?
   a. 90%
   b. 80%
   c. 60%
   d. 30%

3.90 Which of the following chemotherapy agents is known to cause fluid retention that may manifest as abdominal ascites, as a pleural effusion, or as a combination?
   a. Mitoxantrone
   b. Megestrol acetate
   c. Docetaxel
   d. Paclitaxel

3.91 Andrea has ovarian cancer and complains of abdominal fullness. In this patient the presence of shifting dullness during percussion would be indicative of which of the following?
   a. Abdominal carcinomatosis
   b. Liver enlargement
   c. Ascites
   d. All of the above

3.92 Malignant peritoneal effusion (ascites) is caused by which of the following?
   a. Obstruction of diaphragmatic lymphatics
   b. Tumor seeding of the peritoneum
   c. Humoral factors that cause increased capillary leakage of proteins
   d. All of the above

3.93 Your patient with ascites has had a paracentesis and removal of 1–2 liters repeatedly in the past and is calling now with a request for another tap because the fluid has come back and she is uncomfortable. Your response is based on knowledge of which of the following?
   a. Sclerosis with instillation of chemotherapy is the most effective treatment.
   b. Draining the peritoneum only makes fluid accumulate faster.
   c. Repeated paracentesis can lead to severe protein depletion.
   d. Paracentesis can lead to tumor seeding.

ALTERATIONS IN ELIMINATION

Incontinence

3.94 Risk factors for urinary incontinence following radical prostatectomy include
   a. Age over 65
   b. Development of anastomatic stricture
   c. Stage T1a or T1b disease
   d. All of the above

3.95 A patient's prostate cancer has recurred, and he is receiving radiation to a portal including the prostate, periprostatic tissue, and pelvic lymph nodes. Possible complications of radiation to this area include *all but* which of the following?
   a. Constipation and bowel narrowing
   b. Urinary incontinence
   c. Lower extremity edema
   d. Cystitis

3.96 Laser therapy is an option for small superficial bladder tumors. The advantages of this procedure include *all but* which of the following?
   a. An indwelling catheter is necessary for only a short time period.
   b. Dissemination of disease in the bladder is less likely compared to fulguration.
   c. It can be performed under local anesthesia.
   d. The risk for bladder perforation is minimal.

3.97 Late complications of the continent urinary diversion include
   a. Urinary leakage
   b. Difficult catheterization
   c. Ascending infection
   d. a and b

3.98 Mr. Benson presents with some pain and frequency of urination. During a rectal palpation, the examiner detects a diffuse enlargement of the prostate. There seems to be no mass, however. With no other information, one might infer that Mr. Benson is *most likely* to have
   a. Nephritis
   b. Cancer of the prostate
   c. Cancer of the bladder
   d. Benign prostatic hypertrophy

3.99 Your patient is being prepped for a radical prostatectomy and is concerned about urinary incontinence. Your best advice to him is which of the following?
   a. Urinary incontinence is a major problem in only about 50% of patients.
   b. Stress incontinence occurs in about 25% of patients but is manageable.
   c. Some 92% of patients achieve urinary control following radical prostatectomy.
   d. He should talk to his doctor.

3.100 Following transurethral resection of the prostate (TURP) your patient experiences dribbling and stress incontinence. He asks you about his treatment options. The most appropriate response would include which of the following?
   a. Surgery to relieve urethral obstruction or stricture
   b. Kegel exercises to strengthen the pelvic floor muscles
   c. Alpha-adrenergic agonist drugs to increase sphincter resistance
   d. All of the above

Constipation

3.101 A patient is receiving cyclophosphamide, doxorubicin, and vincristine for lung cancer. He also is receiving opioid analgesics for pain. He normally has a bowel movement every day. He reports that he has not had a bowel movement in 3 days but does not feel the urge and has not been eating normally. Appropriate nursing assessment and management include which of the following?
   a. He has not had a normal routine so it is a good idea to increase fiber and fluids and call if there is no bowel movement in 24 hours.
   b. He should take a laxative, such as milk of magnesia, and call if he has no bowel movement in 48 hours.
   c. Elderly patients often have a decrease in colonic transit time, and with time he will have results.
   d. He should take a laxative and a suppository and call if there are no results in 24 hours.

3.102 Which of the following chemotherapeutic agents is *least likely* to cause constipation?
   a. Vinorelbine
   b. Vincristine
   c. Vinblastine
   d. Carmustine

3.103 A patient is receiving vinorelbine and complains of colicky abdominal pain and abdominal distention. Physiologically, the patient's symptoms are *most likely* caused by
   a. The effect of the vinorelbine on the gastrointestinal mucosa
   b. Decreased colonic transit time with vinorelbine
   c. Diminished effectiveness of afferent and efferent nerve pathways
   d. Cramping and gas pains, which are common with vinorelbine

3.104 Twenty-four hours after taking a laxative, a patient calls and complains of nausea and inability to pass gas. He has not had a bowel movement in 4 days. The most appropriate approach to this situation includes which of the following?
   a. The patient needs to have an enema.
   b. A stool softener and a laxative should be recommended.
   c. The patient should have a physical exam and a flat plate of the abdomen because he could be obstipated.
   d. An oil retention enema and milk of magnesia should be given and repeated if there are no results in 24 hours.

3.105 Opioids affect the gastrointestinal (GI) tract, contributing to constipation by which of the following mechanisms?
   a. Activation of opioid receptors in the GI tract and on the central nervous system
   b. Increased water absorption due to increased transit time
   c. Insensitivity to rectal distention
   d. All of the above

3.106 Which of the following statements regarding vincristine-induced constipation is *not* true?
   a. Vincristine may damage the myenteric plexus of the colon.
   b. Vincristine is more likely to cause constipation than is vinblastine.
   c. Bowel effects usually occur with peripheral nerve dysfunction.
   d. Severe constipation may occur in up to 35% of patients.

3.107 Your patient with prostate cancer is scheduled to undergo brachytherapy. Part of his preprocedural preparation includes instructions on a low residue diet and antidiarrheal agents. The primary purpose of these instructions is which of the following?
   a. Prevent gastrointestinal irritation to the gastrointestinal mucosa
   b. Prevent diarrhea from the radiation
   c. Prevent bowel movements while implants are in place
   d. Prevent contamination of the operative field

3.108 Chemotherapy-related constipation is associated with which of the following?
   a. Colicky abdominal pain
   b. Peripheral nerve dysfunction
   c. Decreased colonic transit time
   d. Reduced rectal emptying due to spinal cord compression

3.109 Opioid-induced constipation is best managed by which of the following approaches?
   a. Increase fiber to 3–4 grams per day
   b. Increase fluid intake to eight 8-ounce glasses of fluid per day
   c. One senokot tablet + 100-mg tablet of colace per 30-mg tablet of MS Contin
   d. All of the above

Diarrhea

3.110 Radiation-induced enteritis can cause significant diarrhea. Which of the following interventions is *not* appropriate management of this problem?
   a. A liquid diet high in milk and milk products
   b. Sandostatin given subcutaneously
   c. Anticholinergics
   d. Paragoric elixir

3.111 Physiologically, the etiology of chemotherapy-induced diarrhea involves which of the following?
   a. Shortening or denuding of the intestinal villa
   b. The destruction of the actively dividing epithelial cells
   c. Microvilli flattening and reducing the absorptive surface
   d. All of the above

3.112 A patient is receiving 5-fluorouracil and leucovorin weekly for 4 weeks. He reports abdominal cramping, rectal urgency, and diarrhea that awaken him at night. On questioning he reports four diarrhea stools on each of the past 3 days, each with a volume of about 1 cup. Appropriate nursing action would include which of the following?
   a. Encourage him to take loperamide with each loose stool and to push fluids and delay treatment for 1 week.
   b. Diarrhea is expected with 5-fluorouracil, and he should receive his chemotherapy with instructions to take loperamide with each loose stool.
   c. Myelosuppression is the dose-limiting toxicity of 5-fluorouracil, so if the counts are good he should receive treatment.
   d. Assess the patient for dehydration, including orthostatic blood pressures.

3.113　A patient receiving chemotherapy complains of severe diarrhea for 6 days and agrees to come to the outpatient clinic to be evaluated. Appropriate nursing action would include which of the following?
a.　Monitor the patient for orthostatic hypotension, lethargy, and weakness.
b.　Monitor fluids and electrolytes.
c.　Notify the physician for fluid replacement and evaluation.
d.　All of the above

3.114　5-Fluorouracil is commonly given with leucovorin to treat gastrointestinal malignancies. This combination of drugs results in which of the following?
a.　Manipulation of the metabolism of the 5-fluorouracil
b.　Potentiate the effect of 5-fluorouracil
c.　Decrease diarrhea occurrence
d.　a and b

3.115　Which of the following chemotherapy agents is *least likely* to cause diarrhea?
a.　Bleomycin
b.　Irinotecan
c.　Docetaxel
d.　Methotrexate

3.116　A patient reports diarrhea 2 weeks after paclitaxel therapy. He had a fever 5 days after his treatment and was placed on antibiotics empirically. He states that he feels well, but he has no appetite and the diarrhea is not slowing down. Appropriate nursing action includes which of the following?
a.　Encourage the patient to take antidiarrheal agents and to push fluids.
b.　Monitor the fluids and electrolytes and give results to the physician.
c.　Send a stool culture for *Clostridium difficile*.
d.　b and c

3.117　In general, antidiarrheal agents should *not* be given to patients as treatment for diarrhea that might be caused by an infectious agent. What is the rationale for this?
a.　The antidiarrheal agent would slow the passage of stool.
b.　The antidiarrheal agent increases the exposure of the mucosa to the infectious agent.
c.　The risk of systemic absorption is increased.
d.　All of the above

3.118　The *most common* injury to the large bowel that occurs following radiotherapy is
a.　Increased bowel motility
b.　Proctosigmoiditis
c.　Abdominal cramping
d.　Loose watery stools

3.119　Mr. Brown has had a bone marrow transplant and suffers from chronic diarrhea. A cause for his diarrhea is *most likely* which of the following?
a.　Viral infection
b.　Graft-versus-host disease
c.　Herpes simplex
d.　Varicella zoster

Bowel Obstruction

3.120 Which of the following clinical manifestations typically occur in patients with a cancer of the sigmoid colon?
a. Anemia and a vague, dull, persistent pain in the upper right quadrant
b. Abdominal pain and melena
c. Sensations of incomplete evacuation and tenesmus
d. Bright red bleeding through the rectum

3.121 Assessments completed on a patient with cancer of the right colon usually find which of the following?
a. A palpable mass
b. Polyps in the rectum
c. Anemia
d. High levels of carcinoembryonic antigen

3.122 During Ms. Harris' rectal examination for complaints of abdominal distention and pain, you detect a stony hard mass in the cul-de-sac. What does this indicate?
a. Ms. Harris has small amounts of intra-abdominal fluid forming a "puddle sign" on the pelvic floor.
b. Ms. Harris has pancreatic or hepatic lesions pressing on the pelvic floor.
c. Ms. Harris has a carcinoma that has metastasized to the pelvic floor.
d. Ms. Harris has metastasis at Virchow's node.

3.123 Which of the following is contraindicated for a patient with constipation due to structural blockage by a tumor?
a. Increase fiber in the diet to greater than 6 grams per day
b. Administer magnesium citrate as needed
c. Administer soap suds enemas
d. All of the above

3.124 Your patient has recurrent intermittent bowel obstruction due to advanced cancer. Which of the following is (are) an appropriate option(s) to offer this patient as management strategies for nausea and vomiting due to bowel obstruction?
a. Nasogastric intubation to avoid a surgical procedure in a patient with advanced cancer
b. Surgical placement of a gastrostomy tube
c. Percutaneous endoscopic gastrostomy
d. b and c

3.125 Your patient has a bowel obstruction complicated by intractable hiccups. Which of the following medications for hiccups is contraindicated?
a. Metoclopramide
b. Chlorpromazine
c. Cisapride
d. Amitriptyline

3.126 Biliary vomiting is indicative of which of the following?
a. Intermittent bowel obstruction
b. Obstruction in the upper part of the abdomen
c. Obstruction in the lower ileus
d. Progressive constipation

3.127 Katrina has end-stage cancer with a bowel obstruction and is currently in hospice care. Which of the following would be an appropriate intervention to minimize her discomfort?
  a. Placement of a nasogastric tube to manage nausea and vomiting
  b. Enemas every other day to promote evacuation
  c. Avoiding the use of opioids, because they will only make it worse
  d. Octreotide acetate to minimize secretions

Ostomies, Urinary Diversions

3.128 Mr. James is scheduled for a radical cystectomy with urinary diversion. He is especially concerned about the possibility of being impotent following surgery. Your responses are based on which of the following?
  a. Because the surgery involves removal of the bladder, attached peritoneum, the prostate, and seminal vesicles, impotence is unavoidable in many cases.
  b. It is possible that the nerves crucial to achieving penile erection may be spared, and he should be encouraged to talk to his surgeon.
  c. Refer him to an enterostomal therapist for information about a penile prosthesis and placement of the urinary diversion.
  d. All of the above

3.129 Which of the following procedures will the surgeon usually perform when a lesion involves the middle and left transverse colon?
  a. A right hemicolectomy that includes the related lymphatic and circulatory channels
  b. A one-stage procedure involving resection of the lesion and a primary anastomosis
  c. A two-stage procedure involving a temporary colostomy or ileostomy
  d. A three-stage procedure involving a diverting colostomy, a resection of the tumor, and takedown of the colostomy

3.130 For upper and mid-rectal adenocarcinomas, the treatment approach of choice is
  a. Low anterior resection, preserving external anal sphincter control
  b. Abdominoperineal resection with a temporary colostomy
  c. Laser therapy to the tumor bed through a colonoscope or flexible sigmoidoscope
  d. Prophylactic oophorectomy

3.131 The primary complications of a cystectomy and urinary diversion are related to *all but* which of the following?
  a. Stoma construction and placement
  b. Wound dehiscence
  c. Long-term kidney damage
  d. Stoma stenosis

3.132 A continent urinary diversion is a surgical method substituting bowel to function like the original bladder. Which of the following is *not* a correct description of this procedure?
  a. A continent urinary diversion provides control of voiding.
  b. One-way valves prevent urinary reflux.
  c. An intra-abdominal pouch is created for storage of urine.
  d. All continent urinary diversions are constructed from terminal ileum.

3.133   Following a radical cystectomy, the nurse is instructed to irrigate the pouch regularly to maintain patency. The patient expresses dismay, stating that he does not feel he can learn to do this. The nurse's best response is which of the following?
   a.   "Has your doctor told you it will be necessary for you to irrigate the pouch?"
   b.   "Most of the time, the mucus becomes very thin and easy to pass."
   c.   "Mucous production will decrease over time and irrigation will become unnecessary."
   d.   "Irrigation is necessary to prevent urinary reflux."

3.134   Mr. Makela has an ileal conduit placed following cystectomy for advanced bladder cancer. Which of the following is considered normal?
   a.   A delay of urinary output for 4–5 hours after surgery
   b.   Protrusion of the stoma 3 inches above the skin surface
   c.   A stoma that is dark red in color and slightly edematous
   d.   A small amount of leakage from the appliance

3.135   If the urine passing from a stoma is cloudy, it may be that
   a.   The patient is dehydrated
   b.   The stoma was formed from intestinal tissue
   c.   A leak in the stoma pouch has occurred, allowing air and bacteria to enter a sterile area
   d.   Antispasmodics are indicated

3.136   In a study of primary carcinoma of the rectum assessing sexual function after total mesorectal excision with autonomic nerve preservation, which of the following outcome(s) were (was) reported?
   a.   More men than women reported sexual dysfunction.
   b.   There was no difference between men over 60 years of age and men under 60 years of age in terms of maintaining potency.
   c.   Men and women reported the same ability to achieve orgasm.
   d.   All of the above

3.137   Which of the following postoperative assessments of stoma viability is a matter of concern that should be brought to the surgeon's attention?
   a.   Persistent peristalsis in the bowel
   b.   Bleeding of the stoma when rubbed
   c.   A dusky or gray stoma
   d.   Protrusion of the stoma

3.138   Postoperative care and teaching of the patient undergoing abdominoperineal resection (APR) for rectal cancer is *most likely* to be influenced by which of the following?
   a.   The type of colostomy to be performed
   b.   The patient's age, sex, and physical condition
   c.   The extent of hepatic invasion
   d.   The type of closure of the perineal wound to be used

Renal Dysfunction

3.139   Nephrotic syndrome is a paraneoplastic syndrome characterized by which of the following?
   a.   The presence of lesions in the renal glomerulus
   b.   A secondary benign disorder resulting from a primary glomerular disease
   c.   Impaired renal function due to obstruction of the glomerulus by tumor products
   d.   All of the above

3.140 As you take the history of a patient with nephrotic syndrome, what signs and symptoms would you expect to see or hear reported?
  a. Brown foamy urine
  b. "Gaunt" face and generalized weight loss with anorexia
  c. Mild hypotension
  d. a and b

3.141 Multiple myeloma is associated with renal failure precipitated by numerous factors. Which of the following contributes *most* to renal failure in multiple myeloma?
  a. Infection
  b. Hypercalcemia
  c. Dehydration
  d. Any of the above

3.142 Several years ago a patient was given concomitant radiation therapy and chemotherapy for cancer of the bladder. Recently, she developed cystitis. If this condition is a late effect of her cancer treatment, which agent is *least likely* to have been the responsible one involved?
  a. Cyclophosphamide
  b. Ifosfamide
  c. Methotrexate
  d. Cisplatin

3.143 Management of tenesmus, cystitis, and urethritis that may result when radiation is given to the pelvic area involves several nursing options, including all of the following *except*
  a. Administering gastrointestinal and urinary antispasmodics
  b. Administering antibiotics if there is evidence of infection
  c. Encouraging high fluid intake by the patient
  d. Providing sitz baths if the perineal area is being irradiated

3.144 Mr. Prang is at high risk for developing hemorrhagic cystitis in response to conditioning therapy for bone marrow transplantation. You propose to help prevent this development with the use of
  a. Hydration
  b. A Foley catheter
  c. The uroprotectant mesna
  d. All of the above

3.145 Kidney cancer has been consistently linked to which of the following risk factors?
  a. Cigarette smoking
  b. Caffeine ingestion
  c. Heredity
  d. Asbestos

3.146 Prolonged diarrhea without adequate management can lead to all of the following *except*
  a. Renal failure
  b. Dehydration
  c. Circulatory collapse
  d. Nutritional malabsorption

3

Gastrointestinal and
Urinary Function

ANSWER EXPLANATIONS

3.1   **The answer is d.** All management is directed at symptom relief and supportive care. This is best accomplished through dietary manipulation, topical anesthesia, and systemic analgesia when needed.

3.2   **The answer is c.** The most common early symptoms of esophagitis include dysphagia (difficulty swallowing), odynophagia (painful swallowing), and epigastric pain. Esophageal pain that worsens and becomes continuous and substernal indicates progressing esophagitis.

3.3   **The answer is a.** Sucralfate suspension is used to treat radiation- and chemotherapy-induced esophagitis. Some suggest that it promotes comfort and possibly healing by binding to proteinaceous exudate in exposed mucosa.

3.4   **The answer is b.** Prior or concurrent radiation may augment the severity and extent of mucosal injury. Some drugs, such as dactinomycin and doxorubicin, potentiate radiation injury to the esophagus and others, including 5-fluorouracil, hydroxyurea, procarbazine, and vinblastine, produce an additive toxic effect with irradiation.

3.5   **The answer is d.** Esophageal fistula, stricture, hemorrhage, radiation pneumonitis, and pericarditis are all possible complications of radiotherapy for esophageal cancer. Side effects to be expected are swallowing difficulties, including burning, pain, dryness, and skin reactions.

3.6   **The answer is b.** Because carcinoma of the thyroid can rapidly invade surrounding structures, symptoms may occur that are related to compressive effects of the enlarging mass on adjacent structures. Patients may experience dyspnea or stridor when the trachea is compressed or infiltrated. Compression of the esophagus may cause dysphagia. Hoarseness can result from malignant infiltration or destruction of the laryngeal or vagus nerves.

3.7   **The answer is b.** Dysphagia and weight loss are classic symptoms of esophageal carcinoma.

3.8   **The answer is a.** Scopolamine is used to manage excessive salivation and respiratory tract secretions.

3.9   **The answer is c.** Liquids are the most difficult to manage and are tried last. Semisolids stay together as a bolus and are easier to swallow. These patients do not have a feeding tube, so they must begin a swallowing program as soon as their nasogastric tube is removed.

3.10 **The answer is c.** Cancer-associated cachexia can be differentiated into primary and secondary types. Primary cachexia results from tumor-produced metabolic abnormalities or host responses. Secondary cachexia results from mechanical effects of the tumor or treatment.

3.11 **The answer is c.** Preparations that may be useful in prevention of disease do not always have a salutary effect when the disease already exists. For example, saw palmetto reduces prostate size, possibly through phytoestrogenic action, and may alter the effectiveness of hormonal drug treatment in prostate cancer.

3.12 **The answer is d.** Cytokines have been proposed to decrease the response to lowered glucose levels resulting in less appetite. There is also support for an effect of serotonin and tryptophan on appetite suppression.

3.13   **The answer is b.** Effective doses of megestrol acetate range from 160 to 1,600 mg per day, with an optimal dose of 800 mg per day to promote weight gain. Benefits include increased appetite, increased caloric intake, weight gain (due mostly to fat gain), and a sensation of well-being. Side effects include edema and thromboembolic events. It may be used for metastatic breast or endometrial cancer but the question concerns weight gain.

3.14   **The answer is c.** Anorexia may occur among individuals receiving radiotherapy, regardless of the treatment site. Anorexia is probably related to the presence in the patient's system of the waste products of tissue destruction.

3.15   **The answer is d.** Anorexia or loss of appetite and declining food intake involves alterations in food perception, taste, and smell that result from the effects of chemotherapy. Abnormalities of carbohydrate, protein, and fat metabolism are central features of anorexia. Visceral and lean body mass depletion are common, along with muscle atrophy, visceral organ atrophy, and hypoalbuminemia.

3.16   **The answer is a.** Anorexia can lead to compromised immune status as manifested by decreased macrophage mobilization, depressed lymphocyte function, and impaired phagocytosis. Hypoalbuminemia occurs, but it is not as sensitive of an indicator of nutritional or immune status.

3.17   **The answer is d.** A loss of more than 10% of body weight within the previous 6 months or an unintentional weight loss of more than 1 kilogram per week is considered a significant risk factor. A macrobiotic diet places the cancer patient at risk for malnutrition.

3.18   **The answer is a.** Although all the other answers are appropriate, anorexia and cancer cachexia are common manifestations of lung cancer; other factors are contributory.

3.19   **The answer is a.** Because the family wants to force feed the patient is not an appropriate rationale since the patient's Living Will requests no life-saving measures. All the other selections are reasons why we should not force feed.

3.20   **The answer is d.** Anorexia-cachexia can result from tumor byproducts causing loss of appetite and decreased food intakes and from multiple metabolic and physiologic abnormalities.

3.21   **The answer is d.** The frequency of oral care should increase with the severity of the symptoms. Any solution is useful to remove debris from the mouth. A basic solution such as sodium bicarbonate or salt cleanses the mouth and creates a basic environment.

3.22   **The answer is a.** Mucositis is observed more often with 5-FU when combined with other mucositis-producing drugs such as methotrexate and doxorubicin and when 5-FU is given concurrently with leucovorin to augment its cytotoxicity.

3.23   **The answer is d.** Management of stomatitis in the cancer patient includes all these choices.

3.24   **The answer is d.** All three choices are risk factors that contribute to stomatitis in the cancer patient.

3.25   **The answer is c.** Gentle frequent mouth care with soothing solutions can be helpful. Care should be taken, however, not to dislodge the plaque-like formations of mucositis and cause bleeding.

3

Gastrointestinal and
Urinary Function

3.26 **The answer is d.** Areas of the oral cavity adjacent to metal tooth fillings are at greater risk for increased reaction due to radiation scatter from the metal fillings. Mucositis is enhanced and prolonged in patients who have preexisting poor oral or dental hygiene, continue to smoke, use chewing tobacco, consume alcohol, and have poorly fitting dentures.

3.27 **The answer is b.** The dose-limiting side effect for 5-FU when given as an intravenous bolus is myelosuppression, but when the drug is given by continuous intravenous infusion the dose-limiting side effect is mucositis.

3.28 **The answer is c.** The incidence of oral herpes simplex virus infection in cancer patients receiving chemotherapy is approximately 50%. In the bone marrow transplantation population, the incidence approaches 80%.

3.29 **The answer is d.** Gingival hypertrophy is the result of infiltration of the gums by leukemic cells. Chemotherapy will treat the underlying cause. The other measures may reduce infection and add to comfort.

3.30 **The answer is a.** Direct stomatotoxicity results from the cytotoxic action of drugs on the cells of the oral basal epithelium, causing a decrease in the rate of cell renewal. The sequelae include a thinned atrophic mucosa and initiation of an inflammatory response (stomatitis).

3.31 **The answer is d.** The radioprotectant amifostine has been shown to be effective in reducing mucositis and dysphagia following radiation therapy. It has also been shown to reduce acute and chronic xerostomia, especially when the radiation field is limited.

3.32 **The answer is a.** Xerostomia is a transient dysfunction of the salivary gland that occurs following chemotherapy. It is a decrease in the quality and quantity of saliva.

3.33 **The answer is c.** Oral care before meals helps to freshen the mouth and stimulate appetite. Increasing fluid intake during meals and snacks helps to lubricate food and ease swallowing. Butter or cooking oil placed in the mouth may be a cost-effective alternative for artificial lubrication. Lemon glycerin is contraindicated as a mouthwash because it dries and irritates the mucosa and can decalcify the teeth.

3.34 **The answer is b.** Specific agents for dissolving and breaking up thick saliva include papain (found in papaya) and amylase (found in pineapple). Sialagogues stimulate the secretion of endogenous saliva and include gustatory stimulants such as sugar-free lemon candy and masticatory stimulants such as sugar-free gum. Pilocarpine to increase saliva should be used with caution for those with cardiovascular disease.

3.35 **The answer is a.** Mucositis is an inflammatory response of the oral mucosa to radiation therapy. The oral cavity appears inflamed, and white patchy areas may be seen. The patient complains of a sore throat and mouth. Xerostomia is a drying of the oral mucosa resulting from loss of saliva due to damage that occurs to the salivary glands subsequent to radiation therapy to the head and neck; it manifests in a thicker saliva. Trismus or jaw hypomobility may occur if the posterior mandible is included in the irradiated field.

3.36 **The answer is b.** Oral pilocarpine has been approved for use as a stimulant to the exocrine glands. This results in diaphoresis, salivation, lacrimation, and gastric and pancreatic secretion. Symptomatic improvements of xerostomia are found in 87% of users.

3.37   **The answer is d.** Radiotherapy to the head and neck region destroys taste buds and cells responsible for saliva secretion, resulting in xerostomia. A person who is experiencing this effect produces little saliva, and the saliva that is produced is viscid, acidic, and high in organic content. Affected individuals often complain of decreased taste perception and difficult mastication.

3.38   **The answer is b.** Saliva provides lubrication for oral tissues and protection from bacterial infections. Saliva also inhibits enamel decalcification and provides an important excretory route for blood-borne urea, uric acid, and ammonia.

3.39   **The answer is d.** Cisplatin causes delayed nausea, and a 5-HT$_3$ antagonist plus a corticosteroid is the most effective treatment.

3.40   **The answer is d.** Nausea and vomiting have been effectively treated with stress-reduction and distraction methods, acupuncture and acupressure, and educational support.

3.41   **The answer is d.** Although cisplatin is most commonly associated with delayed nausea, doxorubicin, cyclophosphamide, and ifosfamide can also produce delayed nausea.

3.42   **The answer is c.** Anticipatory nausea and vomiting occur in 25% of patients as a result of classic operant conditioning from stimuli associated with chemotherapy.

3.43   **The answer is c.** Drug sequencing does not predict the degree and severity of nausea and vomiting. Characteristics that affect the occurrence of nausea and vomiting include susceptibility to motion sickness, poor previous emetic control, and being young.

3.44   **The answer is a.** Vincristine has a very low (<10%) emetogenic potential.

3.45   **The answer is d.** 5-HT$_3$ antagonists are associated with minimal toxicity and work both peripherally and centrally to prevent nausea and vomiting.

3.46   **The answer is d.** Nausea and vomiting following chemotherapy and total body irradiation is a consistent problem. Protracted nausea and vomiting also may be caused by GVHD, CMV esophagitis, or gastrointestinal infections.

3.47   **The answer is d.** The recommendation is to administer a drug she has not received or to significantly change the regimen. She did not receive aprepitant so that is the first choice, especially because her symptoms were delayed. Intravenous and oral agents are equal in efficacy. Doubling the dose of the ondansetron could be effective, but it is not the best answer.

3.48   **The answer is c.** Emesis occurs through several mechanisms, including stimulation of enterochromaffin cells in the duodenum, leading to release of serotonin. Serotonin binds and stimulates the vagus nerve, which in turn stimulates the spinal cord, medulla oblongata, and then the brain's vomiting center.

3.49   **The answer is c.** Vomiting as a sign of increased intracranial pressure may be preceded by nausea, or it may be sudden, unexpected, and projectile. It is not related to food ingestion. Paclitaxel and carboplatin are not usually associated with the sudden onset of nausea and vomiting, especially when it has not been a problem before. Dexamethasone is an appropriate choice for either problem, but the patient's symptoms can progress quickly, and he needs to be evaluated.

3.50   **The answer is c.** Younger patients are more sensitive to the extrapyramidal effects of the prochlorperazine, but this does not mean they are allergic to it. The combination of diphenhydramine and prochlorperazine can prevent extrapyramidal symptoms and dystonia.

3.51   **The answer is b.** Taste loss during radiation therapy is expected, given the role of saliva as a mediator of taste. Taste acuity is partially restored within 60 days and is almost completely restored by 4 months postradiation. A burning tongue (glossodynia) is triggered after contact with spicy or acidic foods.

3.52   **The answer is c.** Chemotherapy does interfere with specific metabolic and enzymatic reactions and causes excitation of the true vomiting center, alteration of intestinal absorptive surface, and, indirectly, food aversions.

3.53   **The answer is d.** Terms commonly used to describe conditions that result from cancer treatment include hypogeusia (decreased taste sensitivity), dysgeusia (perverted taste perception), odynophagia or dysphagia (painful swallowing), and hyposmia (diminished ability to smell).

3.54   **The answer is c.** Altered taste and smell sensors, with loss of taste and olfactory cues, change the normal references that are part of appetite and intake. Changes may be caused by direct tumor invasion; cancer-induced deficiencies in zinc, copper, nickel, vitamin A, and niacin; or cancer-associated circulating factors.

3.55   **The answer is a.** Physiological increases in the recognition thresholds for sweet, sour, and salt and decreases in the recognition levels for bitter are common. These threshold changes can lead to meat and other food aversions.

3.56   **The answer is d.** Alterations in taste are reported during the second week of treatment. Doses in the 50- to 65-Gy range cause maximum taste loss. The most severely affected taste qualities are salt and bitter. Sweet taste is generally least affected.

3.57   **The answer is c.** Choices **a**, **b**, and **d**, along with excessive lacrimation and swelling of the cheeks or orbit, are all clinical manifestations of carcinoma of the nasal cavity and paranasal sinus.

3.58   **The answer is b.** Normal eating is possible after use of a nasogastric tube for nutrition in the immediate postoperative period. Speech is affected by the excision of the vocal cords—esophageal speech or use of a handheld artificial larynx is necessary. Hyposomia and decreased taste acuity are also noted postlaryngectomy.

3.59   **The answer is b.** A common complaint during intravenous administration of drugs such as nitrogen mustard, cisplatin, and cyclophosphamide is that they cause a metallic taste. Some individuals become so sensitized to this taste they become nauseated in anticipation of their administration.

3.60   **The answer is a.** Complementary and alternative therapies are being studied and used more extensively. Nurses and doctors need to teach patients about importance of moderation, given that patients will pursue alternative approaches.

3.61   **The answer is b.** Cisplatin frequently causes hypomagnesemia, which manifests as shaking. Daily magnesium supplementation is indicated during cisplatin therapy, and electrolyte levels should be monitored frequently.

3.62   **The answer is d.** Although properly constructed diets are adequate, many alternative approaches to nutrition do not provide balanced diets. Potential hazards of macrobiotic diets include protein, calorie, iron, vitamin D, and vitamin B_{12} deficiencies. Colitis is more common with a macrobiotic diet.

3.63   **The answer is d.** Although the scientific information is far from complete, in general most clinicians agree that megadose vitamins are harmful because they can cause cardiac abnormalities and especially liver damage. Kidney stones and coagulation abnormalities are common with high doses of vitamins.

3.64   **The answer is d.** Besides its usefulness as a diagnostic tool, fluid removal by paracentesis alone is of little therapeutic value. It is usually reserved until a large volume of fluid has accumulated and the patient is profoundly symptomatic because the fluid accumulates rapidly.

3.65   **The answer is b.** Platinum-based chemotherapy can cause a specific nutritional deficiency, resulting in hypomagnesemia. The deficiency is highly specific to the particular drug.

3.66   **The answer is d.** Hyperuricemia involves a release of uric acid in the plasma during the process of tumor lysis. Urate crystals may be deposited in the kidney, causing damage and perhaps renal failure.

3.67   **The answer is b.** Skinfold thickness measurements are used to determine subcutaneous fat stores. Mid-arm muscle circumference is used to estimate muscle mass and protein stores. Traditional assessments of nutritional status include serum albumin, thyroxine-binding pre-albumin (transtyretin), and transferrin.

3.68   **The answer is d.** Because all muscle produces creatinine, the proportion of creatinine produced is directly proportional to the amount of muscle in the body. In individuals with cancer and in other malnourished individuals, creatinine excretion is decreased as muscle protein is degraded for use as energy.

3.69   **The answer is d.** Surgery can increase energy requirements by 1.5 times the normal dietary requirements. Betty can be somewhat reassured that her cancer is not in the aerodigestive or gastrointestinal tract because she is likely to have nutritional problems resulting from the surgery only in the immediate perioperative period.

3.70   **The answer is a.** A classic triad is apparent with cancer of the head of the pancreas: progressive jaundice, profound weight loss, and pain. Jaundice, which is precipitated by common bile duct obstruction, is the presenting symptom in 80% of all cases of cancer of the head of the pancreas and is the symptom that inevitably leads individuals to seek medical attention.

3.71   **The answer is a.** Most women on CMF gain approximately 15 pounds during the course of their treatment. They often have difficulty losing the weight after the treatment and benefit from counseling before treatment. Women who gain weight during chemotherapy have an increased risk of disease recurrence.

3.72   **The answer is c.** The skinfold measure, if taken in all seven sites, can produce a fairly accurate measure of body composition. However, if fewer than five of the sites are measured, the accuracy is lowered.

3.73   **The answer is d.** The degree of weight loss and the time period over which the loss occurs are important factors in predicting adverse outcomes. An involuntary weight loss of greater than or equal to 10% of usual body weight over a 6-month period or greater than or equal to 5% over 1 month have been used as parameters to define substantial weight loss and have been associated with poorer outcomes.

3.74   **The answer is d.** Because Carlos' eating habits have changed considerably and because he is not going to be staying in the hospital for most of his treatment, both the calorie count method and the 24-hour recall method are inappropriate. Food frequency reporting is not ideal because Carlos has a hard time remembering what he ate. A diet diary would provide an extended record of Carlos' eating habits that would rely on his cooperation and honesty—both of which you believe you can count on.

3.75   **The answer is b.** Hemorrhage, hypovolemia, and hypotension pose the greatest threats to the individual who has just undergone surgery for cancer of the pancreas. As soon as possible after pancreatectomy, small feedings will be started with a diet that is usually bland, low in fat, and high in carbohydrates and protein. Restrictions include caffeine, alcohol, and overindulgence. The stool should be examined daily for the characteristic signs of steatorrhea: frothy foul-smelling stool with fat particles floating in the water.

3.76   **The answer is c.** From 40% to 70% of women with breast cancer who receive adjuvant chemotherapy gain weight, and some become obese.

3.77   **The answer is b.** Corticosteroids are not indicated in William's case because he is a diabetic, and both metoclopramide and tetrahydrocannabinol are indicated for patients experiencing chemotherapy-induced nausea—which William is *not* experiencing. Even though diabetics taking megestrol acetate must monitor themselves closely, the drug is indicated in this case because it increases appetite, causes weight gain, and improves quality of life.

3.78   **The answer is d.** Treatment-induced nutritional problems are often successfully handled by medication and self-care actions. Cancer-associated nutritional problems are best resolved by successful treatment of the malignancy.

3.79   **The answer is d.** The interaction between active cancer cells and their host causes several overlapping metabolic and neuroendocrine syndromes. Proinflammatory cytokines and tumor-derived cachetic glycoproteins play a prominent, if not a causative, role in these syndromes. Cytokines promote numerous physiologic adaptations in the host by promoting metabolic abnormalities in proteins, lipids, and carbohydrates. Cachectin, a cytokine, promotes metabolic losses of protein and contributes to anorexia. Other cytokines affect gastrointestinal functioning, including altered gastric emptying, decreased intestinal blood flow, and changes in small bowel motility.

3.80   **The answer is b.** Cancer-induced sepsis initiates an increase of energy needs, which may or may not bring about an increase of appetite but which would *not* contribute to loss of appetite. All of the rest of these factors—bombesin, cytokines, and psychological distress—could produce a loss of appetite.

3.81   **The answer is a.** Ravi is suffering from primary cachexia resulting from tumor-produced metabolic abnormalities and host responses to cancer. Secondary cachexia is caused by mechanical effects of the tumor or treatment—unlikely in Ravi's case because he is suffering from lung cancer. Simple starvation and marasmus are not indicated when hepatic glucose production is at normal levels.

3.82   **The answer is d.** Cachexia is a condition of advanced protein-calorie malnutrition, characterized by involuntary weight loss, tissue wasting, anorexia, poor performance, and, ultimately, death. The incidence is generally thought to range from 15% to 40% at the initial diagnosis of cancer, 24% early at the diagnosis of advanced cancer, and more than 80% at the terminal stages.

3.83   **The answer is c.** Anorexia leads to cachexia; it is not the same thing. Cachexia does not result from the tumor preferentially consuming the ingested nutrients, and the degree of cachexia is unrelated to tumor burden. It is not reversible with appropriate feeding.

3.84   **The answer is c.** Inanition is progressive deterioration with muscle wasting and energy loss. Cachexia is a general term meaning ill health. It can occur in nonneoplastic diseases but is characterized by anorexia, weight loss, skeletal muscle atrophy, and asthenia.

3.85   **The answer is a.** Cancer cachexia is characterized by anorexia, weight loss, skeletal muscle atrophy, and asthenia (loss of strength). Marasmus is simple starvation with protein-calorie malnutrition.

3.86   **The answer is a.** Malignant peritoneal effusion (ascites) is most common in patients with ovarian cancer.

3.87   **The answer is d.** Ascites can become severe in advanced disease. Palliative measures to control ascites include fluid and sodium restriction, diuretic therapy, paracentesis, and albumin administration.

3.88   **The answer is b.** Ascites is found at presentation in 33% of these patients, and over 60% develop ascites at some time before death.

3.89   **The answer is c.** Over 60% of women with ovarian cancer develop ascites at some time before death. The appearance of ascites in patients with advanced disease is prognostically grim, and palliation is usually all that can be offered. Life expectancy is a few months.

3.90   **The answer is c.** A side effect of docetaxel is fluid retention. The incidence is related to the cumulative dose, which can be disabling and worsens with higher doses. Fluid retention is exhibited peripherally as abdominal ascites, as a pleural effusion, or as a combination.

3.91   **The answer is c.** The physical examination to test for ascites includes percussion to assess for shifting dullness to ascertain the presence of fluid and shifting of fluid as the patient changes positions.

3.92   **The answer is d.** The most common cause of ascitic fluid buildup is tumor seeding of the peritoneum, resulting in obstruction of the diaphragmatic and abdominal lymphatics. The tumor itself may elaborate humoral factors that cause increased capillary leakage of proteins and fluids into the peritoneum.

3.93   **The answer is c.** Removal of 2–3 liters of fluid and repeated paracentesis can lead to severe protein depletion, postural hypotension, and electrolyte abnormalities. Although sclerosing therapy is effective in treating pleural effusions, it is less successful with ascites.

3.94   **The answer is d.** Risk factors identified for postoperative incontinence following radical prostatectomy include age over 65, development of anastomatic stricture, and T1a or T1b disease.

3.95   **The answer is a.** Radiation therapy side effects include impotence, urinary incontinence, bone marrow depression, lower extremity edema, cystitis, urethral strictures, diarrhea, proctitis, and rectal bleeding. Diarrhea can be problematic, because a part of the colon and rectum lie within the irradiated pelvic field.

3.96   **The answer is a.** Outpatient photodynamic therapy, laser therapy, can be done while the patient is under local anesthesia through a small cystoscope, without causing bleeding or the stimulation of the obturator nerve. An indwelling catheter is not necessary following the procedure.

3.97   **The answer is d.** Late complications usually involve problems with continence or catheterization, such as urinary leakage at the stoma or through the urethra, difficult catheterization, electrolyte abnormalities, pyelonephritis, hydronephrosis, and stone formation. A clinical advantage of the continent urinary diversions is that ascending infections are rare.

3.98   **The answer is d.** The normal prostate on palpation is usually a rounded structure about 4 cm in diameter that feels firm. Cancer of the prostate typically appears as a stony hard nodule, whereas benign hypertrophy usually results in a diffuse enlargement of the prostate without masses.

3.99   **The answer is c.** After radical prostatectomy, 92% of patients achieve urinary control, 8% experience stress incontinence, and 6% wear one or fewer incontinence pads per day. Approximately 1% of men are incontinent after a transurethral resection of the prostate.

3.100   **The answer is d.** Sphincter incompetence presents as dribbling and stress incontinence. Treatment includes alpha-adrenergic agonist drugs and surgery. The drugs increase sphincter resistance. Repeat surgery may be needed to relieve urethral compression or stricture.

3.101   **The answer is d.** If a bowel movement does not occur every other day, a laxative must be taken. His risk factors are high for constipation, and it should be stressed to the patient never to wait more than 3 days without a bowel movement before calling the physician.

3.102   **The answer is d.** Vincristine, vinblastine, and vinorelbine are the most common chemotherapy agents to cause neuropathies that can result in constipation.

3.103   **The answer is c.** Rectal emptying is specifically diminished as a result of chemotherapy-induced neuropathies that disrupt the autonomic nervous system.

3.104   **The answer is c.** The fact that he is nauseated and not passing gas means he could be obstipated and needs to be evaluated immediately.

3.105   **The answer is d.** Opioids affect the bowel by activation of specific opioid receptors in both the GI tract and the central nervous system. Increased tone and nonpropulsive motility in the ileum and colon result in increased transit time and water absorption. Morphine-induced insensitivity to rectal distention further contributes to constipation.

3.106   **The answer is c.** Bowel effects of the vinca alkaloids may be unaccompanied by peripheral nerve dysfunction.

3.107   **The answer is c.** Constipation is sometimes induced intentionally among patients undergoing brachytherapy for gynecologic or prostate cancers. In these situations a low residue diet and antidiarrheal agents are prescribed to prevent bowel movements while implants are in place.

3.108   **The answer is a.** Chemotherapy agents cause constipation as a result of autonomic nerve dysfunction manifested as colicky abdominal pain. Rectal emptying is diminished because nonfunctional afferent and efferent pathways from the sacral cord are interrupted.

3.109   **The answer is d.** Combining the softening action with the peristaltic stimulant effect lessens constipation.

3.110   **The answer is a.** Management of severe diarrhea in patients with radiation-induced enteritis includes all of these choices *except* a liquid diet high in milk products.

3.111   **The answer is d.** When these cells are destroyed, atrophy of the intestinal mucosa and shortening of the intestinal villa with flattening and reduction of the absorptive surface results in a "slick gut." Thus the intestinal contents move rapidly through the gut, reducing absorption of nutrients.

3.112   **The answer is d.** Patients may experience abdominal cramps and rectal urgency with 5-fluorouracil, which can evolve into nocturnal diarrhea or fecal incontinence leading to lethargy, weakness, orthostatic hypotension, and fluid/electrolyte imbalance.

3.113   **The answer is d.** Nocturnal diarrhea or fecal incontinence leads to lethargy, weakness, orthostatic hypotension, and fluid/electrolyte imbalance. Without adequate management, prolonged diarrhea causes dehydration, nutritional malabsorption, and circulatory collapse.

3.114   **The answer is d.** The leucovorin potentiates the antitumor effect of the 5-fluorouracil, but it also increases the diarrhea.

3.115   **The answer is a.** Bleomycin can cause some mucositis, but not like the others, which cause mucositis plus potentially severe diarrhea.

3.116   **The answer is d.** Performing a stool culture, giving fluids, monitoring the electrolytes, and reporting results to the physician are all appropriate. Giving antidiarrheal agents to a patient who has recently had antibiotics is not.

3.117   **The answer is d.** If a patient has diarrhea that is due to an infectious agent such as *Clostridium difficile*, the use of antidiarrheal agents can increase risk for sepsis by increasing exposure to the mucosa and subsequent absorption of the toxin because antidiarrheal agents decrease colonic transit time.

3.118   **The answer is b.** The most common injury to the large bowel that occurs after radiotherapy is proctosigmoiditis. Another commonly encountered side effect is increased bowel motility, which creates abdominal cramping and loose watery stools.

3.119   **The answer is b.** After allogeneic bone marrow transplant, diarrhea is a prominent manifestation of intestinal involvement with graft-versus-host disease.

3.120   **The answer is b.** Cancers of the sigmoid colon are most often manifested by abdominal pain and melena. The manifestations in choice **a** are those of a tumor of the right colon; manifestations in choices **c** and **d** are those of rectal cancer.

3.121   **The answer is a.** Because the transverse colon is the most anterior and movable part of the colon, tumors here are more accessible to detection by palpation. Other possible symptoms that might have been determined by inspection, auscultation, palpation, and percussion of the abdomen include distention of the abdomen, enlarged and visible abdominal veins, occult blood in the stool, and enlarged lymph nodes or organs (especially the liver). Diagnostic examination by fiberoptic colonoscopy confirms the presence of the tumor. Anemia is more likely to occur with cancer of the right colon. Polyps in the rectum may be present and may indicate the patient was at high risk for colorectal cancer. Carcinoembryonic antigen, although useful in evaluating the efficacy of treatment, is of limited value in the detection of colon cancer.

3.122   **The answer is c.** On palpation during a rectal exam, the examiner may feel a stony hard mass in the cul-de-sac. The shelf indicates a carcinoma that has metastasized to the pelvic floor, initiating obstruction and pain, and therefore is a sign of advanced malignancy.

3.123   **The answer is d.** High-fiber diets are contraindicated in patients whose constipation results from structural blockage of the bowel, because increasing bulky intraluminal contents may increase the obstruction. Do not give magnesium citrate with bowel obstruction because of a high risk of perforation. Soap suds enemas are contraindicated because of the risk of acute colitis.

3.124   **The answer is d.** If the obstruction continues for more than a few days or is recurrent, a gastrostomy tube is a much more acceptable and well-tolerated route for decompression than nasogastric intubation. Intermittent venting of the gastrostomy tube allows the patient to continue oral intake and maintain an active life-style. The two options currently available are surgically placed gastrostomy and percutaneous endoscopic gastrostomy.

3.125   **The answer is a.** Metoclopramide is particularly useful in treating hiccups due to gastric stasis or distention and gastroesophageal reflux; however, it is contraindicated in patients with bowel obstruction because it stimulates gastric emptying and opposes retrograde peristalsis of retching.

3.126   **The answer is b.** Biliary vomiting is almost odorless and indicates an obstruction in the upper part of the abdomen. The presence of foul-smelling fecaloid vomiting can be the first sign of an ileal or colonic obstruction.

3.127   **The answer is d.** A gastrostomy tube or a percutaneous endoscopic gastrostomy (PEG) would be chosen over a nasogastric tube, which is uncomfortable. Enemas are contraindicated and lead to cramping pain. Opioids are important, because over 90% of patients have continuous abdominal pain.

3.128   **The answer is d.** A radical cystectomy with urinary diversion, particularly if accompanied by a lymphadenectomy, can affect many aspects of sexual functioning. Erectile impotence that results after radical cystectomy may be helped by the insertion of a penile prosthesis. When the nerves crucial to the mechanisms of penile erection are spared, erectile potency has been preserved.

3.129   **The answer is b.** When a malignant lesion involves the middle and left transverse colon, the standard procedure involves resection of the lesion and a primary anastomosis. The two- and three-step procedures are riskier and less often performed. A right hemicolectomy is performed on the cecum or ascending colon.

3.130   **The answer is a.** For upper and mid-rectal adenocarcinomas, the treatment approach of choice is low anterior resection. This preserves external anal sphincter control, thus eliminating the need for a permanent colostomy. Abdominoperineal resection is usually used for poorly differentiated adenocarcinoma and more advanced disease. Laser therapy to the tumor bed through a colonoscope or flexible sigmoidoscope is used for smaller tumors of the colon and rectum, and prophylactic oophorectomy is recommended for only some women diagnosed with adenocarcinoma of the colon and rectum.

3.131   **The answer is b.** Wound dehiscence is not primarily related to cystectomy. Complications are related to stoma construction and placement and to the possibility of long-term kidney damage. Other complications include stomal stenosis.

3.132 **The answer is d.** There are several types of continent urinary diversions. They differ largely in the specific portion of intestine used to create the pouch.

3.133 **The answer is c.** Continent urinary reservoirs and bladder substitutes produce much mucus. They should be irrigated regularly in the early postoperative period to prevent mucous accumulation. Mucous production decreases over time, and irrigation becomes unnecessary.

3.134 **The answer is c.** A urinary diversion should produce urine from the time of surgery, and flow should be more or less continuous. The stoma should protrude 0.5 to 0.75 inches above the skin to allow the urine to drain into the aperture of an appliance. Leakage from the appliance is abnormal and could lead to skin breakdown. The stoma itself should be deep pink to dark red in color.

3.135 **The answer is b.** The intestine normally produces mucus, and mucus is almost always present in diversions using segments of the bowel, causing the urine to appear cloudy. Excessive mucous may clog the urinary appliance outlet, and if this occurs an appliance with a larger outlet may be used.

3.136 **The answer is c.** In a study of primary carcinoma of the rectum assessing sexual function after total mesorectal excision with autonomic nerve preservation, 86% of men younger than 60 years of age and 67% of men older than 60 years of age reportedly maintained potency, with 87% of men retaining their ability to achieve orgasm. The same study found that 85% of women treated with this nerve-sparing surgery experienced arousal with vaginal lubrication and 1% maintained the ability to achieve orgasm.

3.137 **The answer is c.** An important postoperative nursing function is assessment of stoma viability to identify early signs of compromised circulation to the stoma. A stoma that is dusky, gray, or black indicates an inadequate blood supply and is documented and brought to the surgeons's attention. A stoma with necroses sloughs and generally leads to stomal stenosis. The postoperative occurrences in choices **a**, **b**, and **d** all are normal.

3.138 **The answer is d.** Because APR requires a combined surgical approach through the abdomen and perineum, a major complication of APR is the occurrence of perineal and abdominal wound infections. The type of closure used—primary closure, partial closure with an incisional drain, or leaving the wound open and packing it—determines the necessary postoperative care and teaching.

3.139 **The answer is d.** Nephrotic syndrome is impaired renal function resulting in severe proteinuria due to obstruction. It is caused by the presence of paraneoplastic lesions in the renal glomerulus and is a secondary benign disorder resulting from a primary glomerular disease.

3.140 **The answer is a.** Signs and symptoms of nephrotic syndrome include massive proteinuria and brown foamy urine as well as facial and peripheral edema, which may progress to anasarca or edema of all body tissues. The combined water and electrolyte retention may cause mild to moderate hypertension, not hypotension.

3.141 **The answer is d.** Infection, hypercalcemia, and dehydration are all possible contributing factors to the renal failure associated with multiple myeloma.

3.142 **The answer is c.** Nephritis and cystitis are the major long-term renal toxicities that result from cancer treatment. Damage to the nephrons and bladder has been documented in patients treated with cyclophosphamide, ifosfamide, and cisplatin.

3.143 **The answer is d.** Sitz baths are contraindicated if the perineal area is being irradiated.

3.144 **The answer is d.** Prevention of hemorrhagic cystitis is the key to success, including aggressive use of hydration, use of a Foley catheter, and administration of the uroprotectant mesna.

3.145 **The answer is a.** The only risk factor that has been linked persistently to kidney cancer by both cohort studies and epidemiologic studies is cigarette smoking. The links to occupational exposures (lead, asbestos) and genetics are less frequent.

3.146 **The answer is a.** The degree and duration of diarrhea depend on the agent, dose, nadir, and frequency of chemotherapy administration. Patients may experience abdominal cramps and rectal urgency with 5-FU–leucovorin therapy, which can evolve into nocturnal diarrhea or fecal incontinence, leading to lethargy, weakness, orthostatic hypotension, and fluid/electrolyte imbalance. Without adequate management, prolonged diarrhea causes dehydration, nutritional malabsorption, and circulatory collapse. Renal failure does not result from untreated diarrhea.

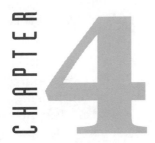

CHAPTER 4

Cardiopulmonary Function

ALTERATIONS IN VENTILATION

Anatomical or Surgical Alterations

4.1 A patient has recently returned from the operating room with a tracheotomy. He has a high-humidity oxygen collar with orders to suction the trachea every 2 hours as needed. The need for the continuous high-humidity collar is best explained by which of the following?
    a. The collar provides necessary oxygen to the lungs.
    b. The collar provides humidity to the air normally supplied by the nose.
    c. The collar protects the airway.
    d. The collar provides humidified air to a permanently altered airway.

4.2 Which of the following is *not* a problem postoperatively for the patient who has had a laryngectomy?
    a. Wound dehiscence
    b. Flap failure
    c. Aspiration
    d. Stomal infection

4.3 The primary purpose of a laryngectomy tube postoperatively is which of the following?
    a. To prevent tracheal trauma
    b. To prevent tracheal closure
    c. To maintain adequate stomal size
    d. a and c

4.4 Individuals with advanced esophageal cancer are considered at high risk for the development of
    a. Other gastrointestinal cancers
    b. Superior vena cava syndrome
    c. Aspiration pneumonia
    d. Xerostomia

4.5 Your patient is newly diagnosed with lung cancer and is scheduled to undergo a pneumonectomy. You schedule a preoperative teaching session to instruct the patient and family on smoking cessation. The rationale for this action is based on which of the following?
    a. Patients who quit smoking before surgery have less immunosuppression and less infection postoperatively.
    b. Smoking cessation strategies are for the family, because the patient should not be around smoke postoperatively.
    c. Risk of death is significantly higher in patients who continue to smoke within 4 weeks of surgery.
    d. There is no benefit at this point to encourage smoking cessation.

4.6 Stan has a well-differentiated tumor on his true vocal folds that seems to be growing slowly. Stan's tumor is most likely to be which kind of tumor?
    a. Subglottic
    b. Supraglottic
    c. Glottic
    d. Either a or c

4.7 Most small cell lung cancer (SCLC) tumors
    a. Are not associated with necrosis
    b. Are responsible for 55% of all lung cancers
    c. Are centrally located, developing around a main bronchus, and eventually compressing the bronchi externally
    d. Have a longer doubling time than that of any other lung cancer type

4.8 In the presence of a known bone tumor, symptoms such as hemoptysis, cough, fever, weight loss, and malaise may indicate
    a. Pulmonary metastases
    b. Pernicious anemia
    c. Radiotherapy toxicity
    d. Infection

4.9 After surgery a patient develops aspiration pneumonia. Which of the following symptoms may have caused this?
    a. Difficulty in swallowing
    b. Mechanical obstruction from cancer
    c. Excessive sedation
    d. All of the above

4.10 In the early postoperative period following pneumonectomy your patient experiences a cardiac arrhythmia. He has a history of a myocardial infarction and is currently on cardiac medications. Nursing action would include which of the following?
    a. Administer oxygen and encourage the patient to cough and deep breathe.
    b. Notify the physician immediately because he may be experiencing atrial fibrillation or another myocardial infarction.
    c. Ensure he has received his cardiac medication on schedule.
    d. Arrhythmias are common in the postoperative period and should be monitored.

Pulmonary Toxicity Related to Cancer Therapy

4.11 Mrs. Alexander has metastatic breast cancer. She presents today with dyspnea, orthopnea, weakness, tachypnea, and jugular venous distention. Echocardiogram reveals a pleural effusion and a slight reduction in ventricular function. This patient is *most likely* suffering from which of the following complications of cancer?
   a. Chemotherapy-induced myocardial dysfunction
   b. Lymphatic obstruction of the mediastinum
   c. Cardiac tamponade
   d. Pulmonary metastases

4.12 Ms. Daniels, who had an allogeneic bone marrow transplantation, develops certain pulmonary complications. You are mindful that because of prolonged periods of immunosuppression caused by her medication, she is at greater risk for developing
   a. Interstitial pneumonia
   b. Cytomegalovirus (CMV) pneumonia
   c. Idiopathic pneumonia
   d. Respiratory syncytial virus pneumonia

4.13 Davis has received prior irradiation to his chest; therefore his doctor would be particularly cautious prescribing which of the following?
   a. Bleomycin
   b. Cytarabine
   c. Mitomycin C
   d. All of the above

4.14 Your patient with disseminated testicular cancer has just completed three full courses of bleomycin, etoposide, cisplatin treatment and is scheduled for surgery to remove a residual retroperitoneal mass. Which of the following is appropriate to emphasize in your teaching of this patient?
   a. Aggressive pulmonary hygiene measures are needed postoperatively because of his increased risk for respiratory failure.
   b. This treatment is designed to be curative.
   c. This treatment is not curative but will significantly increase his survival.
   d. a and b

4.15 Which of the following describes the features of chemotherapy-induced pulmonary toxicity?
   a. The site of damage is the endothelial cells of the lungs.
   b. There is an inflammatory-type reaction.
   c. It is a drug-induced pneumonitis.
   d. All of the above

4.16 The pulmonary function test *most likely* to detect chemotherapy-induced pulmonary toxicity before the onset of clinical symptoms is
   a. The carbon monoxide diffusion capacity measurement
   b. Pulmonary blood gases
   c. CO_2 binding capacity
   d. A chest x-ray

4.17   The best method to establish a histopathological diagnosis of chemotherapy-induced pulmonary toxicity is
    a.   A sputum specimen
    b.   Fiberoptic bronchoscopy
    c.   Thoracotomy
    d.   Needle biopsy

4.18   The earliest symptom of chemotherapy-induced pulmonary toxicity is
    a.   Bilateral basilar rales
    b.   Hypoxia with hypocapnia
    c.   Productive cough
    d.   Hyperthermia

4.19   Risk factors for pneumothorax with placement of a central line in the bone marrow transplant patient includes *all but* which of the following?
    a.   High-dose steroids
    b.   Total body irradiation
    c.   Recent weight loss
    d.   Bed rest

4.20   Pulmonary edema due to fluid overload can occur in the first few days following marrow or blood cell transplant. Which of the following factors increases the risk of pulmonary edema in this population?
    a.   Previous anthracycline therapy
    b.   Previous cyclophosphamide therapy
    c.   Total body irradiation
    d.   All of the above

4.21   Spontaneous pneumothorax has been noted to occur in the acute phase of blood cell transplantation. Which of the following is *not* considered to be a risk factor for spontaneous pneumothorax in this population?
    a.   Prior treatment with antitumor antibiotics
    b.   High-dose steroids
    c.   Total body irradiation
    d.   Poor nutrition with recent weight loss

4.22   Which of the following best explains the mechanism for bleomycin-induced pulmonary fibrosis?
    a.   Pressure necrosis
    b.   Allergic reaction with scarring
    c.   Formation of free radicals and lipid peroxidation
    d.   Damage to type III pneumocytes

Anemia

4.23   Studies involving the use of erythropoietin in patients receiving myelosuppressive chemotherapy resulted in which of the following treatment indications?
    a.   Erythropoietin is indicated for the treatment of iron or folate deficiencies.
    b.   Erythropoietin is used to correct chemotherapy-related anemia.
    c.   Erythropoietin is indicated to prevent anemia in the cancer patient.
    d.   Erythropoietin is used to return the hemoglobin to normal levels following cytotoxic therapy.

4.24   Vascular endothelial growth factor (VEGF) stimulates endothelial cell growth. Which of the following is considered to be the primary trigger for activation of VEGF?
a. Apoptosis
b. Anemia
c. Thrombocytopenia
d. Tumor hypoxia

4.25   The etiology of anemia of malignancy is complicated but is *most likely* related to which of the following?
a. Tumor secretion of cytokines that affect red blood cell metabolism
b. Protein-calorie malnutrition
c. Chronic hemorrhage
d. All of the above

4.26   Your patient with leukemia is severely immunosuppressed and experiencing a coagulopathy. She frequently experiences hemoptysis, dyspnea, and fatigue. She is *most likely* suffering from which of the following?
a. Lung cancer
b. Pneumonia
c. Alveolar hemorrhage
d. Cardiac tamponade

4.27   Management of hemoptysis due to alveolar hemorrhage includes which of the following?
a. Thoracentesis to relieve dyspnea
b. Codeine or hydrocodone for cough suppression
c. Antianxiety medications
d. All of the above

4.28   Which of the following best describes tumor angiogenesis?
a. A process whereby tumor cells are able to divide despite low hemoglobin
b. A response to tumor hypoxia
c. A process whereby tumors are deprived of a vascular network
d. A process whereby tumors create their own vascular network

4.29   Which of the following chemotherapeutic agents causes anemia by inhibiting the maturation of the erythroid lineage cells in the bone marrow?
a. Cyclophosphamide
b. Nitrogen mustard
c. Cisplatin
d. Carboplatin

4.30   A 72-year-old patient with lung cancer complains of extreme fatigue. He is not very active, but with a hemoglobin of 7.7 g/100 mL the decision is made to bring him into the outpatient infusion center to be transfused with 3 units of packed red blood cells. The primary problem associated with a low hemoglobin and the reason to transfuse is which of the following?
a. Risk for hemorrhage
b. Risk for angina
c. Risk for stroke
d. Risk for hypovolemia

4.31   Your patient complains of extreme fatigue, headache, irritability, and dizziness. You suspect he is suffering from which of the following disorders?
a. Iron deficiency
b. Hypercalcemia
c. Anemia
d. Low magnesium

4.32   As a treatment for anemia, erythropoietin is meant to do what?
a. Replenish and stimulate iron stores
b. Increase reticulocytosis
c. Increase erythropoiesis
d. Decrease reticulocytosis

4.33   Anemia of chronic illness is associated with which of the following?
a. Erythroid hypoplasia of the bone marrow
b. A decrease in reticulocytosis
c. Hypoferremia
d. All of the above

4.34   Chronic anemia is associated with cognitive dysfunction. Which of the following has been shown to protect against cognitive decline in women receiving chemotherapy for breast cancer?
a. Vitamin therapy
b. Blood transfusion therapy
c. Epoetin alfa
d. Kava therapy

Pleural Effusions

4.35   Malignant pleural effusions are often associated with a poor prognosis. Which of the following is an accurate description of median survival times of patients with malignant pleural effusions?
a. Breast cancer patients with evidence of a malignant pleural effusion have a median survival time of 14 months.
b. Lung cancer patients with evidence of a malignant pleural effusion have a median survival time of 6 months.
c. Patients with mesothelioma with evidence of malignant pleural effusion have a median survival time of 3 months.
d. a and b

4.36   During a thoracentesis procedure your patient is placed in an upright sitting position. As the fluid is being removed the patient becomes diaphoretic, pale, and appears to be fainting. As you administer care to your patient you realize her symptoms are due to what?
a. Reexpansion pulmonary edema
b. Needle phobia
c. A vasovagal reaction
d. Pneumothorax

4.37   Janis frequently experiences dyspnea due to recurrent pleural effusions. Her doctor has suggested that she have a more permanent device placed into her pleural space to make it easier to drain the fluid from her lung. Which of the following is an accurate description of this device?
   a.   A pleuroperitoneal shunt can be inserted to divert fluid from the chest cavity to the abdomen.
   b.   A pleural port can be implanted underneath the skin just below the ribs, with the catheter resting in the pleural space. The port is accessed with a 19-gauge Huber-point needle whenever she complains of difficulty breathing.
   c.   A small-bore catheter may be placed into the pleural space and allowed to drain through a one-way valve by gravity drainage.
   d.   All of the above

4.38   Thoracentesis involves fluid removal from
   a.   The pericardial sac
   b.   The pleural cavity
   c.   The abdominal cavity
   d.   The spinal column

4.39   The first and most common means of obliteration of the pleural cavity in a patient with chronic recurrent malignant pleural effusions is
   a.   Pleuroperitoneal shunt
   b.   Pleural stripping
   c.   Sclerosis
   d.   Local radiation

4.40   Which of the following chemotherapy agents is known to cause fluid retention that may manifest as abdominal ascites, as a pleural effusion, or as a combination?
   a.   Mitoxantrone
   b.   Megestrol acetate
   c.   Docetaxel
   d.   Paclitaxel

4.41   Cytarabine and mitomycin C can cause diffuse alveolar damage, resulting in which of the following pulmonary disorders?
   a.   Pneumonia
   b.   Capillary leak syndrome
   c.   Obliteration of alveoli
   d.   Pleural effusion

4.42   Mr. Eliot, age 64 and a smoker for 47 years, has an undifferentiated neoplasm arising in the proximal right bronchus. On examination of Mr. Eliot, you hear a dullness on percussion. What might this indicate?
   a.   Tumor in the main bronchus
   b.   Bagpipe sign
   c.   Bronchophony
   d.   Pleural effusion

4.43   Your patient is immediate post-op following a right hepatectomy. He is most at risk for which of the following non–liver-related complications?
   a.   Pneumonia and pleural effusion
   b.   Deep vein thrombosis
   c.   Hemorrhage
   d.   Subphrenic abscess

4.44   What percentage of pleural effusions are malignant?
    a. 100%
    b. 75%
    c. 50%
    d. <25%

4.45   Which of the following tumor-related pathologies is *not* known to cause pleural effusion?
    a. Disseminated intravascular coagulopathy
    b. Superior vena cava syndrome
    c. Postobstructive pneumonitis
    d. Pericardial constriction

4.46   Which of the following differentiates a malignant pleural effusion from a nonmalignant pleural effusion?
    a. Malignant effusions are almost always grossly bloody.
    b. Malignant effusions are almost always an exudate.
    c. Nonmalignant effusions are almost always a transudate.
    d. All of the above

4.47   Which of the following is the most commonly reported symptom of pleural effusion?
    a. Fever
    b. Sharp pleuritic chest pain
    c. Dry irritating cough
    d. Dyspnea

ALTERATIONS IN CIRCULATION

Lymphedema

4.48   Which of the following is *not* considered a risk factor for lymphedema?
    a. Axillary irradiation
    b. Infection
    c. Weight lifting
    d. Breast reconstruction

4.49   Which of the following conditions is benign and iatrogenic in origin and is usually secondary to radical cancer surgery?
    a. Pericardial effusion
    b. Lymphedema
    c. Pleural effusion
    d. Anasarca

4.50   Although the incidence of lymphedema has decreased because breast surgeries have become less radical, the percentage of women who experience lymphedema following a modified radical mastectomy is approximately
    a. 5%
    b. 10%
    c. 15%
    d. 20%

4.51   A woman who is about to have a modified radical mastectomy for diffuse multicentric breast cancer states, "Having a lymph node dissection is all right with me. I want all the cancer cells taken out if they are there." The most appropriate nursing response is which of the following?
a.   The axillary dissection could cause lymphedema depending on the number of nodes removed.
b.   The purpose of the lymph node dissection is staging; it is not a therapeutic procedure.
c.   Because her disease is all over the breast, it is a good idea that she is having a more extensive dissection under her arm.
d.   If any nodes are left behind, radiation can always be used.

4.52   A woman is more at risk for lymphedema if she has which of the following risk factors?
a.   Obesity
b.   Inflammation or infection
c.   Radiation therapy
d.   All of the above

4.53   A woman with a history of modified radical mastectomy with axillary dissection and radiation therapy completed chemotherapy 6 months ago and calls concerned about slight swelling and redness in her affected arm. On questioning her you learn that she has recently been to Europe. What is the appropriate nursing action and why?
a.   She should keep the arm elevated. Slight swelling is common following exposure to compression changes in an airplane. Wear a sleeve.
b.   The swelling is probably due to the flight and the fact that she probably carried a suitcase. The redness is a problem. She should be on antibiotics, so she should see her doctor as soon as possible.
c.   Keep the arm elevated. If it is not better in a week, call back.
d.   She needs a diuretic and an antibiotic, so she should see her doctor.

4.54   The physiological reason for lymphedema is best explained by which of the following?
a.   An increased resistance to venous flow occurs.
b.   A disturbance in oncotic pressure occurs because of protein accumulation.
c.   Lymphatic obstruction causes backflow of fluid.
d.   a and b

4.55   The mainstay of symptomatic lymphedema treatment is
a.   Redirection of fluid
b.   Manual lymphatic drainage
c.   Stimulation of the dermal lymphatomes
d.   All of the above

4.56   Complex decongestive physiotherapy for the management of lymphedema involves all but which of the following?
a.   Deep massage
b.   Compression garments
c.   Exercises
d.   Bandaging

4.57   Following treatment for ovarian cancer, your patient calls to complain that her legs feel heavy, painful, and slightly numb. Nursing management includes which of the following?
a.   Inform her to elevate her legs and restrict fluids.
b.   Instruct her to come into the emergency room to rule out a deep vein thrombosis.
c.   Inform her that her symptoms are likely due to obstruction of lymph drainage in her abdomen, and she needs to be evaluated.
d.   Reassure her that her symptoms are likely due to chemotherapy and will improve over time.

Cardiovascular Toxicity Related to Cancer Therapy

4.58   Approximately what percentage of persons who receive mediastinal irradiation for Hodgkin's disease experience pericardial toxicity?
a.   20%
b.   30%
c.   50%
d.   70%

4.59   Althea has received both extensive mediastinal radiation and chemotherapy. Short- and long-term side effects to anticipate include
a.   Pericarditis and hemodynamic compromise
b.   Chest pain, edema, and cardiac tamponade
c.   Coronary artery disease and cardiomyopathy
d.   All of the above

4.60   Chronic cardiotoxic effects can occur months after treatment with certain chemotherapeutic agents. Patients are routinely monitored for
a.   Nonproductive cough, dyspnea, and pedal edema
b.   Biventricular congestive heart failure
c.   Low-voltage QRS complex
d.   All of the above

4.61   An individual is admitted with congestive heart failure. Medical records indicate a history of acute leukemia, which was treated 10 years ago with anthracyclines. The most probable long-term late effect of this treatment is
a.   Angina
b.   Pulmonary fibrosis
c.   Pericarditis
d.   Cardiomyopathy

4.62   Cardiotoxicity associated with doxorubicin can be minimized by the administration of which of the following cardioprotective agents?
a.   Calcium gluconate
b.   Digitalis
c.   Amifostine
d.   Dexrazoxane (Zinecard)

4.63   Which of the following is considered to be a significant risk factor for cardiotoxicity?
a.   An ejection fraction of 45% or less at rest
b.   Anthracycline cumulative dose of 300 mg/m^2
c.   Combination of doxorubicin and paclitaxel chemotherapy
d.   Total body irradiation

4.64   Which of the following is not considered to be a significant risk factor for cardiac tamponade?
a.   Lung cancer
b.   Radiation to the pericardium
c.   Pericardial fluid accumulation of 300 cc
d.   Increased catecholamine production

4.65   In a blood cell transplant patient who receives cyclophosphamide, the most critical risk factor for cardiac toxicity is
    a.   Dose
    b.   Prior anthracycline therapy
    c.   Bolus versus continuous infusion
    d.   Mediastinal radiation

4.66   Delayed radiation injury to the heart can manifest as which of the following?
    a.   Pericardial disease
    b.   Myocardial disease
    c.   Coronary heart disease
    d.   All of the above

4.67   The mechanism of cardiac damage following anthracycline therapy includes *all but* which of the following?
    a.   Overexpression of genes encoding for cardiac muscle protein
    b.   Binding to membranes rich in cardiolipin
    c.   Formation of free radicals
    d.   Inhibited expression of genes encoding for cardiac muscle protein

4.68   The mechanism of cardiac damage from radiation therapy primarily involves which of the following?
    a.   Microvascular thrombosis
    b.   Rupture of the endothelial cells
    c.   Swelling of the cells of the myocardial capillaries
    d.   All of the above

Fluid and Electrolyte Imbalances

4.69   What side effects may a patient experience as a direct result of pheresis?
    a.   Fever—especially localized fever—from rapid movement and return of large volumes of blood to the body
    b.   Hypercalcemia from high volumes of intravenous calcium gluconate
    c.   Hypovolemia, especially for patients with a history of cardiac problems
    d.   a and c

4.70   A patient receiving mitomycin and 5-FU develops a 15-pound weight gain, decreased hemoglobin, thrombocytopenia, ascites, encephalopathy, and elevated bilirubin and serum glutamic-oxaloacetic transaminase (SGOT) lab values. You recognize these as classic symptoms of
    a.   Liver failure
    b.   Severe dehydration
    c.   Venoocclusive disease
    d.   Intractable ascites

4.71   Control of extracellular calcium levels within a narrow range is achieved through the action of several agents, including all of the following *except*
    a.   Parathyroid hormone (PTH), which controls renal regulation of calcium
    b.   1,25-dihydroxyvitamin D, which controls intestinal calcium absorption
    c.   Calcitonin
    d.   Glucocorticoids, which control osteoclast activity

4.72 How does the body typically respond to elevated levels of extracellular calcium?
    a. By reducing parathyroid hormone secretion
    b. By increasing bone resorption
    c. By increasing renal synthesis of 1,25-dihydroxyvitamin D
    d. By decreasing urinary calcium excretion

4.73 Bone remodeling activity is controlled by all of the following *except*
    a. Prostaglandins, regulatory proteins, and constituents of the organic matrix
    b. Mechanical factors such as weight bearing
    c. Calcium ingestion, which is needed to couple bone resorption and bone formation
    d. Osteotropic hormones, especially parathyroid hormone and 1,25-dihydroxyvitamin D

4.74 Third spacing is
    a. The normal fluid distribution in the extracellular and intravascular compartments
    b. An excess of interstitial fluid accumulation
    c. Fluid retention in sites that normally have very little or no fluid
    d. Lack of normal osmotic pressures

4.75 Choose the statement that most accurately describes the degree of subjective symptoms produced by malignant pericardial and pleural effusions.
    a. Symptoms tend to be related more to the rate of fluid accumulation than to the volume collected.
    b. Symptoms tend to be related more to the volume of fluid collected than to the rate of the collection.
    c. Symptoms are related more to the underlying disease and length of time the patient has been diagnosed with cancer.
    d. Symptoms correspond directly to whether the metastatic disease is from microscopic seeding of the cavities or from local extension.

4.76 Acute renal failure secondary to tumor lysis syndrome is primarily due to
    a. Hyperuricemia and hyperkalemia
    b. Hyperkalemia and hyperphosphatemia
    c. Hyperuricemia and hyperphosphatemia
    d. Hyperuricemia and hypokalemia

4.77 The cardiac conduction abnormalities related to tumor lysis syndrome are due to
    a. Intracellular hypokalemia
    b. Extracellular hyperkalemia
    c. Intracellular hypercalcemia
    d. Extracellular hypercalcemia

4.78 In a patient whose calcium is 11.8 mg/dL and serum albumin is 2.5 g/dL, a formula is needed to determine the total serum calcium. Why is this formula necessary?
    a. When a patient has less serum albumin to bind with calcium, a greater portion of the total serum calcium must be ionized.
    b. Ionized calcium and calcium bound to albumin are inversely related.
    c. Albumin binds calcium, precipitating hypocalcemia.
    d. Low albumin levels drive calcium to abnormally high levels.

Thrombotic Events

4.79 Vaginal cancer is generally treated with surgery and radiation. Complications following treatment include *all but* which of the following?
   a. Venous thrombosis and vaginal engorgement
   b. Vaginal fibrosis and scarring
   c. Constriction in blood supply
   d. Loss of vaginal elasticity

4.80 Mr. Archer has had an implanted port for 4 weeks and recently complained of pain in his right neck and shoulder, just above the catheter insertion site. On examination you notice slight swelling over the neck, face, shoulder, and arm. He also complains that his arm is cold at times and there is some tingling in his arm and shoulder. What is the most appropriate action to take?
   a. These symptoms are normal following port placement and should resolve in 2–3 weeks. Have him return to the clinic in a week if he is not better.
   b. Flush the line with heparin to make sure it is not clotted.
   c. Notify the physician to examine the patient. A venogram will probably demonstrate a venous thrombosis.
   d. Notify the physician to obtain an order for urokinase. The patient probably has a fibrin sheath formation around the tip of the catheter.

4.81 Thromboembolism (TE) is most frequently seen with which of the following?
   a. Small cell lung cancer
   b. Non–small cell lung cancer
   c. Mucin-secreting bladder carcinoma
   d. Mucin-secreting adenocarcinoma of the gastrointestinal tract

4.82 The etiology of thromboembolism is
   a. Tumor secretion of cytokines, such as interleukin-1, affecting red cell metabolism
   b. The ability of tumor cells to affect systemic activation of coagulation and cause platelet dysfunction
   c. Chronic hemorrhage
   d. Bone marrow failure

4.83 Tumor cells may precipitate paraneoplastic thromboembolism by
   a. Activation of the coagulation pathway
   b. Damage to the endothelial lining of blood vessels
   c. Protein-calorie malnutrition
   d. a and b

4.84 The prognosis for a patient with colorectal cancer is probably poorest if which of the following exists?
   a. Venous and lymph node invasion
   b. High blood pressure
   c. Location of the tumor above the peritoneal reflection
   d. Squamous cell involvement

4.85 Mrs. Mura has chronic myeloma and has recently begun to complain of blurred vision, headache, drowsiness, and occasional confusion. These symptoms may be caused by which of the following?
   a. A high concentration of proteins that increases serum viscosity
   b. Chronic effects of steroid use
   c. Hyperviscosity syndrome
   d. a and c

4.86 On inspection, you note that Ms. Harris exhibits edema and a bluish tint to the face and that her neck veins seem too prominent. What might be causing these symptoms?
   a. Blockage of the inferior vena cava
   b. Nodular umbilicus
   c. Distention
   d. Intra-abdominal fluid

4.87 The primary pathology of disseminated intravascular coagulation that leads to increased morbidity and mortality is
   a. Uncontrolled and diffuse bleeding
   b. Uncontrolled and diffuse thrombosis
   c. Diffuse pulmonary embolus
   d. Intracranial hemorrhage

4.88 Cancers most likely to be associated with thromboembolism include *all but* which of the following?
   a. Lung cancer
   b. Colon cancer
   c. Pancreatic cancer
   d. Melanoma

4.89 Thromboembolic disease that is refractory to anticoagulation therapy is often indicative of underlying cancer.
   a. True
   b. False

4.90 Which of the following tests is considered most useful in diagnosing disseminated intravascular coagulation (DIC)?
   a. Antithrombin III level and fibrinopeptide A level
   b. Platelet count
   c. Plasminogen level
   d. D-dimer and fibrinogen degradation products/fibrinogen split products (FDP/FSP) assay

4.91 The major complication related to thrombocythemia includes which of the following?
   a. Bleeding
   b. Thrombosis
   c. Pulmonary embolism
   d. All of the above

ANSWER EXPLANATIONS

4.1   **The answer is b.** Patients with a tracheotomy have lost the functions of the nose in warming, moistening, and filtering the air when breathing. A tracheotomy is not permanent.

4.2   **The answer is c.** Patients who have a laryngectomy no longer have communication between the mouth and throat so aspiration is not physically possible.

4.3   **The answer is d.** The tube will help prevent trauma to the tracheal mucosa due to suctioning and, most important, will maintain an adequate stoma size. Because the laryngectomy stoma is permanent, the tube may be removed and cleaned without fear of stomal closure.

4.4   **The answer is c.** When an esophageal tumor gets so large that it causes saliva, food, and liquids to spill over into the lungs, affected individuals are at high risk for the development of aspiration pneumonia. Because of this potential, pulmonary hygiene and aspiration precautions should be a focus of nursing care for the person with esophageal cancer.

4.5   **The answer is c.** Risk of death is significantly higher in patients who are still smoking within 1 month of pneumonectomy. There is higher morbidity and mortality for smokers who continue to smoke before surgery. Patients who stop smoking within 10 weeks of surgery have the same risk as those who had never smoked.

4.6   **The answer is c.** The glottic area includes the true vocal folds and the anterior and posterior glottic commissures. Tumors in this area tend to be well differentiated, grow slowly, and metastasize late. Lesions that lie superior to a horizontal plane passing through the floor of the ventricles and including the epiglottis, aryepiglottic folds, arytenoids, and ventricular bands (false cords) are classified as supraglottic.

4.7   **The answer is c.** Most SCLC tumors are centrally located, developing around a main bronchus as a whitish-gray growth that invades surrounding structures, eventually compressing the bronchi externally. Necrosis is frequently seen, and SCLC is responsible for 25% of all lung cancers, not 55%. Its doubling time is shorter, not longer, than that of any other lung cancer type.

4.8   **The answer is a.** Metastatic spread in bone cancer occurs primarily to the lungs by the hematogenous route. Symptoms of pulmonary metastases include weight loss, malaise, hemoptysis, cough, chest pain, and fever.

4.9   **The answer is d.** Aspiration pneumonia in the surgical oncology patient may be caused by difficulty in swallowing, mechanical obstruction from the cancer, or excessive sedation.

4.10 **The answer is b.** Atrial arrhythmias are common in the patient who has undergone a lung resection because of irritation to the vagus nerve. Stroke is a complication of atrial fibrillation. Patients are monitored closely during the postoperative period, and beta-blockers are initiated if atrial fibrillation persists. Patients who have had a myocardial infarction within 3 months of resection are at risk of another one, and the mortality from this complication rises with increasing age.

4.11   **The answer is c.** Symptoms of pericardial effusion include dyspnea, cough, chest pain, orthopnea, fever, edema, fatigue, weakness, and dizziness. Cardiac tamponade is the term used to describe the severe decrease in cardiac output caused by pericardial effusion. Physical findings include tachycardia, cyanosis, tachypnea, jugular venous distention, peripheral edema, and irregular heart rate.

4.12   **The answer is b.** CMV pneumonia is the leading cause of infectious pneumonia after bone marrow transplantation. The incidence of CMV pneumonia may be higher in allograft versus autograft recipients, specifically because of prolonged periods of immunosuppression caused by medication.

4.13   **The answer is d.** Agents associated with pulmonary toxicity include, among others, bleomycin, cytarabine, mitomycin C, cyclophosphamide, carmustine, and methotrexate. Prior irradiation to the chest enhances risk for toxicity.

4.14   **The answer is d.** Men who receive bleomycin at a cumulative dose of greater than 200 mg/m^2 are at greater risk of pulmonary fibrosis with subsequent respiratory failure or death during the postoperative recovery period. Individuals with even mild bleomycin toxicity demonstrate some degree of arterial oxygen desaturation with high concentrations of inspired oxygen (as in those given at surgery under normal conditions) and an abnormal carbon monoxide diffusion capacity. Goal of treatment is cure.

4.15   **The answer is d.** Pulmonary toxicity usually is irreversible and progressive as a result of chemotherapy administration. The initial site of damage seems to be the endothelial cells, with an inflammatory-type reaction resulting in drug-induced pneumonitis.

4.16   **The answer is a.** The most sensitive pulmonary function test is the carbon monoxide diffusion capacity measurement that becomes abnormal before the onset of clinical symptoms.

4.17   **The answer is b.** The best method to establish a histopathologic diagnosis is to obtain involved tissues by means of an open-lung biopsy or a fiberoptic bronchoscopy.

4.18   **The answer is a.** Pulmonary toxicity usually presents clinically as dyspnea, unproductive cough, bilateral basilar rales, and tachypnea.

4.19   **The answer is d.** Predisposing factors for pneumothorax include high-dose steroids, total body irradiation, and poor nutrition with recent weight loss.

4.20   **The answer is d.** Pulmonary edema can be seen in the first few days following marrow or blood cell transplant and is the result of fluid overload. Previous exposure to anthracyclines and the use of cyclophosphamide and total body irradiation during conditioning can exacerbate this complication.

4.21   **The answer is a.** Spontaneous pneumothorax may occur in the acute phase of transplant. Predisposing factors for pneumothorax include high-dose steroids, total body irradiation, and poor nutrition with recent weight loss.

4.22   **The answer is c.** The mechanisms of bleomycin injury include formation of free radicals and lipid peroxidation of phospholipid membranes. Subsequently, interstitial edema and damage to type I pneumocytes occur.

4.23   **The answer is b.** Erythropoietin is indicated for chemotherapy-induced anemia in patients with nonmyeloid malignancies. It has not been used to prevent anemia, and it is not intended to be used to return the hemoglobin to normal or pretreatment levels. The goal of erythropoietin is to reduce transfusion requirements and to raise the hematocrit to 36%. Epoetin alfa is not indicated for the treatment of anemia in cancer patients due to factors such as iron or folate deficiencies, hemolysis, or gastrointestinal bleeding.

4.24   **The answer is d.** The angiogenic switch refers to the ability of tumor cells to release angiogenic factors and convert the tumor cell to an angiogenesis inducer. This switch correlates with an increased production of VEGF, which is known to induce angiogenesis. A primary trigger of the angiogenic switch is tumor hypoxia, which turns on the VEGF tyrosine kinase signaling pathway.

4.25   **The answer is d.** Tumor secretion of cytokines, such as interleukin-1, affect red blood cell metabolism and function and is a factor associated with anemia of malignancy. Patients with protein-caloric malnutrition often have insufficient iron and folic acid stores, leading to anemia. Bone marrow failure can occur in heavily treated patients who have received multiple courses of chemotherapy, and, finally, chronic microscopic bleeding in patients with primary or metastatic diseases can result in anemia as a result of chronic hemorrhage.

4.26   **The answer is c.** Patients who are severely immunosuppressed and have a coagulopathy are most likely to bleed into the alveoli. These individuals are usually bone marrow transplant recipients or have leukemia. The alveoli fill with blood, prohibiting gas exchange and leading to hypoxia.

4.27   **The answer is d.** Hemoptysis is usually very scant and will stop spontaneously within a short period of time. Cough suppression might help because coughing is an aggravating factor. For treating substantial hemoptysis, the individual needs to be kept calm and on bed rest, lying on his or her side, with the side of hemorrhage dependent so as not to cause asphyxiation by draining the blood into the other lung.

4.28   **The answer is d.** Tumor angiogenesis is a complex multistep process that enables tumors to develop a new blood supply from a preexisting vascular network.

4.29   **The answer is c.** Cyclophosphamide and nitrogen mustard are alkylators and quite toxic but generally do not cause significant anemia. Carboplatin is platelet sparing.

4.30   **The answer is b.** Anemia manifests as pallor, hypotension, headaches, irritability, and fatigue. Tachycardia and tachypnea may be present due to the hypoxic effects on the heart.

4.31   **The answer is c.** Anemia manifests as pallor, hypotension, headaches, irritability, and fatigue.

4.32   **The answer is c.** Erythropoietin is a growth factor for erythroid progenitor cells that promotes proliferation and maintains their survival.

4.33   **The answer is d.** Anemia of chronic disease is associated with erythroid hypoplasia of the bone marrow. This results in a slight decrease in reticulocytosis, hypoferremia, and a decrease in serum erythropoietin.

4.34   **The answer is c.** Researchers have found that epoetin alfa has neuroprotective effects. Studies of systematically administered epoetin alfa have demonstrated that the drug crosses the blood–brain barrier and has significant cognitive-enhancing effects. Epoetin alfa raises the erythropoietin levels in the brain and central nervous system and protects neurons from damage.

4.35   **The answer is d.** Median survival times of patients with mesothelioma with evidence of malignant pleural effusion is 16 months.

4.36   **The answer is c.** Symptoms of a vasovagal reaction include diaphoresis and feeling as if loss of consciousness is imminent. Complications of the thoracentesis may include bleeding, vasovagal reaction, pain from reexpansion of the lung and apposition of pleural surfaces, and, in approximately 5% of cases, pneumothorax requiring tube thoracostomy.

4.37   **The answer is d.** Pleural fluid removal through an implanted port and intrapleural catheter can be performed by the nurse on an outpatient basis. New technology using small-bore needles may permit management of malignant pleural effusions on an outpatient basis. These radiologically placed small-bore catheters are connected to a plastic bag with a one-way valve system for gravity drainage. In cases of recurrent effusion, a pleuroperitoneal shunt can be inserted to divert fluid from the chest cavity to the abdomen.

4.38   **The answer is b.** Relief of pleural effusion symptoms such as dyspnea, cough, and dull aching chest pain is a short-term treatment goal that is usually achieved when the pleural fluid is mechanically drained. Thoracentesis involves pleural fluid removal by needle aspiration through the chest wall. Fluid tends to reaccumulate when it is not possible to control the underlying cancer. Long-range treatment goals are directed toward the obliteration of the pleural space so that pleural fluid cannot reaccumulate.

4.39   **The answer is c.** Sclerosis with chemical agents is the most common method used to obliterate the pleural space in patients with malignant pleural effusions. Chemical sclerosing does not prolong the patient's life but may enhance quality of life by relieving symptoms and reducing the time a patient spends in the hospital. Shunts and stripping are surgical methods that become options after other approaches have been tried and the pleural effusion remains uncontrolled. Although external beam radiation may be used as local treatment for mediastinal tumors, hemithoracic radiation is not recommended as a first-line management of malignant pleural effusions because of the hazard of pulmonary fibrosis.

4.40   **The answer is c.** A side effect of docetaxel is fluid retention. The incidence is related to the cumulative dose, which can be disabling and worsens with higher doses. Fluid retention is exhibited peripherally as abdominal ascites, as a pleural effusion, or as a combination.

4.41   **The answer is b.** A capillary leak syndrome, involving primarily the lung, occurs 2–21 days after the first dose of cytarabine, resulting in pulmonary edema and respiratory failure. Mitomycin C damage to the lung presents as diffuse alveolar damage with capillary leak and pulmonary edema.

4.42   **The answer is d.** Dullness on percussion indicates either pleural effusion or a consolidated lung. Lung cancer is the most common cause of hemorrhagic pleural effusion in middle-aged and elderly male smokers. Mr. Eliot has smoked since he was 17.

4.43   **The answer is a.** Pleural effusion is common following liver resection and is most often seen after right hepatectomy.

4.44   **The answer is c.**

4.45   **The answer is a.** Tumor-related pathologies that can cause pleural effusion include superior vena cava syndrome, endobronchial obstruction with atelectasis, postobstructive pneumonitis, and pericardial constriction.

4.46   **The answer is d.**

4.47   **The answer is d.** Dyspnea caused by the accumulating effusion is the most commonly reported symptom. Sharp pleuritic chest pain may or may not be accompanied by a pleural rub. Other symptoms include fever, dry irritating cough, and hypoxia.

4.48   **The answer is d.** The most common causes of chronic or late lymphedema are prior axillary irradiation, infection, and tumor recurrence or tumor enlargement in the axilla. Heat, strenuous exercise, or lifting objects weighing more than 5–10 pounds contribute to lymphedema.

4.49   **The answer is b.** Lymphedema is a benign iatrogenic problem caused by radical cancer surgery. Arm lymphedema often developed after the most common treatment for all types of breast cancer in the past: radical mastectomy with axillary node dissection followed by radiation. It now occurs much less frequently. Lymphedema of the leg may develop after groin dissection that is performed for the treatment of metastatic disease from primary tumors. Mechanical interruption (surgical technique) and radiation often produce lymphatic obstruction, the most common cause of lymphedema.

4.50   **The answer is b.**

4.51   **The answer is b.** A lymph node dissection stages disease. It is not a therapeutic procedure.

4.52   **The answer is d.** Factors that contribute to the development of lymphedema are obesity, insufficient muscle contraction, inflammation, trauma, formation of fibrosclerotic tissue within the lymph vessel, and scarring secondary to radiation therapy or infection.

4.53   **The answer is b.**

4.54   **The answer is d.** Lymphatic obstruction is a factor, but it is an anatomic reason for lymphedema, not a physiological one.

4.55   **The answer is d.** The mainstay of symptomatic lymphedema treatment is manual lymphatic drainage performed by a physical therapist trained in lymphedema management. It is light stimulation of the dermal lymphatomes and the lymphatic vessels to redirect the protein-rich fluid and is not to be confused with deep massage.

4.56   **The answer is a.** Complex decongestive physiotherapy consists of skin care, manual lymphatic drainage, bandaging, exercises, and wearing a compression garment.

4.57   **The answer is c.** Obstruction of lymphatic drainage from the abdomen due to ovarian cancer results in bilateral lower extremity swelling. It can be painful, and the legs feel heavy and painful.

4.58   **The answer is d.** Ultimately, 76% of patients who receive mediastinal radiotherapy develop pericardial toxicity. A retrospective review of patients who underwent mediastinal irradiation and required valve replacement concluded that radiation injury was a major factor responsible for the development of mitral valve disease and was a contributing factor in aortic valve disease.

4.59 **The answer is d.** Toxic effects include acute and chronic pericarditis, along with a spectrum of symptoms ranging from cough and chest pain to edema, paradoxic pulse, cardiac tamponade, and hemodynamic compromise. Coronary artery disease and cardiomyopathy are also seen following extensive mediastinal radiation.

4.60 **The answer is d.** Chronic cardiotoxic effects include a nonproductive cough, dyspnea, and pedal edema and involve irreversible cardiomyopathy presenting as a classic biventricular congestive heart failure with a characteristic low-voltage QRS complex.

4.61 **The answer is d.** One of the most serious side effects of anthracyclines is cardiac toxicity, which typically presents as cardiomyopathy with clinical signs of congestive heart failure. Evidence indicates that structural damage can occur in the absence of clinical signs and that cardiac failure may occur many years after completion of therapy.

4.62 **The answer is d.** Zinecard interferes with the intracellular process responsible for anthracycline-induced cardiomyopathy.

4.63 **The answer is a.** Further doses of chemotherapy are not recommended if the ejection fraction drops to 45% or less at rest or deteriorates more than 5% from baseline.

4.64 **The answer is d.** Catecholamine production results in an increase in heart rate, which is a compensatory mechanism.

4.65 **The answer is a.** The dose of cyclophosphamide is a major risk factor in the development of cardiac toxicity. The contribution of prior anthracycline therapy or mediastinal radiation therapy is unclear.

4.66 **The answer is d.**

4.67 **The answer is a.** The mechanism of cardiac damage following anthracycline therapy includes inhibited expression of genes encoding for cardiac muscle protein, binding to membranes rich in cardiolipin, and the formation of free radicals.

4.68 **The answer is d.** Cardiac damage following radiation primarily involves the endothelial cells of the myocardial capillaries. The injury causes swelling, microvascular thrombosis, or rupture.

4.69 **The answer is d.** Chilling and fever can occur because of the large volume of blood being returned to the patient. A large volume of the anticoagulant sodium citrate can cause hypocalcemia. Intravenous calcium gluconate may be needed if the hypocalcemia becomes severe. Hypovolemia may be a problem, especially for patients with a history of cardiac problems. Thrombocytopenia is problematic with some types of equipment.

4.70 **The answer is c.** Signs of chemotherapy-induced venoocclusive disease have been described as (1) unexplained thrombocytopenia refractory to platelets, (2) sudden weight gain, (3) sudden decrease in hemoglobin, (4) increase in liver enzymes, (5) intractable ascites, and (6) encephalopathy.

4.71 **The answer is d.** Glucocorticoids, including prednisone and hydrocortisone, are used to treat hypercalcemia. They are not part of the body's normal homeostatic mechanism that regulates serum calcium. PTH and 1,25-dihydroxyvitamin D exert their effects by controlling movement of calcium across bone, kidney, and small intestine. PTH's action on the kidney occurs through the formulation and action of NcAMP, which acts as a second messenger influencing calcium transport.

4.72   **The answer is a.** The body's homeostatic response to increased calcium loads involves suppression of parathyroid hormone, which decreases bone resorption and inhibits intestinal calcium absorption. This inhibitory effect occurs as a result of decreased renal synthesis of 1,25-dihydroxyvitamin D and increased urinary calcium excretion. The calcium load is cleared principally by the kidney.

4.73   **The answer is c.** Bone remodeling, the process of bone formation and resorption, involves three types of bone cells: osteoblasts, osteocytes, and osteoclasts. Incitement of bone remodeling is thought to be directed at the osteocyte. Bone remodeling continues throughout life and is coupled; that is, bone resorption at a particular site equals bone formation at that site. Uncoupling refers to the failure of bone formation to follow the resorption process. Bone remodeling activity is influenced by mechanical factors such as weight bearing, by the activity of osteotropic hormones, and by local factors such as prostaglandins, regulatory proteins, and constituents of the organic matrix.

4.74   **The answer is c.** The distribution pattern of body water is termed *fluid spacing. First spacing* describes a normal distribution of fluid in both the extracellular and the intracellular compartments. *Second spacing* refers to an excess accumulation of interstitial fluid (edema), and *third spacing* is fluid retention in sites that normally have no fluid or a minimum of fluid (effusion).

4.75   **The answer is a.** Common presenting signs and symptoms of malignant effusions are distressing to most patients. The degree of subjective symptoms produced by a pleural effusion depends less on the amount of fluid involved than on the rapidity with which it accumulates. If fluid accumulation is gradual, the heart and lungs can accommodate, but rapid accumulation can trigger an oncologic emergency.

4.76   **The answer is c.** Acute renal failure secondary to tumor lysis syndrome is primarily due to hyperuricemia and hyperphosphatemia.

4.77   **The answer is b.** When cell lysis occurs, potassium is released from the intracellular compartment to the extracellular compartment and serum potassium levels increase, depressing cardiac function.

4.78   **The answer is a.** Ionized calcium and calcium bound to albumin are in equilibrium. Therefore when a patient has less serum albumin to bind with calcium, a greater portion of the total serum calcium portion must be ionized. Conversely, when serum albumin is high, less calcium is in the ionized form.

4.79   **The answer is a.** For women receiving radiation therapy to the vagina, vaginal fibrosis and scarring with a loss of blood supply and elasticity is a major adverse effect.

4.80   **The answer is c.** Signs and symptoms of a venous thrombosis are related to impaired blood flow and include edema of the neck, face, shoulder, or arm; prominent superficial veins; neck pain; tingling of the neck, shoulder, or arm; and skin color or temperature changes. A venogram with contrast media is used to assess for a venous thrombosis.

4.81   **The answer is d.** The type of cancer most often implicated in incidence of TE is mucin-secreting adenocarcinoma of the gastrointestinal tract. Other malignancies primarily associated with TE include small cell lung cancer, non–small cell lung cancer, and colon and pancreatic cancers. To a lesser extent, TE-associated cancers include breast, prostate, ovarian, and bladder carcinomas.

4.82   **The answer is b.** The etiology of thromboembolism is the ability of tumor cells to affect systemic activation of coagulation and cause platelet dysfunction. Anemia is caused by the other choices given: the tumor secretion of cytokines, such as interleukin-1, affecting red cell metabolism; chronic hemorrhage; and bone marrow failure.

4.83   **The answer is d.** Tumor cells may remotely precipitate paraneoplastic thromboembolism by activation of the coagulation pathway, damage to the endothelial lining of blood vessels, or platelet activation. Choice **c**—protein-calorie malnutrition—is involved in the etiology of anemia of malignancy.

4.84   **The answer is a.** Poor prognosis has been associated with obstructing or perforating carcinomas, occurrence in young people, location of the tumor below the peritoneal reflection, lymph node involvement, venous invasion, hepatic metastasis, and invasion of the bowel wall.

4.85   **The answer is d.** The patient's symptoms could be caused by hyperviscosity syndrome, a rare occurrence in myeloma patients caused by a high concentration of proteins that increases the serum viscosity.

4.86   **The answer is a.** Venous distention is caused by blockage of the inferior vena cava, which can occur from spread of cancer. With this condition there is edema of the eyelids, a bluish face and lips, prominent neck veins, and pitting edema of the arms and large veins over the upper portions of the chest and shoulders.

4.87   **The answer is b.** Diffuse thrombosis leads to ischemia, impairment of blood flow, and end-organ damage. Diffuse bleeding is a symptom of the underlying thrombosis.

4.88   **The answer is d.** Mucin-secreting adenocarcinomas of the gastrointestinal tract are most often associated with a thromboembolism. The malignancies primarily associated with thromboembolism include small cell lung cancer, non–small cell lung cancer, colon and pancreas and, to a lesser extent, breast, prostate, ovarian, and bladder carcinomas.

4.89   **The answer is a.** Several prospective studies have confirmed a relationship between recurrent, episodic, idiopathic deep vein thrombosis and the subsequent development of malignancy.

4.90   **The answer is d.** D-dimer and FDP/FSP assay are two of the more reliable tests used to support the diagnosis of DIC. Although platelets usually are decreased in the presence of DIC, a platelet count is neither sensitive nor specific to DIC.

4.91   **The answer is d.** Thrombocythemia and thrombocytosis are a result of overproduction of platelets. The major complications related to an increased platelet count are bleeding and thrombosis. Thrombosis may result in symptoms associated with venous thrombosis pulmonary embolism, transient cerebral ischemia, myocardial infarction, and angina.

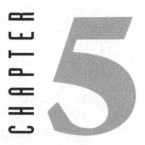

CHAPTER 5

Oncologic Emergencies

METABOLIC

Disseminated Intravascular Coagulation (DIC)

5.1   Platelet dysfunction in the individual with cancer is related to many factors. Which of the following chemotherapeutic agents is known to disturb normal platelet function?
   a.   L-asparaginase
   b.   Vinca alkaloids
   c.   Anthracyclines
   d.   All of the above

5.2   Sepsis is an important cause of bleeding. Which of the following conditions most accurately describes how sepsis causes bleeding?
   a.   Sepsis and bleeding occur simultaneously in patients who are immunosuppressed.
   b.   Sepsis causes viruses to thrive, and viruses cause bleeding.
   c.   Endotoxins released from bacteria activate the coagulation cascade.
   d.   Antiangiogenesis factors are released during periods of sepsis, which leads to bleeding.

5.3   The symptoms of DIC seem paradoxical because
   a.   Both platelet function and platelet numbers are implicated in DIC.
   b.   Patients may experience fever at the same time their bodies are hypothermic.
   c.   DIC may be both the cause and effect of malignancy.
   d.   Thrombosis and hemorrhage may occur simultaneously.

5.4   Therapy for DIC often involves the administration of several substances. Which of the following is *not* a common treatment for DIC?
   a.   Heparin
   b.   Epsilon-amino caproic acid (EACA or Amicar)
   c.   Vitamin K
   d.   Platelet replacement

5.5   Patients with cancer may have bleeding, despite normal platelet counts and coagulation factors. An example of this problem is bleeding caused by
   a.   Platelet sequestration
   b.   DIC
   c.   Decreased platelet adhesiveness
   d.   Hypocoagulability

5.6   Which of the following statements best describes the physiologic characteristics of DIC?
   a.   All clotting factors are prolonged.
   b.   In contrast to what would be expected, the international normalized ratio, prothrombin time, and PTT are elevated.
   c.   The platelet count is decreased, the plasma fibrinogen is low because of consumption of fibrinogen by the clotting cascade, and the prothrombin time is prolonged.
   d.   There is an absence of coagulation, and therefore there is widespread hemorrhage.

5.7   The most common cause of acute DIC associated with cancer is
   a.   Thrombopoiesis
   b.   Infection and sepsis
   c.   Tumor products
   d.   Anaphylaxis

5.8   The major and only definitive treatment for DIC is
   a.   Aggressive antibiotic therapy
   b.   Treatment of the underlying cancer
   c.   Administration of platelets and fresh frozen plasma
   d.   Reversing the clotting cascade by the administration of heparin

Syndrome of Inappropriate Antidiuretic Hormone Secretion (SIADH)

5.9   Which of the following drugs has been found to be effective in the treatment of SIADH?
   a.   Docetaxel
   b.   Demeclocycline
   c.   Arginine sulfide
   d.   Immunoglobulin

5.10   Which of the following is *not* considered diagnostic for SIADH?
   a.   Increased levels of blood urea nitrogen, uric acid, creatinine, and albumin
   b.   Serum sodium less than 130 mEq/L
   c.   Absence of edema
   d.   Normal renal, adrenal, and thyroid function

5.11   Mr. Bradford, a patient with small cell lung cancer, develops anorexia, weakness, and fatigue. At first these are attributed to the cancer itself. As his condition worsens Mr. Bradford's wife, who is caring for him through a hospice arrangement, calls you in tears, reporting that he has suddenly become combative. You tell her that he must have a serum chemistry as soon as possible because you suspect
   a.   Hypercalcemia
   b.   Hyponatremia
   c.   Paraneoplastic adrenotropic hormone (pACTH) syndrome
   d.   End-stage cancer

5.12 The incidence of clinically evident SIADH in small cell lung cancer is approximately
    a. 5%
    b. 10%
    c. 35%
    d. 50%

5.13 Which of the following is indicative of SIADH?
    a. Increased plasma sodium and decreased urine output
    b. Hyponatremia with high serum osmolality and high urine osmolality
    c. Hypernatremia with high serum osmolality and high urine osmolality
    d. Hyponatremia with low serum osmolality, high urine sodium, and high urine osmolality

5.14 The problem with ectopic antidiuretic hormone (ADH) secretion as a paraneoplastic syndrome in cancer compared to normal ADH secretion is which of the following?
    a. Ectopic ADH is not regulated.
    b. Ectopic ADH acts on cardiac tissue.
    c. Ectopic ADH does not respond to dehydration.
    d. Ectopic ADH is not related to mental status changes.

5.15 Mr. Lindy has a history of small cell lung cancer and returns for his 6-month checkup. He has felt well except for some nausea, weakness, and, at times, confusion, headache, and lethargy. His lab values reveal hypokalemia, hyponatremia, low blood urea nitrogen, and low creatinine. His clinical symptoms are suspicious for which of the following?
    a. Metastatic disease to the brain
    b. Metastatic disease to the liver
    c. SIADH secretion
    d. Adrenal insufficiency

5.16 Which of the following is *not* considered a therapeutic approach to the management of SIADH?
    a. Water restriction to less than 1000 mL/day
    b. Water load test
    c. Hypertonic saline infusions
    d. Demeclocycline

Septic Shock

5.17 Which of the following is considered the most important prognostic indicator for septic shock?
    a. Polymicrobial infections
    b. Prolonged neutropenia
    c. The presence of multiple organ dysfunction syndrome
    d. Sepsis-induced hypotension

5.18 Major fluid volume depletion occurs in patients with septic shock because of which of the following pathophysiological mechanisms characteristic of shock?
    a. Third spacing of fluid
    b. Vascular pooling and capillary leak
    c. Decreased venous tone
    d. All of the above

5.19 Which of the following variables does *not* influence the incidence of sepsis?
   a. Concurrent radiotherapy and chemotherapy
   b. Length of myelosuppressive therapy
   c. Absolute granulocyte count less than 500/mm^3
   d. Duration of granulocytopenia

5.20 Septic shock is the most common cause of circulatory collapse in patients with cancer. The predominant hemodynamic feature(s) of this condition is (are)
   a. Arterial vasodilation
   b. Normal to decreased cardiac output
   c. Mild hypotension
   d. a and c

5.21 Once treatment for septic shock has been initiated, the nurse needs to monitor the patient for complications of shock, which include
   a. Disseminated intravascular coagulation
   b. Hepatic abnormalities
   c. Below-normal temperature
   d. a and b

5.22 Granulocytopenia is the single most important risk factor for sepsis in individuals with cancer. Which of the following is a common cause of granulocytopenia?
   a. Leukemia
   b. Chemotherapy
   c. Total body irradiation
   d. All of the above

5.23 Septic shock ultimately causes death due to which of the following?
   a. Fever
   b. Coagulopathy
   c. Tissue ischemia
   d. Hypotension

Tumor Lysis Syndrome

5.24 Acute TLS is a complication of cancer therapy that occurs most commonly in patients with tumors that have a high proliferation index and are highly sensitive to chemotherapy. Acute TLS is *least likely* to be seen in which of the following cases?
   a. Colon cancer
   b. Lymphoma
   c. Acute myelogenous leukemia
   d. Non-Hodgkin's lymphoma

5.25 Non-Hodgkin's lymphoma patients with big, bulky, high-grade disease are at high risk for acute TLS. One important aspect of the nursing care for such patients is
   a. Looking for signs of motor incoordination and cognitive deficits
   b. Monitoring urine output for signs of renal failure
   c. Discontinuing vinca alkaloid treatment if signs of severe jaw pain occur
   d. Providing oral or intravenous agents that keep blood and urine acidic

5.26   Mr. James has chronic myelogenous leukemia in blastic transformation. He is considered to have a high tumor burden and has evidence of lymphadenopathy and splenomegaly. Which of the following laboratory tests indicates that he is experiencing acute TLS?
  a. Acute hyperuricemia
  b. Hypokalemia
  c. Hypercalcemia
  d. All of the above

5.27   The primary physiologic complication of acute TLS is
  a. Tumor cell obstruction of microvasculature, causing disseminated intravascular coagulation
  b. Liver failure caused by a venoocclusive disease
  c. Uric acid crystallization in the renal tubules, causing obstruction and acute renal failure
  d. Tumor lysis, causing release of tissue, which produces pulmonary emboli

5.28   The most effective means of preventing acute TLS includes which of the following?
  a. Sodium bicarbonate and vigorous hydration
  b. Heparinization
  c. Maintaining a urine pH of less than 7
  d. a and c

5.29   TLS results in a release of a large amount of phosphorus into the blood and a proportional decrease in what other serum electrolyte?
  a. Magnesium
  b. Calcium
  c. Potassium
  d. Sodium

5.30   Which of the following is a key element in the prevention of TLS?
  a. Aggressive hydration
  b. Diuresis
  c. Allopurinol
  d. All of the above

5.31   Mr. Clay has lymphoma and received chemotherapy 4 days ago. He has been doing well but comes in complaining of fatigue, dizziness, and a "fluttering" feeling in his chest. Chemistries reveal potassium, 6 mEq/L; creatinine, 2.7 mg/dL; and calcium, 6 mg/dL. Your assessment is which of the following?
  a. He is dehydrated and needs fluids.
  b. He could have a life-threatening arrhythmia and should be admitted.
  c. He is probably anemic and needs blood.
  d. He is losing calcium and needs magnesium.

Anaphylaxis

5.32   Mr. Stevens has just begun his first treatment with rituximab. One hour into the infusion he complains of fever, chills, rigors, and nausea. Appropriate nursing action is based on which of the following?
  a. This is an anaphylactic reaction, and the medication should be permanently discontinued.
  b. The infusion should be maintained; these symptoms are expected and signal a good response to therapy.
  c. The symptoms are expected and will lessen with each subsequent treatment.
  d. Monitor the blood pressure because rituximab can significantly raise the blood pressure, requiring the drug to be discontinued.

5.33   Measures to prevent a hypersensitivity reaction to a monoclonal antibody include *all but* which of the following?
  a.   Speed up the infusion to decrease the amount of time the infusion takes.
  b.   Administer an antihistamine before beginning the infusion.
  c.   Administer a steroid the evening before and morning of the infusion.
  d.   Administer epinephrine 1:1000 as directed.

5.34   Mrs. Howe has just arrived for her first treatment with Herceptin, a monoclonal antibody. As you plan her teaching about her medication, you are careful to include which of the following?
  a.   She should report any difficulty breathing, chills, or cough because her medication could cause an anaphylactic reaction.
  b.   If she does have a reaction, the medication will be stopped temporarily and restarted after her symptoms subside.
  c.   Diphenhydramine and acetaminophen are often given before the first infusion to minimize risk of an infusion-related reaction.
  d.   All of the above

5.35   Alex has an infection of his vascular access device and is beginning vancomycin therapy. Twenty minutes into a 60-minute infusion, you notice his face and upper torso are flushed and he is wheezing slightly. Appropriate nursing action includes which of the following?
  a.   Stop the infusion; he is having an allergic reaction.
  b.   Administer decadron and benadryl immediately.
  c.   Slow the infusion and administer morphine.
  d.   This is not an antigen antibody reaction; slow the infusion to 90 minutes.

5.36   Allison is receiving a loading dose of Herceptin therapy. The infusion is to be administered over 90 minutes. Shortly after the infusion begins, she complains of hives, rash, and itching all over. She has a fever of 102°F and chills. Appropriate nursing action includes which of the following?
  a.   Stop the infusion, administer steroids, and monitor vital signs.
  b.   Stop the infusion, monitor vital signs, and administer diphenhydramine and benadryl. Resume the infusion.
  c.   Slow the infusion and administer morphine for the chills.
  d.   Stop the infusion, administer epinephrine, and monitor vital signs.

5.37   Which of the following drugs is *not* commonly associated with a hypersensitivity reaction?
  a.   Paclitaxel
  b.   Cytarabine
  c.   L-asparaginase
  d.   Docetaxel

5.38   Of the patients who experience a hypersensitivity reaction to paclitaxel, what percentage experience symptoms within 10 minutes of initiating the drug, after only a few milligrams had been infused?
  a.   20%
  b.   40%
  c.   60%
  d.   80%

Hypercalcemia

5.39   Which of the following types of malignancies is *least likely* to be associated with hypercalcemia?
a. Lung cancer
b. Breast cancer
c. Multiple myeloma
d. Colon cancer

5.40   Among the common early symptoms in hypercalcemic patients are all of the following *except*
a. Nausea and vomiting
b. Diarrhea
c. Hypertension
d. Polyuria

5.41   The most important initial treatment for hypercalcemia is
a. Improving renal calcium excretion
b. Treating the primary tumor
c. Inhibiting osteoclast function
d. Inhibiting bone resorption

5.42   The pathophysiology of hypercalcemia involves a combination of two factors: bone resorption and
a. Decreased renal calcium clearance
b. Increased osteoclast activity
c. Increased glomerular function
d. Decreased availability of ionized calcium

5.43   Factors produced by tumors have been implicated in malignancy-associated hypercalcemia. Probably the most important of these humoral circulating factors is
a. Prostaglandin
b. Parathyroid hormone–like factor
c. Bisphosphonate
d. Osteoclast-activating factor

5.44   A patient is found to have a large tumor mass associated with high levels of parathyroid hormone–related protein but normal levels of 1,25-dihydroxyvitamin D and normal intestinal absorption rates. Bone absorption is found to exceed bone formation. The most likely diagnosis is
a. Primary hyperparathyroidism
b. Multiple myeloma
c. Humoral hypercalcemia of malignancy (HHM)
d. Hodgkin's disease

5.45   The symptoms of hypercalcemia in cancer patients are best described as
a. Similar to those of acute renal failure
b. Easily identified but difficult to treat
c. Distinct from those of end-stage disease
d. Numerous, vague, and nonspecific

5.46   A patient develops confusion, disorientation, and hallucinations with an elevated serum calcium and occasional bradycardia. Therapeutic interventions might include which of the following?
   a.   Saline diuresis
   b.   Intravenous pamidronate
   c.   Aggressive cancer therapy
   d.   All of the above

STRUCTURAL

Cardiac Tamponade

5.47   Malignant pericardial effusions
   a.   Are extremely rare
   b.   Are easily detected by tachycardia, low blood pressure, and shortness of breath
   c.   Occur in 50% of all patients with cancer, especially the hematologic malignancies
   d.   Are not easily detected because patients are asymptomatic

5.48   The patient who is experiencing a cardiac tamponade shows signs and symptoms that include
   a.   Chest pain, confusion, nausea, and vomiting
   b.   Confusion, nausea, vomiting, and hypertension
   c.   Hypertension, bradycardia, and increased cardiac output
   d.   Decreased cardiac output, dyspnea, cough, and chest pain

5.49   Which of the following tumor types is *not commonly* associated with pericardial effusion and tamponade?
   a.   Lung cancer
   b.   Gastrointestinal carcinoma
   c.   Breast cancer
   d.   Leukemia

5.50   Which of the following statements about cardiac tamponade is *false*?
   a.   An echocardiogram is the most precise method for visualization of a malignant pericardial effusion.
   b.   Hypotension is an early and common objective symptom for cardiac tamponade.
   c.   Pericardiocentesis is both therapeutic and diagnostic.
   d.   The clinical picture in cardiac tamponade is caused by a buildup of pressure around the heart.

Spinal Cord Compression

5.51   You will soon begin work in a clinic that specializes in the detection and treatment of spinal cord tumors. You are aware that the *most common* presenting symptom of a spinal cord tumor is
   a.   Weakness
   b.   Cold, numbness, and tingling
   c.   Pain
   d.   Uncoordinated ataxic gait

5.52 Spinal cord compression occurs by which of the following mechanisms?
   a. Direct extension of the tumor into the epidural space
   b. Vertebral collapse
   c. Displacement of bone into the epidural space
   d. All of the above

5.53 Mrs. Johnson has complained of back pain for 6 months and now presents with weakness. Which of the following helps to explain her symptoms?
   a. Pain is rarely a symptom of spinal cord tumors.
   b. Weakness is a classic symptom of spinal cord tumors.
   c. Back pain and weakness are likely caused by her chronic steroid use.
   d. a and b

5.54 Mark is being discharged from the hospital. His prostate cancer involves some bone metastasis. Which of the following developments is likely to indicate a need for radiation therapy?
   a. Worsening back pain
   b. Weakness of the lower extremities
   c. Sensory deficits
   d. All of the above

5.55 A woman with breast cancer and known bone metastasis is currently on pamidronate. Her primary complaint is weakness in both arms. She has back pain, but it is unchanged from the previous week. The most logical explanation for her symptoms and the correct nursing action is which of the following?
   a. Weakness in arms and legs is common with pamidronate, and she should increase her use of the arms to avoid losing muscle strength.
   b. She has known bony metastasis that is no worse; the pamidronate will help the bone to heal, so it is appropriate to monitor her symptoms.
   c. If she has bony disease in her spine, she should have an emergency magnetic resonance image to rule out spinal cord compression.
   d. She should be encouraged not to cough, strain, or lift heavy objects because she could have osteoporosis and is at risk for disc disease.

Superior Vena Cava Syndrome

5.56 A man with a history of lung cancer calls his doctor to report the following symptoms: headache, swollen face and neck, and shoulders and chest are covered with a lacy venous pattern. Which of the following best identifies what he is describing?
   a. Telangiectasia and complications of prior radiation therapy
   b. Possible pneumothorax
   c. Possible local recurrence with brain metastasis
   d. Possible superior vena cava obstruction

5.57 Mrs. Ruthe recently had a Port-a-cath placed for long-term chemotherapy administration, and her doctor advised her to take coumadin 1 mg a day for as long as she has the port. She is inquiring why she needs the coumadin. The most appropriate response is which of the following?
   a. People with cancer are more prone to clotting disorders, and she is at increased risk for blood clots in her legs.
   b. Coumadin is used in place of the heparin flushes to maintain port patency.
   c. She needs the coumadin for only about a week until she is completely healed and then she can stop it.
   d. The coumadin is necessary to prevent clot formation around the port and possible venous thrombosis.

5.58 Which of the following is *not* characteristic of SVCS?
  a. As the superior vena cava is compressed, there is reduced venous return to the right atrium.
  b. An increase in venous pressure causes venous hypertension.
  c. Late symptoms include cough and dyspnea.
  d. Initial symptoms include hoarseness and edema in the face, neck, and arms.

5.59 What is the most likely initial treatment of choice for quickly progressing SVCS caused by non–small cell lung cancer?
  a. Radiation therapy
  b. Chemotherapy
  c. Surgical resection
  d. Administration of anticoagulants

5.60 Surgical management of chronic SVCS generally includes which of the following procedures?
  a. The portion of the vena cava that is being compressed is repositioned surgically following resection of the tumor.
  b. A bypass graft or stent is placed into the superior vena cava to dilate and expand the narrowed lumen of the vessel.
  c. A bypass graft is fashioned to redirect blood flow around the obstruction.
  d. b and c

5.61 Which of the following cancers is responsible for more than 70% of all cases of SVCS?
  a. Breast cancer
  b. Lung cancer
  c. Hodgkin's disease
  d. Kaposi's sarcoma

5.62 Which of the following is a primary cause of SVCS?
  a. External compression by primary tumor
  b. Direct invasion by tumor
  c. Thrombus formation within the vessel
  d. All of the above

Increased Intracranial Pressure

5.63 In most instances of central nervous system tumors, the first, earliest, and most sensitive indicator of dysfunction is a change in
  a. Level of consciousness
  b. Cognitive ability
  c. Motor and sensory function
  d. All of the above

5.64 After tumor resection, a patient suffers postoperative cerebral edema. This *most likely* results from
  a. Surgical manipulation of the surrounding brain tissue
  b. Changes in regional blood flow
  c. Brain injury caused by excessive retraction
  d. Any of the above

5.65   Jeffrey's intracranial pressure is acutely elevated. In acute situations like his, the drug of choice is
    a. Mannitol
    b. A corticosteroid
    c. Vincristine
    d. Vinblastine

5.66   Which of the following statements regarding brain tumors is *not* accurate?
    a. Metastatic brain tumors are the most common type of brain tumor.
    b. The incidence of metastatic brain tumors is decreasing because of advances in cancer care.
    c. Tumors in the lung are the most likely of all solid tumors to metastasize to the brain.
    d. Radiation therapy is the primary mode of treatment and is palliative.

5.67   In balancing intracranial pressure, the mechanism that specifically maintains a normal intracranial pressure despite fluctuations in arterial pressure and venous drainage is
    a. Autoregulation
    b. Compensation
    c. Cerebrospinal fluid displacement
    d. Cerebral blood flow

ANSWER EXPLANATIONS

5.1   **The answer is d.** The chemotherapeutic drugs mithramycin, carmustine, and the anthracyclines are associated with abnormal platelet aggregation and other coagulopathies. Vinca alkaloids such as vincristine and vinblastine are also associated with platelet dysfunction. L-asparaginase inhibits the synthesis of clotting factors and can lead to either hemorrhage or thrombosis. Mitomycin can cause a thrombotic microangiopathy, manifested as hemolytic uremic syndrome.

5.2   **The answer is c.** Risk of bleeding increases during periods of febrile neutropenia. This is due to the activation of the coagulation cascade by complement. DIC is a dangerous sequelae of sepsis. This is most frequently seen in gram-negative sepsis due to the endotoxins released from the bacteria.

5.3   **The answer is d.** DIC always results from an underlying disease process that triggers abnormal activation of thrombin formation. Thrombin is both a powerful coagulant and an agent of fibrinolysis. Thus small clots may be formed in the microcirculation of many organs at the same time that clots and clotting factors are being consumed. The result is hemorrhage because the body is unable to respond to vascular or tissue injury.

5.4   **The answer is c.** Vitamin K might be administered to a patient experiencing hypocoagulability, but not the hypercoagulability caused by DIC. All the other therapies may provide short-term relief of DIC symptoms. Treatment of the underlying malignancy is vital in treating the patient with DIC, inasmuch as the tumor is the ultimate stimulus.

5.5 **The answer is c.** Choices **b** and **d** are coagulation abnormalities; choice **a** is a quantitative abnormality. Qualitative abnormalities, such as choice **c**, refer principally to alterations in platelet function, which may include a decreased procoagulant activity of platelets, decreased platelet adhesiveness and decreased aggregation in response to adenosine diphosphate, thrombocytosis associated with myeloproliferative disorders, and the coating of platelets by fibrin degradation products as a result of the increased activation of coagulation factors.

5.6 **The answer is c.** DIC represents the most common serious hypercoagulable state in individuals with cancer. Tests generally done to help support the diagnosis of DIC include prothrombin time, platelet count, and the plasma fibrinogen level; all are reduced.

5.7 **The answer is b.** The most common cause of acute DIC is infection and sepsis associated with cancer. It is believed that bacterial endotoxins, which are released from gram-negative bacteremia, activate the Hageman factor. This factor can initiate coagulation as well as stimulate fibrinolysis.

5.8 **The answer is b.** Treatment of the underlying malignancy is vital in the patient with a hypercoagulability abnormality, because the tumor is the ultimate stimulus. All other therapy, although effective on a short-term basis, provides only an interval of symptomatic relief.

5.9 **The answer is b.** Demeclocycline (600–1200 mg daily) is an antibiotic that is most frequently used to treat chronic SIADH. It stimulates diuresis by inhibiting the effect of arginine vasopressin on the renal tubule.

5.10 **The answer is a.** The criteria for the diagnosis of SIADH includes serum osmolality less than 275 mOsm/kg; serum sodium less than 130 mEq/L; urine osmolality greater than serum osmolality; urinary sodium greater than 20 mEq/L; euvolemia; *decreased* levels of blood urea nitrogen, uric acid, creatinine, and albumin; absence of edema; and normal renal, adrenal, and thyroid function.

5.11 **The answer is b.** Mr. Bradford most likely has hyponatremia secondary to SIADH. SIADH is primarily associated with small cell lung cancer. Water intoxication accounts for the signs and symptoms seen with SIADH. The early symptoms, such as nausea, weakness, anorexia, and fatigue, can be easily attributed to the cancer. However, as the hyponatremia worsens, symptoms may progress to include altered mental status, confusion, and combativeness.

5.12 **The answer is b.** SIADH is primarily associated with small cell lung cancer. Although most of these patients (80%) may have some aspects of SIADH, only about 10% have clinical signs and symptoms of SIADH.

5.13 **The answer is d.** SIADH results from ADH secretion by the tumor. The symptoms include hyponatremia and low serum osmolality, characterized by mental status changes, lethargy, seizures, and confusion.

5.14 **The answer is a.** Although structurally identical to normal ADH, ectopic ADH is not regulated. Atrial natriuretic peptide, a hormone arising from cardiac atrial tissue, has been identified as the cause of hyponatremia. Water intoxication accounts for the symptomatology of SIADH.

5.15 **The answer is c.** Serum chemistries frequently show low blood urea nitrogen, creatinine, albumin, and uric acid; this is a dilutional effect in hyponatremia associated with SIADH. SIADH occurs commonly in patients with small cell lung cancer and initially presents as nausea, weakness, confusion, and lethargy.

5.16   **The answer is b.** The water load test is a diagnostic study for SIADH, not a therapeutic approach. Fluids are restricted to less than 1000 mL/day. Hypertonic saline is given intravenously with furosemide to expedite water loss. Demeclocycline is an antibiotic used to treat chronic SIADH. It stimulates diuresis by impairing the effect of argonine vasopressin on the renal tubule.

5.17   **The answer is c.** When sepsis progresses to a state of organ dysfunction, hypoperfusion, or hypotension, severe sepsis is present. Multiple organ dysfunction syndrome, which is defined as the presence of altered organ function in an acutely ill patient such that homeostasis cannot be maintained with intervention, is the final common pathway for the critically ill patients. The presence of multiple organ dysfunction syndrome is an important prognostic indicator for septic shock; in fact, severe prolonged dysfunction of three or more organs correlates with a mortality rate of 70% or more.

5.18   **The answer is d.** Major fluid volume depletion occurs in patients with septic shock due to decreased venous tone, vascular pooling, capillary leak, and third spacing of fluid. The hallmark of septic shock is profound hypotension.

5.19   **The answer is a.** There is a direct relationship between the number of circulating polymorphonuclear neutrophilic leukocytes (PMNs) and the incidence of infection. When the granulocyte count is less than $500/mm^3$, risk of infection is significant. As the length of therapy and the duration of granulocytopenia increase, so does the incidence of sepsis. Although concurrent radiotherapy and chemotherapy might increase the degree of myelosuppression, the incidence of sepsis is not increased.

5.20   **The answer is d.** Septic shock evolves through two phases that, although not always distinct, are characterized by different hemodynamic patterns. The early phase consists of arterial vasodilation, decreased peripheral vascular resistance, normal to increased cardiac output, and mild hypotension.

5.21   **The answer is d.** Once treatment has been initiated, nurses closely monitor for complications of shock, including thrombocytopenia, disseminated intravascular coagulation, renal failure, gastrointestinal bleeding, hepatic abnormalities, and acute respiratory distress.

5.22   **The answer is d.** Granulocytopenia occurs secondary to leukemia, bone marrow infiltration, total body irradiation, and cytotoxic chemotherapy.

5.23   **The answer is c.** The clinical picture of septic shock illustrates the cumulative effects of coagulopathy, hypotension, hypoperfusion, and, ultimately, tissue ischemia involving failure of all body systems.

5.24   **The answer is a.** Acute TLS is most commonly seen in patients with high-grade lymphoma, acute myelogenous leukemia, chronic myelogenous leukemia, and non-Hodgkin's lymphoma.

5.25   **The answer is b.** Acute TLS generally occurs when the patient is initially treated. Tumor cells spill their contents into the general circulation, causing a metabolic disturbance. Renal failure and death may occur. The treatment of choice is prevention, including hydration, sodium bicarbonate, and intravenous or oral allopurinol to prevent hyperuricemic nephropathy.

5.26   **The answer is a.** Acute TLS is most often characterized by the development of acute hyperuricemia, hyperkalemia, hyperphosphatasemia, and hypocalcemia with or without acute renal failure.

5.27   **The answer is c.** Uric acid crystallization in the renal tubules, causing obstruction, decreased glomerular filtration, and/or acute renal failure, is a major complication of acute TLS.

5.28   **The answer is d.** Acute TLS can be prevented by prophylactic alkalinization of urine—maintaining the urine pH at a level greater than 7—with the use of sodium bicarbonate and vigorous hydration.

5.29   **The answer is b.** In TLS there is an inverse relationship between phosphorus and calcium, whereby if one mineral increases, the other decreases in the same proportion.

5.30   **The answer is d.** Aggressive hydration is needed, to at least 3 liters of fluid per day with adequate urinary output and using diuretics to prevent renal tubular damage. Allopurinol inhibits the enzyme xanthine oxidase and prevents the formation of uric acid, which in turn prevents uric acid nephropathy.

5.31   **The answer is b.** An increase in phosphate, potassium, uric acid, blood urea nitrogen, and creatinine or a 25% decrease in calcium within 4 days of chemotherapy is indicative of TLS and places the patient at risk for life-threatening arrhythmias.

5.32   **The answer is c.** An infusion-related symptom complex consisting of fever, chills and rigors, nausea, asthenia, and headache occur in most patients during the first infusion. The symptoms decrease with subsequent infusions. Rituximab causes hypotension, not hypertension.

5.33   **The answer is a.** Anaphylactoid reactions have most commonly occurred with monoclonal antibody therapy. Most of these reactions occurred at the beginning of therapy administration to patients with lymphoma or leukemia or when administered by rapid infusion.

5.34   **The answer is d.** Acute side effects that occur during infusion are most commonly fever, chills, malaise, myalgia, nausea, and vomiting. Dyspnea, cough of a monoclonal antibody, and chest pain can occur during infusion and may be related to the rate of infusion. The symptoms often resolve if the rate is slowed.

5.35   **The answer is d.** Vancomycin causes release of histamine from the mast cells, which causes vasodilation and the appearance of an allergic reaction. The red neck, or red man syndrome, is common with vancomycin and improves with slowing to a 90-minute infusion.

5.36   **The answer is b.** Fever, chills, and rash are common with the first infusion and respond to acetaminophen and diphenhydramine. Stop the infusion temporarily when hives, rash, pruritus, and fever are present. Notify physician and monitor vital signs. Resume the infusion and monitor the patient.

5.37   **The answer is b.** Hypersensitivity reactions due to cytarabine are rare and seen only within the past few years where the doses used are 10–15 times normal. Hypersensitivity reactions are frequent enough with paclitaxel, docetaxel, and asparaginase therapy to be a treatment-limiting toxicity.

5.38   **The answer is d.** Most patients (80%) who have a hypersensitivity reaction develop the reaction within 10 minutes of initiating the drug. The remainder of those who develop a reaction (20%) do so during their second infusion.

5.39   **The answer is d.** Patients with lung and breast cancer account for the highest percentage of malignancy-induced hypercalcemia. However, multiple myeloma, which is relatively rare, is the underlying cause in more than 20% of malignancy-associated hypercalcemia cases.

5.40   **The answer is b.** Constipation, *not* diarrhea, is more likely to be observed during the early stages of hypercalcemia. Elevated extracellular calcium levels depress smooth muscle contractility, leading to delayed gastric emptying and decreased gastrointestinal motility.

5.41   **The answer is a.** Before excessive bone resorption can be treated, impaired renal calcium excretion must be improved, usually by correcting dehydration and removing factors that may exacerbate hypercalcemia, including thiazide diuretics. Oral or intravenous hydration with normal saline may be required.

5.42   **The answer is a.** Hypercalcemia is characterized by excess extracellular calcium. This condition results from bone resorption—the release of skeletal calcium into serum—and from the failure of the kidneys to clear extracellular calcium. As calcium levels rise, symptoms of hypercalcemia appear.

5.43   **The answer is b.** Malignancy-associated hypercalcemia is a complex metabolic complication in which bone resorption exceeds both bone formation and the kidney's ability to excrete extracellular calcium. Humoral circulating factors include a parathyroid hormone–like factor, transforming growth factors (transforming growth factor-alpha) and 1,25-dihydroxyvitamin D. Hypercalcemia that develops in patients with solid tumors but without bone metastases is thought to be caused by parathyroid hormone–like factor.

5.44   **The answer is c.** In humoral hypercalcemia of malignancy (HHM), patients secrete high levels of parathyroid hormone–related protein but have normal levels of 1,25-dihydroxyvitamin D and normal intestinal absorption rates. Osteoblastic and osteoclastic activities are "uncoupled" so that bone resorption exceeds bone formation. Hypercalcemia and hypercalciuria thus occur.

5.45   **The answer is d.** Hypercalcemia symptoms are numerous, vague, and nonspecific, and because many cancer patients with hypercalcemia have large tumor burdens and die in 3–6 months, symptoms of hypercalcemia may be confused with those of end-stage disease.

5.46   **The answer is d.** Paraneoplastic hypercalcemia often presents as confusion, disorientation, and hallucinations with bradycardia. Treatment of hypercalcemia includes vigorous hydration and pamidronate.

5.47   **The answer is d.** Malignant pericardial effusions are not easily detected by routine tests because most patients are asymptomatic. Often, clinical manifestations are vague or attributed to other causes. This uncertainty poses a clinical challenge.

5.48   **The answer is d.** Cardiac tamponade interferes with cardiac function because the fluid burden occupies space and reduces the volume of the heart in diastole. Systemic circulatory effects of decreased cardiac output and impaired venous return lead to generalized congestion. The body tries to compensate in several ways: tachycardia, an increase in systemic and pulmonary venous pressure, and increased ejection fraction.

5.49   **The answer is b.** Gastrointestinal cancer rarely results in pericardial effusion and tamponade, probably because of its natural pattern of metastases to the liver and surrounding organs.

5.50   **The answer is b.** Hypotension occurs, but in only about one-third of patients who have cardiac tamponade.

5.51   **The answer is c.** Pain is the most common presenting symptom of a spinal cord tumor. Weakness is the most readily identified objective finding and may follow the appearance of sensory symptoms. Specific sensory deficits depend on where the tumor is on a cross-section of the spine. A lateral tumor affects pain and temperature, causing cold, numbness, and tingling. Anterior tumors lead to weakness and an uncoordinated ataxic gait.

5.52   **The answer is d.** Spinal cord compression occurs either by direct extension of the tumor into the epidural space or by vertebral collapse and displacement of bone into the epidural space. It can also occur by direct extension through the intervertebral foramina.

5.53   **The answer is b.** Weakness is the most readily identified objective finding for spinal cord tumor. Choice **a** cannot be correct because pain is the most common presenting symptom of a spinal cord tumor. There is no evidence to support choice **c**.

5.54   **The answer is d.** All patients with bone metastasis are at risk for spinal cord compression. Worsening back pain, weakness of the lower extremities, or sensory deficits require immediate medical attention—usually radiation therapy to control tumor impingement on the spinal cord.

5.55   **The answer is c.** Imminent spinal cord compression should be suspected in individuals who have known bone metastases, progressive back pain associated with weakness, paresthesias, bowel or bladder dysfunction, or gait disturbances.

5.56   **The answer is d.** Obstruction of the superior vena cava is a common complication of lung cancer. The clinical picture includes edema of both eyelids, arms, and hands; the face is a dusky blue color; the lips are deeply cyanotic; and the shoulders, chest, and upper abdomen are covered with a lacy collateral venous pattern.

5.57   **The answer is d.** Catheter-induced SVCS, most often the result of thrombosis, is treated with fibrinolytic therapy, such as urokinase. Prevention involves using coumadin 1 mg daily.

5.58   **The answer is c.** Initial symptoms of SVCS include cough; dyspnea; stridor; hoarseness; edema in the face, neck, and arms; and neck and chest vein distention.

5.59   **The answer is a.** Radiation therapy is the treatment of choice for SVCS caused by non–small cell lung cancer because non–small cell lung cancer (NSCLC) does not respond to chemotherapy. Radiation therapy is also the choice in patients without a histologic diagnosis.

5.60   **The answer is d.** One of two approaches, superior vena cava bypass graft or stent placement, may be performed for the patient with a good prognosis who has chronic or recurrent SVCS for whom other treatment options have been exhausted. The graft creates a new vessel that circumvents the obstruction; the stent is inserted into the superior vena cava to dilate and expand its narrowed lumen.

5.61   **The answer is b.** Lung cancer is responsible for 52–81% of all cases of SVCS. Small cell carcinoma of the lung is the most common histologic type, followed by squamous cell carcinoma of the lung.

5.62   **The answer is d.** SVCS may be caused by external compression by primary or metastatic cancer, direct invasion by tumor, or thrombus formation within the vessel.

5.63   **The answer is a.** In most instances the first, earliest, and most sensitive indicator of dysfunction is a change in the level of consciousness. Mental status and cognitive ability, as well as motor and sensory function and cranial nerve function, are assessed.

5.64 **The answer is d.** Postoperative cerebral edema results from the surgical manipulation of the surrounding brain tissue, changes in regional blood flow, or brain injury caused by excessive retraction.

5.65 **The answer is a.** In situations in which intracranial pressure is acutely elevated, corticosteroids alone are insufficient and osmotic diuretics (hyperosmolar agents), usually mannitol, are required.

5.66 **The answer is a.** Gliomas are the most common primary brain tumor in adults.

5.67 **The answer is a.** In balancing intracranial pressure, autoregulation is the mechanism that specifically maintains a normal intracranial pressure, despite fluctuations in arterial pressure and venous drainage.

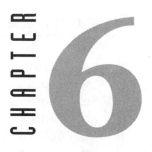

Scientific Basis for Practice

CARCINOGENESIS

6.1 A patient asks, "What are tumor-suppressor genes?" As part of your answer, you explain that tumor-suppressor genes code for proteins that _____ growth-promoting factors.
   a. Enhance
   b. Fuel
   c. Inactivate
   d. Duplicate

6.2 The *p53* gene is
   a. A potent oncogene
   b. The most frequently mutated gene in human cancer
   c. The "guardian of the oncogene"
   d. Protected from DNA viruses

6.3 In clonal selection
   a. Mutation in the genome of a cell may confer a survival advantage on that cell.
   b. A cell becomes weaker with each mutation.
   c. Oncogenes are destroyed.
   d. Telomeres develop, which are completely duplicated during cell division.

6.4 A patient asks you to describe the "types of things that cause cancer." Because of her interest in "types" of causes, you might begin by explaining that cancer is *ordinarily* classified as being caused by a combination of factors that include
   a. Biological, viral, physical, or chemical
   b. Occupational, viral, dietary, or familial
   c. Chemical, viral, physical, or familial
   d. Viral, chemical, familial, occupational, or life-style

6.5   Mr. Henderson's cancer is said to have been induced by familial carcinogenesis. From this, you can assume that in his case certain genes
    a.   Caused cancer by functioning to excess
    b.   Caused cancer by their absence
    c.   Acted as growth promoters
    d.   Lost their ability to prevent malignant growth by their loss of homozygosity

6.6   One encouraging aspect of research into tumor-associated viruses is the discovery of
    a.   Their direct tumor causation
    b.   Their promise for prevention through development of vaccines from animal forms of the viruses
    c.   Their promise for prevention through inactivation
    d.   Similar viruses in animals that have been eliminated by vaccines made from attenuated viruses

6.7   Which of the following is *not* true of carcinogenesis and chemoprevention?
    a.   Chemoprevention is the most promising form of host modification, using nutrients or pharmacological agents to inhibit or reverse carcinogenesis.
    b.   Protooncogenes are most likely involved in initiation and promotion of cancer.
    c.   Chemoprevention has the potential for both secondary and tertiary prevention, but by definition it cannot be useful in primary prevention.
    d.   Agents that inhibit carcinogenesis generally are classified by the point in the process at which they are effective.

6.8   The *ras* oncogenes
    a.   Have a screening usefulness of about 45%
    b.   Function early in the process of carcinogenesis
    c.   Are a late event
    d.   Are not effective as targets for early detection

6.9   Asbestos, the major carcinogenic fiber, is related to which of the following diseases?
    a.   Gastrointestinal cancer
    b.   Bladder cancer
    c.   Mesothelioma
    d.   Renal cancer

6.10 Fat and fiber are two dietary factors that appear to be correlated with the occurrence of colorectal cancer. It is thought that they operate by affecting, in opposite ways, the
    a.   Conversion of ionized bile salts into insoluble compounds
    b.   Rate of uptake of calcium by the gastrointestinal tract
    c.   Breakdown of carcinogenic compounds by digestive enzymes
    d.   Exposure of the gastrointestinal tract to promoters of carcinogenesis

6.11 Mrs. Harris has hepatocellular carcinoma and states she has never drank alcohol in her life and cannot understand how she could have liver cancer. You explain that although the cause is not really known, hepatocellular carcinoma is associated with which of the following?
    a.   Chronic hepatitis B virus infection
    b.   Chronic hepatitis C virus infection
    c.   Macronodular cirrhosis
    d.   All of the above

6.12 One of the most exciting developments in the mechanism of carcinogenesis is the discovery of a relationship between the mucosa-associated lymphoid tissue (MALT) lymphoma and which bacteria?
   a. *Helicobacter pylori*
   b. *Escherichia coli*
   c. *Staphylococcus aureus*
   d. *Pseudomonas aeruginosa*

IMMUNOLOGY

6.13 The macrophage
   a. Manufactures interleukin-3, -4, and -6 and alpha- and gamma-interferon to aid in its ultimate function of target cell wall damage
   b. Is a glycoprotein product that initiates effector defense functions
   c. Is a primary initiator to an inflammatory immune response
   d. a and c

6.14 Diseases such as Kaposi's sarcoma that are common in AIDS are referred to as *opportunistic*. This is because they
   a. Affect any or all organs and tissues in the body
   b. Normally occur in a benign state in most individuals
   c. Occur in patients with preexisting immunodeficiency
   d. Affect only HIV-infected individuals who have other diseases

6.15 Which of the following best describes what cytokines do?
   a. They bind to surface receptors of target cells and act as regulators of cell growth or as mediators of defense functions.
   b. They are capable of nonspecific tumor cell killing.
   c. They are sedentary cells located in the spleen.
   d. They facilitate the attachment of a natural killer cell and other cytotoxic cells.

6.16 Each of the following is an important function of the body's immune system *except*
   a. Protecting the body against injury from foreign substances
   b. Preserving the body's internal environment
   c. Preventing the growth of aberrant cells that might develop into neoplasms
   d. Providing support and nourishment to the body's genetic machinery

6.17 The body can generally respond to a nonself invader cell more quickly and powerfully the second time it encounters such a cell than it did the first time, even if months have passed between invasions. Which of the following cells is *most closely* related to this ability?
   a. Polymorphonuclear granulocytes
   b. Memory B lymphocytes
   c. Natural killer cells
   d. Mononuclear phagocytes

6.18 Antibody is the final product in the differentiation of
   a. B lymphocytes
   b. Helper T lymphocytes
   c. Mononuclear phagocytes
   d. Suppressor T lymphocytes

GENETICS

6.19 Genes that predispose for the development of cancer are generally transmitted in an autosomal dominant fashion. What does this mean for the risk of cancer?
   a. Individuals who harbor a mutated gene have a 50% chance of passing the mutated gene on to their children.
   b. Every affected person in a pedigree has an affected parent.
   c. The pattern of transmission is usually vertical, meaning successive generations are affected.
   d. All of the above

6.20 Which of the following statements best describes the significance of the *BRCA1* gene?
   a. It is an inherited gene that identifies women who are ensured of having breast cancer during their premenopausal years.
   b. It is an inherited gene mutation that identifies families at significant risk for breast cancer and ovarian cancer.
   c. It is an inherited gene mutation that identifies women likely to have breast cancer in their postmenopausal years.
   d. It is an inherited gene that is present in over 90% of women with breast cancer.

6.21 Approximately what percentage of people with cancer have an increased risk for cancer due to a hereditary predisposition?
   a. 15%
   b. 25%
   c. 33%
   d. 50%

6.22 Which of the following statements regarding our understanding of the genetic susceptibility in breast cancer and ovarian cancer is *not* correct?
   a. The *BRCA1* gene is associated with increased susceptibility to both breast and ovarian cancer.
   b. The *BRCA2* gene is associated only with an increased susceptibility to ovarian cancer.
   c. One of the genes is estimated to be present in approximately 15% of breast cancer cases.
   d. The genes are associated with breast cancer diagnosed at an early age.

6.23 Which of the following statements regarding genetic susceptibility to colon cancer is *not* correct?
   a. Individuals who have a first-degree relative with colorectal cancer have double the risk for developing colon cancer.
   b. Adenomatous polyps are considered to be precursors of colorectal carcinoma.
   c. An inheritable autosomal dominant trait is found in families with a high incidence of colon cancer.
   d. Individuals who have familial adenomatous polyposis (FAP) syndrome are at a 50% risk for developing cancer of the colon.

6.24 Knudson observed that acquired retinoblastoma occurs as a single tumor, whereas children with hereditary retinoblastoma had multiple primary tumors. What does this observation suggest about retinoblastoma?
   a. Retinoblastoma must result from a protooncogene left permanently in the "on" position.
   b. All cells in the retinal tissue of an affected eye are genetically predisposed to retinoblastoma.
   c. Retinoblastoma must be the result of recessive inheritance.
   d. None of the above

6.25   Which of the following variables appears to be the best descriptive determinant of cancer risk?
  a.   The mortality rates for Japanese Americans with stomach cancer are significantly higher than for the white American population.
  b.   As more women smoke, more women are developing lung cancer.
  c.   A study of Johns Hopkins medical students found that 55 students who later developed cancer perceived themselves as less close to their parents than did their healthy counterparts.
  d.   Familial aggregates of cancer have been found to occur.

6.26   Which of the following cancer-causing mutations is transmitted to the next generation at birth?
  a.   Oncogene mutations
  b.   Germ cell mutations
  c.   Somatic mutations
  d.   Antioncogene mutations

SPECIFIC CANCERS

Pathophysiology

6.27   Ms. Jantzen will soon begin induction therapy for acute myelogenous leukemia. As her oncology nurse you explain that the goal of therapy is to cause severe bone marrow hypoplasia, using
  a.   Busulfan and hydroxyurea
  b.   Cytosine arabinoside and daunorubicin
  c.   Vincristine, prednisone, L-asparaginase, and daunorubicin
  d.   Chlorambucil and cyclophosphamide

6.28   Which of the following statements about lymphomas is correct?
  a.   Non-Hodgkin's lymphoma (NHL) is distinguished from Hodgkin's disease (HD) primarily on the basis of its different clinical manifestations.
  b.   Lymphomas are predominantly a malignancy of the lymphocyte.
  c.   There seems to be a single malignancy for all stages in the developmental sequence from primitive to mature lymphocyte.
  d.   In general, B-lymphocyte malignancies are more aggressive than T-lymphocyte malignancies.

6.29   The most common form of skin cancer is
  a.   Basal cell carcinoma
  b.   Squamous cell carcinoma
  c.   Malignant melanoma
  d.   Superficial spreading melanoma

6.30   Ms. Smith, who has acute myelogenous leukemia (AML), is in complete remission after two courses of induction therapy. She is beginning postremission therapy, in which she will receive very high doses of the same drugs used for induction therapy. She asks, "What's the point of this? I'm so sick of treatment. I'm in remission, aren't I?" You explain that this type of postremission therapy is

a. Consolidation therapy to prevent leukemic recurrence related to minimal residual disease
b. Intensification therapy to treat substantial toxicities, including extended myelosuppression and cerebellar dysfunction
c. Maintenance therapy, which is used to help prevent a recurrence in some specific cases
d. Central nervous system prophylaxis to prevent leukemic recurrence related to minimal residual disease

6.31   You are the new oncology nurse in a large hospital. On your first day you meet Mr. Jackson. His physician neglects to tell you what type of leukemia Mr. Jackson has, but he says to you, "He still has the Philadelphia chromosome, so we don't exactly have a cure yet." From this you are able to discern that Mr. Jackson has

a. Acute lymphocytic leukemia
b. Acute myelogenous leukemia
c. Chronic lymphocytic leukemia
d. Chronic myelogenous leukemia

6.32   The most common site of metastasis for tumors of the bone is the

a. Gastrointestinal tract
b. Central nervous system
c. Liver
d. Lungs

6.33   All of the following are common metastatic sites for breast cancer *except* the

a. Brain
b. Liver
c. Bone
d. Gastrointestinal tract

6.34   The glioblastoma multiforme

a. Is most common in individuals who are between 30 and 50 years of age
b. Has less necrosis than anaplastic astrocytoma
c. Is the most common adult primary brain tumor
d. a and c

6.35   Which of the following conditions is commonly associated with colorectal carcinoma?

a. Appendicitis or gallbladder disease
b. Hemorrhoids
c. Anal condylomata acuminata
d. Chronic ulcerative colitis

6.36   During the initial workup Mr. Smith, who has testicular cancer, complains of low back pain that has been present for about 1 month. This may indicate

a. Metastatic disease to the lumbar spine
b. That the cancer has spread to the prostate
c. That the cancer has spread into the retroperitoneal lymph nodes
d. a and c

6.37 Multiple myeloma is a cancer of which of the following cell types?
   a. B lymphocyte
   b. Plasma cell
   c. Monoclonal lymphocyte
   d. a and b

Diagnostic Measures

6.38 You are preparing for an initial meeting with Mr. Jennings, who is about to undergo diagnostic screening for a suspected abdominal cancer. In describing this process, you intend to tell him that major goals of the diagnostic evaluation may be to establish, among other things, the
   a. Tissue type of the malignancy
   b. Primary type of the malignancy
   c. Extent of disease within the body
   d. All of the above

6.39 Mr. Phillips has liver cancer. The preferred procedure for imaging the abdomen is usually
   a. Ultrasonography
   b. Computed tomography
   c. Thermography
   d. X-ray

6.40 Mrs. Ellis has stage II breast cancer and is receiving adjuvant doxorubicin and cyclophosphamide. She has no symptoms of bone involvement but asks that a bone scan and a CA-15-3 tumor marker be done. The most appropriate response would be which of the following?
   a. A bone scan would not be useful because Mrs. Ellis has no symptoms.
   b. CA-15-3 is used to monitor metastatic disease and not as an early detection test.
   c. Both tests should have been done before surgery.
   d. a and b

6.41 The diagnosis of either Hodgkin's disease or non-Hodgkin's lymphoma usually is established by
   a. Cytologic examination of the Reed-Sternberg cells
   b. Computed tomography and magnetic resonance imaging of the nodular tissue
   c. Lymph node biopsy
   d. Exploratory laparotomy

6.42 The preferred initial surgical procedure for suspected cutaneous melanoma is
   a. Excisional biopsy
   b. Incisional biopsy
   c. Wide excision
   d. Curettage and electrodesiccation

6.43 Which of the following procedures is considered the standard approach for definitive pathological diagnosis of testicular cancer?
   a. Biopsy
   b. Fine-needle biopsy
   c. Transcrotal approach orchiectomy
   d. Inguinal orchiectomy

6.44   All of the following are commonly used in the diagnosis/staging of cervical cancer *except*
   a. Pap smear
   b. Colposcopy
   c. Biopsy
   d. Laparoscopy

6.45   Adenocarcinomas
   a. Constitute 30% of all lung cancers and are more common in males than in females
   b. Arise from the basal cells of the bronchial epithelium and usually present as masses in large bronchi
   c. Are the most common lung cancer in females and in nonsmokers and account for 40% of all primary tumors
   d. Are the least common type of lung cancer, representing approximately 10–15%

6.46   A sarcoma is a malignant tumor of the connective tissue, whereas a carcinoma is a malignant tumor arising from which of the following tissues?
   a. Epithelium
   b. Endothelial
   c. Mesenchymal
   d. Hematopoietic

6.47   Approximately what percentage of people diagnosed with cancer are diagnosed with a tumor of unknown origin?
   a. 20–25%
   b. 15–20%
   c. 10–15%
   d. 2–4%

Prognosis

6.48   In determining the progression of bladder cancer, the *most important* feature is the
   a. Degree of hematuria present
   b. Presence of bladder neck obstruction
   c. Depth of penetration into the bladder wall
   d. Presence of pain in the suprapubic region

6.49   Carry asks you to explain the relationship among tumor size, node involvement, and prognosis. Which of the following statements is *most accurate*?
   a. Smaller tumors with positive node involvement have the best prognosis.
   b. Larger tumors with negative node involvement have the best prognosis.
   c. Smaller tumors with negative node involvement have the worst prognosis.
   d. Larger tumors with positive node involvement have the worst prognosis.

6.50   The prognosis for a patient with Hodgkin's disease is *most closely* related to
   a. Elevated lactic dehydrogenase level
   b. Histologic type
   c. Abdominal lymph node involvement
   d. Stage at presentation

6.51 Which of the following patients with prostate cancer is *most likely* to be given "watchful waiting" as a treatment choice?
    a. Frank, who is 37, recently married, and still hopes to have children
    b. Harold, who is 76 and enjoying an active retirement with his wife
    c. Byron, who is 56 and has poorly differentiated localized disease
    d. Phil, who is 40 and has a high-grade tumor

6.52 Of the following factors related to cutaneous melanoma prognosis, the one *most closely* correlated with decreased survival rates in patients with stage I cutaneous melanoma (CM) is
    a. Anatomic level of tumor invasion
    b. Tumor location
    c. Clark level
    d. Tumor thickness

6.53 A poor prognosis for survival in a patient with AIDS-related Kaposi's sarcoma includes all of the following *except*
    a. History of fever, night sweats, and weight loss
    b. CD4 cell count >200/mm^3
    c. Karnofsky performance status of <70%
    d. History of opportunistic infection or thrush

6.54 Mr. James has been told by his physician that he has a high-grade seminoma of the testis. His doctor seemed encouraged by this, but your patient is concerned that a high-grade tumor might be associated with a poor prognosis. Which of the following statements might help to clarify the issue for Mr. James?
    a. High-grade seminomas respond poorly to radiation and surgery but are curable with chemotherapy.
    b. High-grade tumors have a brief tumor cell doubling time, which means they are more susceptible to the cell kill effects of chemotherapy.
    c. High-grade seminomas tend to be more like the cell of origin and therefore metastasize infrequently.
    d. A high-grade seminoma is curable by surgery, whereas chemotherapy is used for palliation only.

6.55 The *most favorable* prognostic factor for a patient with small cell lung cancer (SCLC) is
    a. Female gender
    b. Normal serum lactic dehydrogenase
    c. Limited-stage disease
    d. Good performance status

6.56 Alicia is diagnosed with breast cancer and is confused about prognostic indicators and how tests on her tumor will determine the type of treatment she should receive. Which of the following would be appropriate points to clarify for this patient regarding what the test results mean for her treatment and prognosis?
    a. The hormone receptor analysis is used to determine the likelihood of metastases.
    b. The hormone receptor analysis and assessment for the presence or absence of the human growth factor receptor (HER2) gene are used to decide what type of treatment is needed for metastatic disease.
    c. The hormone receptor analysis and assessment for the presence or absence of the human growth factor receptor (HER2) gene are used to determine treatment strategies and prognosis for both local and advanced disease.
    d. Women who have tumors that are positive for the hormone receptor do not require further treatment beyond surgery.

6.57   The prognosis for a patient with colorectal cancer is probably poorest if which of the following exists?
   a. Venous and lymph node invasion
   b. High blood pressure
   c. Location of the tumor above the peritoneal reflection
   d. Squamous cell involvement

CLASSIFICATION

Tumor Classification

6.58   Important features of tumor classification systems include which of the following features?
   a. Allows for tumors to be classified by their biological behavior
   b. Allows for tumors to be classified by their tissue of origin
   c. Provides clinical and prognostic information
   d. All of the above

6.59   A benign tumor
   a. Is well circumscribed or encapsulated and appears to be orderly
   b. Is not made up of cells similar to those of its parent tissue
   c. Invades the organs from which it originated and is made up of cells that vary greatly in size and shape
   d. a and b

6.60   Cervical intraepithelial neoplasia (CIN) stage III is characterized by neoplastic changes involving up to full thickness of the epithelium with no areas of stromal invasion or metastases. CIN III is also known as
   a. Preclinical invasive carcinoma
   b. Carcinoma in situ
   c. Adenocarcinoma
   d. Verrucous carcinoma

6.61   Two patients have been diagnosed with bronchogenic cancer. You know this does not mean that both patients will necessarily have a similar symptomatology or course of treatment because bronchogenic cancers are grouped into two broad categories:
   a. Small cell lung cancer and non–small cell lung cancers
   b. Adenocarcinoma and large cell carcinoma
   c. Heterogeneous and histologic
   d. Hyperplasia and carcinoma in situ

Staging

6.62   The primary objective of classification and staging of malignant tumors is to do which of the following?
   a. To provide the information necessary for treatment planning
   b. To identify individuals who might be candidates for research studies
   c. To provide prognostic information
   d. All of the above

6.63 The *most important* objective of solid tumor staging is which of the following?
   a. Provide information regarding risk factors
   b. Provide the necessary information for individual treatment planning
   c. Identify individuals at high risk for disease recurrence
   d. Determine performance status and eligibility for research protocols

6.64 In the TNM staging system
   a. cTNM indicates that assessment has been obtained clinically.
   b. cTNM indicates whether carcinogenesis has occurred.
   c. rTNM indicates that remission of the cancer is occurring.
   d. aTNM indicates that the cancer has been detected on first assessment.

6.65 Stage groupings involve
   a. Combining the various classification elements of tumor site, regional lymph node involvement, and the presence or absence of metastasis
   b. Two main staging periods: pretreatment and posttreatment
   c. Two main staging periods: clinical diagnostic staging and pretreatment staging
   d. a and b

6.66 After a course of treatment Ms. Trent's treatment response is evaluated. This reevaluation or restaging
   a. Makes possible the redesignation of a more appropriate stage to be referenced throughout the remaining course of the illness, replacing the stage ascribed at the time of diagnosis
   b. Focuses attention on the disease parameters that were positive at diagnosis
   c. Determines whether the patient is eligible to participate in a clinical trial
   d. a and b

6.67 In determining the survival rate for persons with cancer of the renal pelvis, the most important factor seems to be
   a. The stage of the tumor
   b. Whether or not radiotherapy was used in treatment
   c. Whether or not the tumor is hormone sensitive
   d. The age and physical condition of the patient at diagnosis

6.68 The American Joint Committee on Cancer (AJCC) staging system for lung cancer uses
   a. Eight stages, each of which is distinct relative to treatment and 5-year survival statistics
   b. The TNM letters
   c. The simple two-stage system
   d. Two defining terms—limited-stage disease and extensive-stage disease—to stage lung cancers

6.69 Which of the following statements about the staging of Hodgkin's disease (HD) is correct?
   a. Stage II malignancy is determined by a positive bone marrow biopsy.
   b. Stage determination is important because it influences what treatment option will be used.
   c. Stage II presentation is usually indicative of a more aggressive HD type.
   d. HD rarely presents as stage II.

6.70   Accurate staging of a patient with Hodgkin's disease is *least likely* to include which of the following procedures?
   a.   A chest radiograph
   b.   An exploratory laparotomy
   c.   Blood chemistries, including liver and kidney function tests
   d.   A complete blood count

6.71   The phase of cutaneous melanoma tumor growth that is characterized by focal deep penetration of atypical melanocytes into the dermis and subcutaneous tissue is the
   a.   Radial phase
   b.   Vertical growth phase
   c.   Nodular phase
   d.   Acral lentiginous phase

Grading

6.72   Treatment of advanced intermediate/high-grade non-Hodgkin's lymphoma is *most likely* to involve
   a.   Invasive surgery
   b.   High doses of topical radiation
   c.   Combination chemotherapy
   d.   Cyclophosphamide combined with radiation

6.73   A liver tumor may be suspected if laboratory tests reveal elevated levels of
   a.   Gastrin
   b.   Cholesterol
   c.   Alpha-fetoprotein
   d.   Amylase

6.74   A primary tumor is one that is histologically confirmed to arise from a specific site of tumorigenesis, whereas a secondary tumor refers to
   a.   A tumor that arises in another site after the primary tumor has been discovered
   b.   A tumor of unknown origin
   c.   A metastatic tumor resembling the primary tumor histologically
   d.   A second primary cancer that is histologically different from the primary tumor

6.75   Grading a malignant neoplasm is a method of classification based on histopathologic characteristics of the tissue. Which is *not* considered to be a primary objective of grading?
   a.   Establishing the aggressiveness or degree of malignancy of tumor cells
   b.   Providing prognostic information for all cancers
   c.   Quantifying information to assist in treatment planning
   d.   Determining the stage of disease of selected cancers

6.76   Mr. Fleischman's cancer is given an American Joint Committee on Cancer (AJCC) classification of G2. This means his cancer is
   a.   Undifferentiated
   b.   Well-differentiated
   c.   Poorly differentiated
   d.   Moderately well-differentiated

6.77   Histopathologic type refers to
    a. A qualitative assignment given to a lesion at a site other than the orginal site that is of the *same* cell type as the original; this is used to determine metastatic tumors
    b. A quantitative assessment of the extent to which the tumor resembles the tissue of origin
    c. A qualitative assessment whereby a neoplasm is categorized in terms of the tissue or cell type from which it has originated
    d. A qualitative assignment that indicates that a lesion at a site other than the original site is of a *different* cell type than the original tumor; this is used to indicate a second primary cancer

6.78   The *least* threatening prostate cancers are those that
    a. Feature large tumor volume
    b. Have a Gleason grade of 3–5
    c. Originate in the peripheral zone
    d. Are indolent

6.79   The primary application of flow cytometry analysis in solid tumors is to do which of the following?
    a. Determine DNA content (ploidy)
    b. Determine the percentage of cells synthesizing DNA (the S-phase fraction)
    c. Measure tumor markers
    d. a and b

MAJOR TREATMENT MODALITIES

Surgery

6.80   Mr. Vance just had gastric surgery and needs both radiation and chemotherapy. Why would these both be given after surgery?
    a. Sometimes it is difficult for the surgeon to assess before surgery whether invasion has occurred and excision is the best choice.
    b. Most likely, the tumor was found to be invading nearby tissues that could not be surgically resected, and micrometastasis is a potential problem.
    c. Radiotherapy before surgery is appropriate only as a first-line means of defense; the surgery was a second-line treatment that was unsuccessful, so a more aggressive third line—combination therapy—is now being used.
    d. b and c

6.81   You have recently become part of a new interdisciplinary oncology team. You are aware that situations lending themselves best to surgical treatment include such factors as
    a. Slow-growing tumors that consist of cells with prolonged cell cycles
    b. An ability to achieve resection of the entire tumor mass as well as a margin of safety of normal healthy tissue surrounding the tumor
    c. Embedded tumors
    d. a and b

6.82   Stereotactic biopsy is used to accomplish which of the following?
   a.   Several biopsies are obtained from samples of tissue from different locations.
   b.   Radiographic images are used to create three-dimensional views of a tumor.
   c.   "Sound" waves are recorded in stereo to outline a tumor.
   d.   Biopsies are used to diagnose metastatic disease.

6.83   Which of the following lung tumor types is thought to be nonresectable because it is of neuroendocrine origin?
   a.   Small cell lung cancer
   b.   Large cell lung cancer
   c.   Squamous cell lung cancer
   d.   Adenocarcinoma of the lung

6.84   Within a week of surgery for esophageal cancer, contrast studies are likely to be done to check for
   a.   Local edema
   b.   Any signs of residual tumor
   c.   Anastomotic leaks
   d.   Swallowing ability

6.85   All of the following are possible contraindications to hepatic resection for liver cancer *except*
   a.   Jaundice
   b.   Severe cirrhosis
   c.   Chemotherapy failure
   d.   Ascites

6.86   In women, radical cystectomy includes removal of the
   a.   Bladder, urethra, uterus, ovaries, fallopian tubes, and the anterior wall of the vagina
   b.   Bladder, urethra, and anterior wall of the vagina only
   c.   Bladder and urethra only
   d.   Bladder only

6.87   A new patient, Charles, undergoes transurethral resection of the prostate (TURP). He asks if this will cure the disease. You explain that
   a.   TURP is sometimes found to cure prostate cancer, but the chances diminish with increasing tumor involvement.
   b.   TURP is used to treat symptoms of bladder outlet obstruction.
   c.   TURP provides pathologic evidence that a cancer, previously unsuspected, is present.
   d.   b and c

Radiation

6.88   The biological effects on tissue from fractionated radiation therapy depend on the four "Rs" of radiobiology, which are
   a.   Redistribution, reevaluation, reoxygenation, repair
   b.   Repair, resimulation, redistribution, reoxygenation
   c.   Repair, redistribution, repopulation, reoxygenation
   d.   Reoxygenation, redistribution, radiosensitivity, repair

6.89   Breast-conserving radiotherapy after conservative breast surgery is to prevent local recurrence. The treatment techniques utilized include
   a.   Whole breast radiotherapy
   b.   MammoSite Radiation Therapy
   c.   Intrabeam brachytherapy system
   d.   All of the above

6.90   An important advantage of megavoltage equipment over conventional or orthovoltage equipment used in radiotherapy is that it
   a.   Is more effective in treating surface lesions
   b.   Reduces absorption of radiation by bone
   c.   Delivers radioisotopes to the site of the tumor
   d.   Limits release of dangerous heavy ions and negative pi-mesons

6.91   The possibility of contamination of equipment, dressings, and linens is greatest when radioactive isotopes are delivered as
   a.   Implants
   b.   Colloids or solutions
   c.   Molds
   d.   Ovoids separated by a spacer

6.92   Compounds that assist in maximizing the tumor cell kill achieved with radiation while minimizing injury to normal tissues are called
   a.   Radioantagonists
   b.   Radiosensitizers
   c.   Oxygen-enhancement ratios
   d.   Linear energy transfer

6.93   Nurses are often involved with managing the side effects that result from radiotherapy. To minimize the degree of the symptoms experienced, the nurse should schedule to see most patients
   a.   Immediately after the first fractionated dose
   b.   On completion of the scheduled 5-week course
   c.   At the end of the first week
   d.   10–14 days after treatment has begun

6.94   Simulators are used in treatment planning for radiotherapy to localize a tumor and to
   a.   Define the volume to be treated with radiotherapy
   b.   Remove a section of a tumor for a laboratory evaluation
   c.   Reduce the size of a tumor before surgical resection
   d.   Prepare a histopathologic profile of a tumor

6.95   Radiation effects take place primarily at the level of
   a.   Cells
   b.   Tissues
   c.   Organs
   d.   The whole body

6.96   One of the primary goals of dose fractionation is to
   a.   Redistribute cell age within the cell cycle, making normal cells less radiosensitive
   b.   Allow tumor cells to repopulate, making them more vulnerable to the late consequences that occur if new growth was inhibited
   c.   Deliver a dose sufficient to prevent tumor cells from being repaired while allowing normal cells to recover before the next dose is given
   d.   Provide time between treatments for normal cells to reoxygenate, thus making them less radiosensitive

6.97   The late effects of radiation that are often seen 6 months or more after radiotherapy are the result of
   a.   Cell damage in which mitotic activity is temporarily altered in some way
   b.   Acute damage that occurs to tissues and organs outside the treatment field
   c.   The organism's attempt to repair the damage inflicted by ionizing radiation
   d.   Acute site-specific reactions to treatment

6.98   Hank received prostatic brachytherapy with implantation of seeds of iodine-125. Which of the following is *not* included as part of your patient education plan for Hank and his family?
   a.   Implants may be permanent or temporary.
   b.   The urine may be strained to retrieve any dislodged seeds.
   c.   A condom should be worn during sexual intercourse for the first 2 months following implantation.
   d.   Hank must remain hospitalized until the source that emits gamma radiation has completely decayed so he is not a source of radiation to those around him.

Biotherapy

6.99   Which of the following side effects are *most often* associated with cetuximab therapy?
   a.   Hair loss, fatigue, constipation
   b.   Fatigue, hair loss, nausea and vomiting
   c.   Acne-like rash, swelling and redness of the nails, malaise
   d.   Blood clots, disorientation, fever

6.100   The primary mechanism of action of an epidermal growth factor receptor monoclonal antibody (e.g., cetuximab) is which of the following?
   a.   Disruption of mitosis by spindle binding
   b.   By attaching to the receptor it blocks the signaling agents
   c.   By attaching to the signaling agent it prevents attachment to the receptor
   d.   All of the above

6.101   While teaching your patient about cetuximab you would be certain to include which of the following important points?
   a.   Infusion reactions such as tightening in the throat, hoarseness, and rash can occur with the first infusion or with subsequent infusions.
   b.   If a severe infusion reaction occurs, the cetuximab would be discontinued permanently.
   c.   If a reaction does not occur with the first infusion of cetuximab, it will not occur with subsequent infusions.
   d.   a and b

6.102   The primary action of bevacizumab (Avastin) is to accomplish which of the following?
   a.   Increase nitric oxide production, thus regulating vascular tone
   b.   Inhibit blood vessel formation
   c.   Remodeling of blood flow at the tumor site, thereby increasing efficacy of chemotherapy
   d.   b and c

6.103 Patients who receive bevacizumab can complain of headache and experience severe (grade 3) hypertension. The occurrence of these two relatively serious side effects is due to which of the following?
a. Bevacizumab was infused too rapidly.
b. Bevacizumab decreases vascular endothelial growth factor, which decreases nitric oxide production.
c. Bevacizumab reduces nitric oxide production, which results in vasoconstriction.
d. b and c

6.104 Your patient has been on bevacizumab (Avastin) for 3 months and complains that testing his urine for protein results in delay of his treatment, and he believes it can be stopped after all this time. To increase his compliance with therapy and to help him understand his treatment, you would most likely respond with which of the following?
a. These are doctor's orders and must be followed.
b. Vascular endothelial growth factor impairs glomerular endothelial cells.
c. The Avastin can impair the ability of the kidneys to filter proteins.
d. All of the above

6.105 Recombinant humanized monoclonal antibodies directed against vascular endothelial growth factor are effective in impeding tumor growth based on which of the following basic facts regarding how tumors grow?
a. Tumors grow exponentially rather than at the same rate over time.
b. Tumors cannot grow beyond 1–2 mm without establishing a new blood vessel system.
c. Tumors require certain proteins to supply the tumor with nutrients.
d. Tumors invade regional blood vessels to gain blood and nutrients for tumor growth.

6.106 Which of the following substances is *not* a cytokine?
a. Alpha-interferon
b. Interleukin-2
c. Levamisole
d. Tumor necrosis factor

6.107 Flulike syndrome, specifically fever, is common when biological agents are administered. This fever is believed to be due to which of the following physiological mechanisms?
a. Infection causes the fever, and vasoconstriction causes the shivering.
b. Pyrogenic pathogens stimulate the release of endogenous cytokines that act on the thermal brain centers to create an increase in the body's temperature set point.
c. The hypothalamic temperature set point is lowered as the level of endogenous pyrogens increases.
d. Tachyphylaxis is common with biological agents and is a normal physiological response to the antigen–antibody response.

6.108 Allen has non–small cell lung cancer and has begun treatment with gefitinib (Iressa), an epidermal growth factor receptor–tyrosine kinase inhibitor. Which of the following is considered to be a common side effect of this treatment?
a. Anaphylaxis
b. Hypotension
c. Skin rash
d. Pancytopenia

6.109 Biologic response modifiers are
   a. Agents that restore, augment, or modulate host antitumor immune mechanisms
   b. Cells or cellular products that have direct antitumor effects
   c. Biologic agents that have other biologic antitumor effects
   d. All of the above

6.110 Among the therapeutic cellular activities of interferons are all of the following *except*
   a. Antiviral activity—protecting a virally infected cell attack by another virus
   b. Immunomodulatory activity—interacting with T lymphocytes that stimulate the cellular immune response
   c. Antiproliferative activity—directly inhibiting DNA and protein synthesis in tumor cells
   d. Immunoregulatory activity—mediating the proliferation and activation of hematopoietic factors

6.111 Cytokines are glycoprotein products of immune cells that share which of the following properties?
   a. They bind to surface receptors and regulate cell growth.
   b. They mediate and regulate immune defense functions of the body.
   c. They produce synergistic effects in the cytokine network.
   d. All of the above

Antineoplastic Agents

6.112 Your patient is receiving oxaliplatin. He is instructed to avoid cold fluids during therapy and for 5 days after therapy. He also wears gloves and a scarf and covers his mouth when breathing cold air. These precautions are useful to avoid which of the following complications of oxaliplatin?
   a. Palmar-plantar erythrodysesthesia
   b. Acute neurotoxicity
   c. Pancytopenia
   d. All of the above

6.113 When administering capecitabine (Xeloda) to a patient who is also taking warfarin it is important to frequently monitor the international normalized ratio (INR) or prothrombin time (PT). What is the nature of this drug interaction?
   a. Capecitabine interferes with the metabolism of warfarin in the liver.
   b. Capecitabine interferes with absorption of warfarin.
   c. Clinically significant increases in PT and INR occur.
   d. a and c

6.114 Which of the following are important teaching points for prostate cancer patients who are receiving ketoconazole therapy?
   a. Ketoconazole should be taken on an empty stomach with an acidic environment.
   b. Ketoconazole blocks the production of male hormones in the testes and the adrenal glands.
   c. Antacids and cimetidine interfere with absorption of ketoconazole.
   d. All of the above

6.115 The metabolic activation and inactivation or catabolism of drugs is carried out primarily by the
   a. Liver
   b. Spleen
   c. Gastrointestinal system
   d. Kidneys

6.116 Chemotherapy drug resistance occurs primarily because the cancer cell has the ability to do which of the following?
   a.   Increase the number of target enzymes
   b.   Repair DNA lesions
   c.   Modify target enzymes so as to interfere with binding to antagonistic drugs
   d.   All of the above

6.117 Capecitabine is an oral agent used to treat patients with metastatic colorectal or breast cancer. Which of the following statements *best* describes how this drug becomes activated in the body?
   a.   This drug is activated via the cytochrome P-450 system.
   b.   This drug undergoes enzymatic changes before becoming 5-FU.
   c.   Once metabolized in the liver, the metabolic byproducts become cytotoxic.
   d.   Activation is dependent on the presence of leucovorin to enhance tumoricidal effects.

6.118 While teaching your new patient about capecitabine therapy you note that he is also taking folic acid for a folic acid deficiency, dilantin for a chronic seizure disorder, and low-dose coumadin to maintain patency of his implanted catheter. Patient care would include which of the following?
   a.   Monitoring his international normalized ratio and his prothrombin time due to a potential drug interaction with capecitabine.
   b.   Monitoring his dilantin levels because capecitabine could cause elevated dilantin levels.
   c.   Consider increasing the dose of folic acid because it could potentially increase the efficacy of capecitabine.
   d.   a and b

6.119 Mrs. Collins has breast cancer and is about to begin docetaxel. She has taken her decadron as premedication. As you check her lab tests, you notice her liver function test results are elevated. Which of the following statements is important regarding your course of action?
   a.   The docetaxel should be delayed until liver function improves.
   b.   Docetaxel is eliminated by the kidney, so liver function is not important.
   c.   The docetaxel dose may need to be reduced because of elevated liver function results.
   d.   The steroid often causes an elevation of liver functions and can be ignored.

6.120 The rationale for the use of preoperative chemotherapy in patients with osteogenic sarcoma includes *all but* which of the following aspects?
   a.   It treats micrometastases.
   b.   It decreases the size of the primary tumor, possibly facilitating limb salvage surgery.
   c.   It enhances the effect of postoperative radiation.
   d.   It evaluates the effectiveness of the chemotherapy.

6.121 When telling Jeanne about cyclophosphamide, methotrexate, and 5-fluorouracil (CMF), you are careful to give her instructions regarding which of the following potential side effects?
   a.   Severe thrombocytopenia and bleeding
   b.   Symptoms of bladder infection as early signs of hemorrhagic cystitis
   c.   Transient peripheral neuropathies
   d.   All of the above

6.122 Nursing care of patients receiving capecitabine therapy includes teaching patients to discontinue their drug at the first sign of a grade 2 toxicity. Which of the following side effects of capecitabine would warrant discontinuing the drug?
   a. Four bowel movements over their normal or one nocturnal stool in a 24-hour period
   b. Vomiting more than once in a 24-hour period
   c. Fever >100.5°F
   d. All of the above

6.123 Although 5-fluorouracil is the cytotoxic agent of choice for colorectal cancer, it is most commonly administered in combination with
   a. Floxuridine
   b. Capecitabine
   c. Leucovorin
   d. None of the above

6.124 Mrs. Otis has been diagnosed with multiple myeloma and will begin therapy with melphalan and prednisone. You will monitor Mrs. Otis closely for adverse drug effects such as
   a. Decreased blood urea nitrogen and creatinine
   b. Hypercalcemia and bone pain
   c. Bone marrow–suppressive effects
   d. All of the above

6.125 One week into his first treatment with capecitabine, your patient calls to report some redness and slight peeling of the palms of his hands and soles of his feet. He also has some tolerable discomfort. You instruct him to do which of the following?
   a. Continue therapy and report any worsening in symptoms.
   b. Continue therapy but reduce the dose by one-half.
   c. Discontinue therapy until symptoms go away and resume at full dose.
   d. Discontinue therapy until symptoms go away and resume at 50% dose.

Bone Marrow Transplant

6.126 Allogeneic transplant is *most frequently* indicated for which of the following diagnoses?
   a. Breast cancer
   b. Non-Hodgkin's lymphoma
   c. Acute lymphocytic leukemia
   d. Chronic lymphocytic leukemia

6.127 Hematopoietic growth factors (HGFs) are administered to patients undergoing blood cell transplantation just before pheresis. The timing of administration of the HGFs is intended to accomplish which of the following outcomes?
   a. Stimulate pluripotent stem cells to differentiate and mature
   b. Stimulate stem cell receptors to make them more vulnerable to cell kill effects
   c. Mobilization, which makes more stem cells available for collection from the circulation
   d. a and c

6.128 After transplantation Ms. Daniels is monitored for complications. Naturally, you will monitor her for possible relapse and any related complications. Besides relapse, what reaction is the most common life-threatening complication experienced by bone marrow transplantation patients in response to preparative regimen-related toxicity?
   a. Renal complication
   b. Venoocclusive disease
   c. Congestive heart failure
   d. Interstitial pneumonia

6.129 If Ms. Daniels were to acquire chronic graft-versus-host disease (GVHD) as a late complication of bone marrow transplantation, which factor is *most likely* to be a causative risk factor?
a. Mismatched donor and recipient
b. Male-to-female transplant
c. Age under 18
d. Failure to receive methotrexate and cyclosporine as chronic GVHD prophylaxis in chronic myelogenous leukemia

6.130 Mr. Jackson is admitted for marrow infusion. He will receive allogeneic bone marrow transplantation and is about to undergo total body irradiation (TBI). You tell him that TBI
a. Offers optimal tumor cell kill but without penetrating the central nervous system
b. Is given before marrow infusion to prevent graft rejection by the patient's own immune system
c. Is usually given in single doses to reduce toxicities
d. Should not be given as a booster in any form to patients with bulky disease because of the risk of major organ toxicity

6.131 A patient is first considered for bone marrow transplant. However, the physician selects blood cell transplantation as the treatment of choice, using peripheral pluripotent stem cells and progenitor cells obtained from peripheral blood. This procedure
a. Delays recovery of neutrophils and platelets when progenitor cells are used
b. Enables neutrophils and platelets to recover rapidly
c. Involves collecting committed progenitors that are not as far along the differentiation pathway as the PPSCs harvested from the bone marrow
d. b and c

6.132 Mrs. Adams has diseased marrow as a result of leukemia. Her physician plans a bone marrow transplant (BMT) and chooses autologous rather than allogeneic BMT. Mrs. Adams tells you, "I've never heard of using a person's own bone marrow cells. Why would anyone do that when I'm the one with the disease?" You explain that autologous BMT
a. Eliminates the risk of graft-versus-host disease (GVHD) and other toxicities, such as myelosuppression
b. Is less toxic, although there is an increased risk of venoocclusive disease
c. Reduces the risk of tumor contamination seen in allogeneic BMTs
d. Reduces the risk of the graft-versus-leukemic effect (graft-versus-leukemic effect can increase the risk of relapse.)

Unproven/Alternative Therapies

6.133 Homeopathy is best described by which of the following?
a. It is a method of manipulating physical and psychological characteristics of the human body to treat illness.
b. It is a medical system based on the manipulations of similars.
c. It is a theory that purports that a drug that causes symptoms at full strength will cure those symptoms if it is diluted.
d. b and c

6.134 The use of the mind-body technique, psychic energy in cancer includes which of the following?
a. Healing touch
b. Reiki therapy
c. Polarity therapy
d. All of the above

6.135 Which of the following is *not* one of the four basic principles involved in the administration of psychiatric drugs to cancer patients?
   a. The starting dose of the drug is generally lower than that typically given to healthy individuals.
   b. The dosage is increased more slowly.
   c. The therapeutic dose may be significantly higher in cancer patients than in healthy individuals.
   d. Potential side effects are monitored carefully, as antidepressants often affect the same organs as drugs used in cancer treatment.

6.136 There is controversy concerning the use of soy and soy products to manage hot flashes in women who have breast cancer. This controversy is based on which of the following true statements?
   a. Soy, like black cohosh contains phytoestrogens.
   b. Phytoestrogens are steroidal compounds derived from plants.
   c. Soy contains proteins that are bioactive compounds similar to estradiol.
   d. All of the above

ANSWER EXPLANATIONS

6.1 **The answer is c.** Suppressor proteins "turn off" cell growth. Because the genes coding for these proteins have an opposite function to that of oncogenes, they are called antioncogenes. Because they suppress malignant growth, they are also called tumor-suppressor genes.

6.2 **The answer is b.** The *p53* gene is one of the most important of the tumor-suppressor genes. Not only is it the most frequently mutated, but when it is not mutated another abnormal gene blocks the p53 protein. The protein product of *p53* is the "guardian of the genome." DNA viruses produce proteins that inactivate the p53 protein.

6.3 **The answer is a.** In clonal selection mutation in the genome of a cell may confer a survival advantage on that cell. The cell grows stronger, not weaker, with each mutation. The cancer cell is immortal because it seems to lack the "biologic clocks" like *telomeres*, which are not completely duplicated during cell division and thus grow progressively shorter until the chromosome can no longer replicate. In cancer the final common path of action is through oncogenes, the growth-promoting genes: Oncogenes must be mutated or relocated to be activated.

6.4 **The answer is c.** Carcinogenesis is ordinarily classified as chemical, viral, physical, or familial, even though it is likely that human carcinogenesis involves a combination of factors. Carcinogenesis can also be classified as occupational, dietary, environmental, life-style, and so forth.

6.5 **The answer is b.** Familial carcinogenesis is based in large part on a group of genes that, when mutated, cause cancer by their absence; that is, they seem to prevent cancer when they are functioning normally. These protective genes are the cancer-suppressor genes. The loss of the normal copy of a gene by the process of mitotic recombination is referred to as *loss of heterogeneity* or *reduction to homozygosity* because the cell becomes homozygous for the abnormal gene, thus losing its ability to prevent malignant growth.

6.6   **The answer is d.** Tumor-associated viruses probably are necessary but not sufficient for tumor causation. The discovery of cancer-causing viruses in humans shows some promise for cancer prevention in that similar viruses in animals have been eliminated by vaccines made from the attenuated (inactivated) viruses.

6.7   **The answer is c.** Chemoprevention is the most promising form of host modification, using nutrients or pharmacological agents to inhibit or reverse carcinogenesis. Protooncogenes are most likely involved in initiation and promotion of cancer. The theoretical disruption of carcinogenesis at several points provides the rationale for use of chemopreventive agents. Agents that inhibit carcinogenesis generally are classified by the point in the process at which they are effective. Chemoprevention has the potential for primary, secondary, and tertiary prevention.

6.8   **The answer is b.** The *ras* oncogenes appear to function early in the process of carcinogenesis and may be a good target for early detection.

6.9   **The answer is c.** Asbestos is related to about 2000 cases of mesothelioma annually in the United States. Asbestos causes more bronchogenic cancers than mesotheliomas because of its synergism with tobacco smoke. Lung cancer is rare in asbestos workers who do not smoke. There is a long latent period between exposure and the onset of mesothelioma. Data do not support an association between asbestos and gastrointestinal, bladder, or renal cancer.

6.10   **The answer is d.** It is believed that dietary factors affect the exposure of the gastrointestinal tract to promoters of carcinogenesis. Fats increase the production, and change the composition, of bile salts. These altered bile salts are converted into potential carcinogens. Fiber decreases the effects of fatty acids and may actually protect against the disease, even in the presence of a high-fat diet. Fiber may limit the time the colon is exposed to cancer promoters by speeding intestinal transit time.

6.11   **The answer is d.** Hepatocellular carcinoma is associated with chronic hepatitis B and C, viral infection, macronodular cirrhosis, schistosomias and other parasitic infections, environmental carcinogens, and organic materials. Smoking has also been associated with the development of hepatocellular carcinoma.

6.12   **The answer is a.** The relationship between *H. pylori* and MALT lymphoma has been determined, and after treatment with antibiotics to eradicate the bacteria the lymphoma was resolved.

6.13   **The answer is c.** The macrophage is a primary initiator to an inflammatory immune response. It originates in the bone marrow, circulates as a monocyte, and becomes a macrophage when it enters a tissue at a site of infection. The macrophage is also a secretory cell manufacturing key pyrogenic cytokines such as interleukin-1, tumor necrosis factor, and interleukin-6.

6.14   **The answer is c.** AIDS-related diseases such as Kaposi's sarcoma, non-Hodgkin's lymphoma, and primary central nervous system lymphoma are referred to as *opportunistic* because they occur in patients with preexisting immunodeficiency. This immunodeficiency can be the result of HIV infection (which destroys the immune system), therapeutic immunosuppression (e.g., chemotherapeutic agents used in organ transplantation), or primary immunodeficiency (e.g., as the result of a genetic defect). These malignancies normally occur at a low incidence and in a more benign form. An AIDS-related opportunistic disease that is not a malignancy is *Pneumocystis carinii* pneumonia.

6.15 **The answer is a.** Cytokines are glycoprotein products of immune cells. They bind to surface receptors of target cells and act as regulators of cell growth or as mediators of defense functions. Natural killer cells are capable of killing transformed cells. Lymphokine-activated killer cells are a special population of cytotoxic cells used in cancer therapy that comprise primarily natural killer cells, which are capable of nonspecific tumor cell killing. B lymphocytes are sedentary cells located in lymph nodes and spleen.

6.16 **The answer is d.** The classic function of the immune system is that cited in choice **a**, distinguishing self from nonself and destroying foreign substances. Homeostasis and surveillance are other important functions.

6.17 **The answer is b.** B memory cells (memory B lymphocytes), along with T memory cells (memory T lymphocytes), make up the recall component of the immune system. They have memory of antigens previously recognized by the body and deal with a particular antigen each time it is encountered.

6.18 **The answer is a.** B lymphocytes form plasma cells that produce specific immunoglobulins when stimulated by helper T lymphocytes and an encounter with a foreign antigen. Antibody is an antigen-specific immunoglobulin that is synthesized and secreted by a mature plasma cell, the final cell of B-lymphocyte differentiation. Each plasma cell produces only one type of antibody, and each antibody is specific for only one type of antigen.

6.19 **The answer is d.** Genes that predispose for cancer development are generally transmitted in an autosomal dominant fashion, meaning that individuals who harbor a mutated gene have a 50% chance of passing the mutated gene on to their children. Inheritance of the altered gene confers an increased risk for developing cancer. The pattern of transmission seen with cancer susceptibility genes is usually vertical, meaning successive generations are affected; depending on the disease, males and females are generally equally affected.

6.20 **The answer is b.** Inheritance of the *BRCA1* susceptibility gene is associated with a strong likelihood that the effect of the mutation will result in the disease for families with multiple breast and ovarian cancers (90%) as well as for those with breast cancers diagnosed before the age of 45 (70%).

6.21 **The answer is a.** Most people believe cancer risk is increased simply because someone in the family has cancer, which is not true. For example, breast cancer is estimated to have a familial component in only about 10–20% of cases.

6.22 **The answer is b.** The *BRCA2* gene is associated only with an increased susceptibility to breast cancer.

6.23 **The answer is d.** Individuals who have a first-degree relative with colorectal cancer have double the risk for developing adenomatous polyps, which are considered to be precursors of colorectal carcinoma. Persons who have a FAP have 100% risk of developing colorectal cancer.

6.24 **The answer is b.** The inherited form of retinoblastoma, characterized by multiple primary tumors, originates when both copies of the retinoblastoma antioncogene are absent or damaged. Without the protection of this gene, all retinal cells are predisposed to malignant growth.

6.25 **The answer is d.** Data regarding the genetic basis of cancer have been derived from a number of sources, including familial patterns, which have been studied in an attempt to elicit features of the transmission of neoplastic tendencies.

6.26   **The answer is b.** Germ cell mutations are transmitted to the next generation at birth and are responsible for hereditary (familial) cancer. Most human cancers result from a combination of acquired and inherited mutations with alterations of both oncogenes and antioncogenes.

6.27   **The answer is b.** The cornerstone of induction therapy in acute myelogenous leukemia is the cell cycle–specific antimetabolite cytosine arabinoside, plus an anthracycline such as daunorubicin.

6.28   **The answer is b.** Lymphomas are preeminently a malignancy of the lymphocyte. However, there seems to be a separate malignancy for each sequential stage in the developmental sequence from primitive to mature lymphocyte. At each stage of development, the potential exists for the normal maturing lymphocyte to be transformed into a cancer cell. Once transformed, the new clone of malignant cells follows the behavioral pattern of the stage of the lymphocyte at which the transformation occurred. For example, if the function of the maturing cell at the time it is transformed is secretion of an antibody, the tumor cells continue to secrete that normal protein in abnormal quantities. HD and NHL are distinguished on the basis of the Reed-Sternberg giant cells in NHL. The information in choice **d** is reversed.

6.29   **The answer is a.** Basal cell carcinoma is the most common form of skin cancer in whites and outnumbers squamous cell carcinoma by a ratio of 3:1. Nonmelanoma skin cancers, including basal cell carcinoma, have a higher incidence but a lower metastatic potential and mortality rate than malignant melanoma. Malignant melanoma has a much lower incidence but a mortality rate that is triple that of the nonmelanoma cancers. Increased mortality is directly related to its high potential for metastasis.

6.30   **The answer is a.** The purpose of postremission therapies is to prevent leukemic recurrence related to minimal residual disease. The four types of postremission therapies are consolidation therapy, intensification therapy, maintenance therapy, and bone marrow transplant. Consolidation therapy consists of one or two courses of very high doses of the same drugs used for induction (up to 30 times the induction doses of cytosine arabinoside for AML). Intensification regimens use different drugs in the hope that they will not be cross-resistant. Maintenance therapies use lower doses for a prolonged period of time. Maintenance therapy is not currently recommended for the treatment of AML.

6.31   **The answer is d.** Approximately 90% of patients with chronic myelogenous leukemia have the diagnostic marker Philadelphia chromosome *Ph*[1].

6.32   **The answer is d.** Although some bone tumors metastasize to the lymph nodes (e.g., Ewing's sarcoma), few, if any, seem to metastasize to the central nervous system or liver. Most of the more common bone tumors metastasize to the lungs. Whether or not these metastases develop and when depends on the stage and aggressiveness of the disease process.

6.33   **The answer is d.** Breast cancer primarily metastasizes to the bone, liver, lungs, nodes, and brain—but not the gastrointestinal tract.

6.34   **The answer is c.** The glioblastoma multiforme is the most common adult primary brain tumor. It is most common in individuals who are 50 or older. It shares all the characteristics of anaplastic astrocytoma plus necrosis.

6.35 **The answer is d.** A number of predisposing conditions have been associated with an increased risk of colorectal cancer. These include chronic ulcerative colitis, Crohn's disease, familial polyposis, and a strong family history of predisposition to colon cancer and familial adenomatous polyposis.

6.36 **The answer is c.** A complaint of low back pain frequently indicates that the cancer has spread into the retroperitoneal lymph nodes.

6.37 **The answer is d.** In multiple myeloma the malignant cell is the plasma cell, the functional mature cell that differentiates and develops from the B lymphocytes.

6.38 **The answer is d.** The major goals of the diagnostic evaluation for a suspected cancer are to determine the tissue type of the malignancy, the primary site of the malignancy, the extent of disease within the body, and also the tumor's potential to recur in the future.

6.39 **The answer is b.** In the case of liver cancer, computed tomography has been preferred for imaging, but magnetic resonance imaging with contrast may be equivalent. Ultrasound is preferred for differentiating biliary obstruction from hepatic parenchymal disease.

6.40 **The answer is d.** Because Mrs. Ellis displays no symptoms of bone involvement, a bone scan is not appropriate. CA-15-3 is used to monitor metastatic disease, not as an early detection test.

6.41 **The answer is c.** The diagnosis of lymphoma can be established only by a biopsy of involved tissue, usually a lymph node. Because there are many causes of lymphadenopathy, however—including upper respiratory infection, infectious mononucleosis, allergic reactions, and, in older people, cancer of the head and neck—a careful history and physical examination must first determine whether an enlarged lymph node should be biopsied. For persistent lymphadenopathy or when etiology is not known, a biopsy is usually indicated.

6.42 **The answer is a.** Biopsy is the initial surgical procedure for suspected cutaneous melanoma. Because it provides a definitive diagnosis along with microstaging information, an excisional biopsy that entails removal of a few millimeters of normal tissue surrounding the lesion is preferable. An incisional biopsy can be used for lesions in cosmetically sensitive areas or for large lesions. Electrocoagulation, curettage, shaving, and burning are never used to remove a suspicious mole.

6.43 **The answer is d.** Inguinal orchiectomy remains the standard approach for definitive pathological diagnosis. A biopsy or transcrotal approach orchiectomy can cause possible spread of tumor. Both a fine-needle biopsy and a transcrotal approach are contraindicated.

6.44 **The answer is d.** The Pap smear is an effective technique for detecting cervical cancer. When the Pap report shows squamous epithelial lesions, biopsy, colposcopy, and/or treatment is indicated.

6.45 **The answer is c.** Adenocarcinomas are the most common lung cancer, representing 40% of all primary tumors and commonly found in females and in nonsmokers. The squamous cell carcinomas constitute 30–35% of all lung cancers and are more common in males than in females. They are also the ones that arise from the basal cells of the bronchial epithelium and usually present as masses in large bronchi. Finally, the large cell carcinomas, and not the adenocarcinomas, are the least common type of lung cancer, representing approximately 10–15%.

6.46   **The answer is a.** Carcinoma specifies a malignant tumor arising from epithelial tissues. Epithelium covers or lines surfaces within the body and arises from the ectodermal, mesodermal, or endodermal embryonic layer.

6.47   **The answer is d.** The histologic classification most frequently will be adenocarcinoma, but the site of origin may never be determined in 2–4% of cancer patients, even on autopsy.

6.48   **The answer is c.** Although gross hematuria, bladder neck obstruction, and pain in the suprapubic region can all be clinical manifestations of bladder cancer, the most important indicator of disease progression is the depth of tumor penetration into the bladder wall.

6.49   **The answer is d.** The larger the tumor and the more positive nodes involved, the worse the prognosis is.

6.50   **The answer is d.** For Hodgkin's disease, prognosis is most closely related to stage. Age and the total number of lymph node groups involved (independent of stage) are other prognostic factors, whereas for non-Hodgkin's lymphoma prognosis is most closely related to histologic type.

6.51   **The answer is b.** For patients over 70, watchful waiting may be an appropriate option. Research has yet to demonstrate that for those with stage A or B cancer treatment is more beneficial than watchful waiting. For men under 70, a physician may often be reluctant to offer watchful waiting, and there is evidence that for younger men with moderately or poorly differentiated localized prostate cancer, treatment may offer a survival advantage.

6.52   **The answer is d.** Microstaging describes the level of invasion of the CM and maximum tumor thickness. The two parameters that are used in assessing the depth of invasion are the anatomic level of invasion, or the Clark level, and the thickness of tumor tissue, or the Breslow level. The prognosis for patients with metastatic disease at the time of diagnosis is poor, with most dying within 5 years. As CM thickness increases, survival rates decrease. Thus the Breslow level has consistently proved to be a significant prognostic variable in stage I CM.

6.53   **The answer is b.** Factors associated with a poor prognosis in AIDS-related Kaposi's sarcoma (KS) include CD4 cell count <200/mm^3; history of systemic "B" symptoms such as fever, weight loss, and night sweats; history of opportunistic infections; Karnofsky performance status <70%; tumor-associated edema or ulceration; gastrointestinal KS; or KS in visceral organs.

6.54   **The answer is b.** Ninety percent of patients with seminoma are curable by radiation and chemotherapy. Because they are extremely sensitive to radiation and chemotherapy, the stage of the disease at diagnosis is insignificant. High-grade tumors are known to undergo rapid cell division; they double their tumor volume quickly. Because most drugs are active against cells that are undergoing cell division, seminomas are more susceptible to the cell kill effects of chemotherapy.

6.55   **The answer is c.** Limited-stage disease is the most favorable prognostic factor in SCLC. A good ambulatory performance status, female gender, and normal lactate dehydrogenase are also favorable prognostic factors for SCLC. Poor prognostic factors include weight loss, impaired immunocompetence as measured by delayed hypersensitivity skin testing, and Cushing's syndrome.

6.56   **The answer is c.** Hormone receptor analysis reveals whether a tumor is positive for the estrogen and progesterone receptor. If the tumor is positive for hormone receptors, then hormonal manipulation can be used for treatment. Patients with hormone receptor–negative tumors tend to have a poorer prognosis. Women whose tumors are positive for the HER-2 receptor gene are candidates for Herceptin therapy whether they have local or metastatic disease. Presence of the gene indicates a poorer prognosis.

6.57   **The answer is a.** Poor prognosis has been associated with obstructing or perforating carcinomas, occurrence in young people, location of the tumor below the peritoneal reflection, lymph node involvement, venous invasion, hepatic metastasis, and invasion of the bowel wall.

6.58   **The answer is d.** The most relevant classification systems will communicate clinical and prognostic information. The tumors may be classified not only by their biological behavior (benign versus malignant) but also by their tissue of origin.

6.59   **The answer is a.** A benign tumor is well circumscribed or encapsulated; microscopically, it appears orderly and comprises cells similar to those of its parent tissue. A malignant tumor invades both the organs from which it originated and eventually the surrounding tissues, and it is made up of cells that vary greatly in size and shape.

6.60   **The answer is b.** The term *carcinoma in situ* describes a lesion characterized by full-thickness neoplastic change with no evidence of stromal invasion or metastases.

6.61   **The answer is a.** Bronchogenic cancers are grouped into small cell lung cancer and non–small cell lung cancers, which include squamous cell carcinoma, adenocarcinoma, and large cell carcinoma. Many tumors are heterogeneous, containing cells from more than one histologic type. In both types of cancer, both hyperplasia and carcinoma in situ occur.

6.62   **The answer is d.** There are multiple objectives of solid tumor staging, but the most important is to provide the necessary information for individual treatment planning. Other reasons for using a uniform staging system are to give prognostic information, to assist in treatment evaluation, to facilitate the exchange of information and comparative statistics among the treatment centers, and to stratify individuals who may be eligible for clinical trials.

6.63   **The answer is b.** There are multiple objectives of solid tumor staging, but the most important is to provide the necessary information for individual treatment planning.

6.64   **The answer is a.** In the TNM system the extent of the primary tumor (T) is evaluated on the basis of depth of invasion, surface spread, and tumor size. The absence or presence and extent of regional lymph node (N) metastasis are considered, and the presence of distant metastasis (M) is assessed. The system is further classified by whether the assessment is obtained clinically (cTNM or TNM), after pathologic review (pTNM), at the time of retreatment (rTNM), or on autopsy (aTNM).

6.65   **The answer is a.** Stage groupings involve combining the various classification elements of tumor site, regional lymph node involvement, and the presence or absence of metastasis. It involves two main staging periods: pretreatment and retreatment. The two aspects of pretreatment staging of a previously undiagnosed cancer are clinical diagnostic staging, for patients who have had a biopsy, and *postsurgical resection-pathologic* staging, which includes a complete evaluation of the surgical specimen by a pathologist.

6.66   **The answer is b.** Restaging focuses particular attention on the disease parameters that were positive at diagnosis, to signal a search for any remaining evidence that treatment should continue. Restaging does not imply that if a remission is obtained the patient reverts to a lesser disease stage. The stage ascribed at the time of diagnosis is the one referenced throughout the illness.

6.67   **The answer is a.** Five-year survival rates have slowly improved to approximately 62% for all stages of disease, 87% for patients with localized disease, and 9% for stage IV disease.

6.68   **The answer is b.** The AJCC staging system for lung cancer uses the TNM letters. *T* designates primary tumor and is divided into categories relative to size, location, and invasion. *N*, with three categories, represents regional lymph node status. *M* designates the absence or presence of distant metastases. Lung cancer is also divided into eight stages, each of which is distinctive relative to treatment and 5-year survival statistics. Small cell lung cancer is usually staged using a simple two-stage system. Because most small cell lung cancer patients have metastatic disease at the time of diagnosis, this system describes the extent of disease as either "limited" or "extensive."

6.69   **The answer is b.** Determination of the stage of disease in HD is important because it influences which treatment option (radiation therapy or combination therapy) is used. Radiation is very effective for localized HD and is therefore used in early-stage disease. Chemotherapy is more effective than radiation for late-stage disease, when the number of lymph node groups involved is greater, but it also is as effective as radiation in early-stage disease. Non-Hodgkin's lymphoma, on the other hand, is almost always treated with chemotherapy because it usually presents at an advanced stage. A positive bone marrow biopsy indicates a stage IV tumor. A stage II presentation for HD is more likely to indicate a slow-growing malignancy; it is not at all uncommon.

6.70   **The answer is b.** All the other choices, along with a history and physical examination, are standard procedures used in the staging of lymphoma. Other procedures, including a computed tomography of the chest and abdomen, a bone marrow biopsy, a percutaneous liver biopsy, a lower limb lymphangiogram, and an exploratory laparotomy, may be done if there is evidence of lymph node involvement below the diaphragm, hepatomegaly or abnormal liver function, extension of the lymphoma to mediastinal lymph nodes, or splenomegaly. Positive results on these tests often indicate a stage IV disease.

6.71   **The answer is b.** Melanoma has been classified into several types, including lentigo maligna, superficial spreading, nodular, and acral lentiginous. Each type is characterized by a radial and/or vertical growth phase. In the radial phase, tumor growth is parallel to the skin surface, risk of metastasis is slight, and surgical excision is usually curative. The vertical growth phase is marked by focal deep penetration of atypical melanocytes into the dermis and subcutaneous tissue. Penetration occurs rapidly, increasing the risk of metastasis.

6.72   **The answer is c.** Whereas intermediate-grade tumors can be treated with either chemotherapy or radiation therapy, depending on the stage at presentation, advanced intermediate/high-grade lymphoma is treated with combination chemotherapy. Cyclophosphamide, the most active and effective agent, is commonly used in combination with other agents. Initial responses are usually dramatic but are not long-lived; relapse typically occurs in 4–6 weeks following discontinuation of chemotherapy. In addition, treatment-related neutropenia is severe and sometimes precipitates an opportunistic infection.

6.73   **The answer is c.** Alpha-fetoprotein is a tumor marker that is elevated in the serum of 70–90% of individuals with primary hepatocellular carcinoma, but because levels of alpha-fetoprotein are not specific for liver cancer, histologic diagnosis is required.

6.74   **The answer is c.** A secondary or metastatic tumor resembles the primary tumor histologically. A second primary lesion refers to an additional histologically separate malignant neoplasm in the same patient.

6.75   **The answer is b.** For selected tumors the grade is considered more significant than anatomic staging in terms of prognostic value and treatment. In soft tissue sarcomas, the grade is the primary determinant of stage of disease and of prognosis. In other tumors, such as melanoma, testicular cancer, and thyroid cancer, histologic grading has no useful application.

6.76   **The answer is d.** A G2 rating means the tumor is moderately well differentiated. The AJCC recommends the following grading classification:
       GX = grade cannot be assessed
       G1 = well differentiated
       G2 = moderately well differentiated
       G3 = poorly differentiated
       G4 = undifferentiated

6.77   **The answer is c.** Histopathologic type is a qualitative assessment whereby a neoplasm is categorized in terms of the tissue or cell type from which it has originated. Histopathologic *grade* is a quantitative assessment of the extent to which the tumor resembles the tissue of origin. A lesion with the same cell type but at a site other than the original site indicates a metastatic tumor; a different cell type originating from another lesion anywhere in the body indicates a second primary cancer.

6.78   **The answer is d.** Clinically important cancers include features such as large tumor volume, Gleason grades 3–5, an invasive proliferative pattern of growth, elevated PSA, and origination in the peripheral zone. These cancers threaten the patient's life because they progress to fatal metastatic cancers. The vast majority of prostate cancers do not threaten the patient's life and are termed *indolent*.

6.79   **The answer is d.** The primary application of flow cytometry analysis in solid tumors has been to determine DNA content and the percentage of cells synthesizing DNA. Normal DNA is characterized as diploid and contrasts with abnormal disorganized DNA that is aneuploid.

6.80   **The answer is b.** Radiation is usually indicated if the tumor is found to be invading nearby tissues that cannot be surgically resected. Chemotherapy is used to eliminate micrometastasis.

6.81   **The answer is d.** Situations lending themselves best to surgical treatment include such factors as slow-growing tumors that consist of cells with prolonged cell cycles. A surgical procedure intended to be curative must involve resection of the entire tumor mass as well as a margin of safety of normal healthy tissue surrounding the tumor. Superficial and encapsulated tumors are more easily resected than those that are embedded in inaccessible or delicate tissues.

6.82   **The answer is b.** Regional biopsy involves obtaining several samples of tissue from different locations within a tumor. Regional biopsies are used to diagnose metastatic disease in a defined, but not localized, region of the body. Stereotactic biopsy uses radiographic images to create three-dimensional views of a suspected neoplasm.

6.83   **The answer is a.** Small cell lung cancer invades the submucosa and is thought to arise from neuroendocrine cells that secrete peptide hormones. Squamous cell carcinoma, adenocarcinoma, and large cell carcinoma are all examples of non–small cell lung cancer.

6.84   **The answer is c.** Because the esophagus is thin walled and draws upward with each swallow, an anastomosis involving the esophagus has more of a tendency to leak than any other area of the gastrointestinal tract. For this reason contrast studies are performed 4–6 days after surgery to check for patency of the anastomosis. Small leaks usually close spontaneously; larger leaks often require surgical approximation.

6.85   **The answer is c.** Possible contraindications to major hepatic resection for liver cancer include the following: (1) severe cirrhosis; (2) distant metastases in the lung, bone, or lymph nodes; (3) jaundice, which is often indicative of obstruction of the common bile duct; (4) ascites, which is usually indicative of liver failure and an inability to tolerate a surgical procedure; (5) poor visualization on angiographic studies, which may jeopardize the certainty with which the surgeon resects the tumor; (6) certain biochemical changes that indicate poor liver function and lower the probability of survival; and (7) involvement of the inferior vena cava or portal vein, which would make surgical intervention hazardous.

6.86   **The answer is a.** In women a radical cystectomy includes the removal of the bladder, urethra, uterus, ovaries, fallopian tubes, and anterior wall of the vagina. In men the term is synonymous with prostatectomy and includes excision of the bladder with pericystic sac, the attached perineum, the prostate, and the seminal vesicles.

6.87   **The answer is d.** Prostate cancer is not cured by TURP. Rather, TURP is used to treat symptoms of bladder outlet obstruction, and in some patients provides pathologic evidence that a cancer, previously unsuspected, is present.

6.88   **The answer is c.** The four "R"s of radiobiology and their influence on dose fractionation is Repair of damaged cells; Redistribution of cell age so tumor cells will become more radiosensitive; Repopulation, which takes place during cell division; and Reoxygenation, which allows the tumor cells that are in a hypoxic or anoxic state to become oxygenated and radiosensitive.

6.89   **The answer is d.** All three techniques are used in breast-conserving radiotherapy. Whole breast radiotherapy is still used; however, treatment is changing for patients with early-stage breast cancer to include the concept that partial breast irradiation yields similar control. The MammoSite system delivers high-dose radiation directly to the site of tumor excision and targets the area where the cancer would most likely recur. The Intrabeam system uses a single dose of intraoperative radiotherapy in comparison to the fractionated dosing system of MammoSite.

6.90   **The answer is b.** Megavoltage equipment operates at 2–40 million electron volts (MeV), compared to orthovoltage equipment's 40,000–400,000 electron volts (kV). It has the advantages of deeper beam penetration, more homogeneous absorption of radiation (minimizing bone absorption), and greater skin sparing. Megavoltage equipment includes cobalt and cesium units, the linear accelerator, the betatron, and such experimental units as those producing neutron beams, heavy ions, and negative pi-mesons.

6.91 **The answer is b.** In addition to radioactive implantation, some radioactive isotopes are administered orally or intravenously or by instillation. Liquid sources administered as colloids or solutions are adsorbed or metabolized and present a possibility of contamination of equipment, dressings, and linens, depending on the mode of administration and metabolism.

6.92 **The answer is b.** Efforts to improve the therapeutic ratio have resulted in the development of certain compounds that act to increase the radiosensitivity of tumor cells or to protect normal cells from radiation effect. Radiosensitizers are compounds that apparently promote fixation of the free radicals produced by radiation damage at the molecular level.

6.93 **The answer is d.** During a course of radiotherapy, certain treatment-related side effects can be expected to develop, most of which are site specific as well as dependent on volume, dose fractionation, total dose, and individual differences. Many symptoms do not develop until approximately 10–14 days into treatment, and some do not subside until 2 or more weeks after treatments have ended.

6.94 **The answer is a.** Simulator machinery may involve the use of diagnostic x-rays, fluoroscopic examination, transverse axial tomography, computed tomography, and ultrasound, with the goal of localizing a tumor and defining the volume to be treated with radiotherapy. Other aspects of treatment planning include the tattooing of the treatment area, installing various restraining and positioning devices to immobilize the person, shaping the field, and determining what structures are to be blocked and protected from radiation.

6.95 **The answer is a.** The biologic effects of radiation on humans are the result of a sequence of events that follows the absorption of energy from ionizing radiation and the body's attempt to compensate for this assault. Radiation effect takes place at the cellular level, with consequences in tissues, organs, and the entire body.

6.96 **The answer is c.** All of the other choices are opposites of the actual goals of fractionation. Fractionation redistributes cell age within the cell cycle, making tumor cells more radiosensitive. It allows normal cells to repopulate, sparing them from some of the late consequences that occur if new growth is inhibited. It also provides time between treatments for tumor cells to reoxygenate, thus making them more radiosensitive.

6.97 **The answer is c.** Effects of radiation may be acute and immediate (seen within the first 6 months) or may be late (seen after 6 months). Acute effects are due to cell damage in which mitotic activity is altered. If early effects are not reversible, late or permanent tissue changes occur. These late effects are due to the organism's attempt to heal or repair the damage inflicted by ionizing radiation.

6.98 **The answer is d.** After insertion of the source, hospitalization lasts until decay of the source is reduced to 30 millicuries or less. A condom should be worn during intercourse for 2 months after implantation, but the patient poses no danger as a radioactive source.

6.99 **The answer is c.** The most common side effects reported by 774 patients are asthenia/malaise, abdominal pain, fever, headache, nausea, vomiting, diarrhea, acneform rash, and others. Nail disorders are rare, but choice **c** is the best answer. Rarely is alopecia or disorientation seen with cetuximab.

6.100 **The answer is b.** Cetuximab (Erbitux) is a monoclonal antibody that attaches to epidermal growth factor receptor on both normal and tumor cells. When cetuximab attaches to the epidermal growth factor receptor, it blocks the signaling agents from attaching and starting the cell dividing process.

6.101 **The answer is d.** Severe infusion reactions are rare with cetuximab, but they do occur. Approximately 90% of severe infusion reactions were associated with the first infusion despite the use of prophylactic antihistamines. These reactions were characterized by the rapid onset of airway obstruction (bronchospasm, stridor, and hoarseness), urticaria, and/or hypotension. Caution must be exercised with every cetuximab infusion because some patients experienced their first severe infusion reaction during later infusions. Severe infusion reactions require the immediate interruption of therapy and permanent discontinuation from further therapy.

6.102 **The answer is d.** Avastin is an antiangiogenic agent that inhibits blood vessel formation, which starves the tumor. In addition, bevacizumab may have an effect of remodeling existing tumor vasculature to improve drug penetration, thereby enhancing antitumor efficacy of chemotherapeutic agents.

6.103 **The answer is d.** Nitric oxide is a messenger molecule (a molecule that carries signals between cells) that can regulate various physiologic functions, including blood pressure. Some studies suggest that vascular endothelial growth factor increases nitric oxide production, resulting in vasodilation. Reducing nitric oxide production results in vasoconstriction; it has been hypothesized that this process could play a role in hypertension.

6.104 **The answer is c.** Proteinuria can occur with cancer and some cancer therapies. In a clinical setting impairment of the glomeruli that make up the kidney may be a pathologic cause of persistent proteinuria. Inhibition of vascular endothelial growth factor, a key endothelial growth factor, has been shown to impair glomerular endothelial cells that normally filter water and small solutes but not proteins or cells.

6.105 **The answer is a.** Because malignant tumors cannot grow beyond 1–2 mm without establishing a new blood vessel system, agents are being studied that have the capacity to neutralize growth factors, such as vascular endothelial growth factor.

6.106 **The answer is c.** Cytokines (which include lymphokines) are substances released from activated immune system cells that affect the behavior of other cells. They may alter the growth and metastasis of cancer cells by augmenting the responsiveness of T cells to tumor-associated antigens, enhancing the effectiveness of B-cell activity, or decreasing suppressive functions of the immune system, thereby enhancing immune responsiveness. Included among the cytokines are the interferons and interleukins, tumor necrosis factor, and colony-stimulating factors.

6.107 **The answer is b.** Body temperature is controlled by preoptic anterior hypothalamic brain centers in a feedback mechanism. Pyrogenic pathogens, toxins, or drugs stimulate the release of endogenous pyrogenic cytokines, which act on thermal brain centers via prostaglandin release and create an upward reset of the body's temperature set point. Feedback mechanisms now read the body temperature as cold and initiate heat-producing actions such as involuntary muscular contractions or rigors.

6.108 **The answer is c.** The major side effects of gefitinib (Iressa) are skin rash and diarrhea. It rarely causes any allergic type reaction, hypotension, or effect on the bone marrow.

6.109   **The answer is d.** Biologic response modifiers can be classified as agents that restore, augment, or modulate host antitumor immune mechanisms; cells or cellular products that have direct antitumor effects; and biologic agents that have other biologic antitumor effects.

6.110   **The answer is d.** The interferons (IFNs) are a family of naturally occurring complex proteins that belong to the cytokine family. Each of the three major types in humans—alpha-IFN, beta-IFN, and gamma-IFN—originates from a different cell and has distinct biologic and chemical properties. All three types of IFNs exhibit the cellular effects listed in choices **a–c**.

6.111   **The answer is d.** The cytokine network is an overlapping, interactive communication pattern within the immune system. Cytokines share many properties, such as mediating and regulating the immune defense functions of the body. They can influence the stimulation of other cytokines to produce synergistic effects, as in a cytokine network, or to antagonize the actions of other cytokines.

6.112   **The answer is b.** Teach patients that paresthesias may occur in hands, feet, and hypopharynx. Patients should avoid exposure to cold for 1 to 5 days after the drug is given. A scarf wrapped around the neck and mouth prevents inspiration of cold air that could cause pharyngolaryngeal dysesthesia, which is an acute neurotoxicity.

6.113   **The answer is d.** For patients receiving Xeloda and warfarin concomitantly, frequent monitoring of INR or PT is recommended. Clinically significant increases in PT and INR have been observed within days to months after starting Xeloda and infrequently within 1 month of stopping Xeloda. The interaction of Xeloda and warfarin is probably due to an inhibition of cytochrome P-450 by Xeloda and/or its metabolites, whereby warfarin is not metabolized properly.

6.114   **The answer is d.** Ketoconazole is a drug used to treat fungal infections but is also used as a second or third choice hormonal agent to treat prostate cancer. It blocks the production of male hormones in the testes and the adrenal glands, slowing the growth of some prostate cancers. Food, antacids, cimetidine, and rifampin impair absorption, whereas the acidic nature of cola and orange juice has been shown to enhance absorption.

6.115   **The answer is a.** The metabolic activation and inactivation or catabolism of drugs is carried out primarily by the liver.

6.116   **The answer is d.** Cancer cells can overcome the effects of cytotoxic drugs either by increasing the number of target enzymes or by modifying the enzyme so as to interfere with binding to antagonistic drugs. The ability of cells to repair DNA lesions is an important resistance mechanism seen with alkylating agents and cisplatin.

6.117   **The answer is b.** Capecitabine is a prodrug, a chemical precursor of 5-FU. It undergoes three enzymatic changes in the body before becoming 5-FU within the body tissues.

6.118   **The answer is d.** Altered coagulation and bleeding have been reported in patients taking capecitabine and anticoagulants concomitantly. These events occurred within several days and up to several months after initiating capecitabine therapy. The mechanism of interaction between dilantin and capecitabine appears to be the inhibition of the CYP2C9 isoenzyme by capecitabine or its metabolite. This interaction results in toxicities associated with elevated dilantin levels. Folic acid should be discontinued in patients receiving capecitabine because it could potentially increase the toxicity of 5-FU.

Scientific Basis
for Practice

6.119 **The answer is c.** Docetaxel is metabolized by the liver, and elevated liver functions can interfere with metabolism, causing enhanced toxicity of docetaxel. The dose needs to be reduced.

6.120 **The answer is c.** Chemotherapy currently is given preoperatively. The rationale for preoperative chemotherapy is to treat micrometastasis, to decrease the size of the primary tumor (thereby increasing the likelihood of limb salvage surgery), and to assess the effectiveness of the chemotherapeutic agents for 2–3 months. The route of the chemotherapy is either intravenous or intra-arterial.

6.121 **The answer is b.** Side effects associated with CMF include myelosuppression, hair loss, and hemorrhagic cystitis.

6.122 **The answer is d.** Capecitabine is stopped at the first sign of any of the following:

- Four bowel movements over normal
- Nocturnal stool
- Stomatitis with pain or discomfort
- Vomiting more than once in a 24-hour period
- Hand–foot syndrome with pain or discomfort or affecting activities of daily living
- Nausea, loss of appetite, or decrease in food intake over a 24-hour period
- Unexplained bleeding (especially for those on warfarin)

6.123 **The answer is c.** Although 5-fluorouracil is the cytotoxic agent of choice for colorectal cancer, it is most commonly administered in combination with leucovorin. Floxuridine is used in intraportal chemotherapy through the portal vein or hepatic artery into the liver in individuals with metastasis to the liver.

6.124 **The answer is c.** Patients are monitored closely for signs of renal impairment (increased blood urea nitrogen and creatinine, proteinuria), and the dose of melphalan may need to be reduced based on the severity of renal toxicity. It is also important to closely monitor serial blood counts because the bone marrow–suppressive effects of melphalan may be cumulative in older patients. Hypercalcemia and bone pain are symptoms of the disorder itself rather than adverse effects.

6.125 **The answer is c.** On the first occurrence of grade 2 toxicity (hand–foot syndrome with pain or discomfort or affecting activities of daily living) hold therapy until toxicity reaches a grade 0–1 and then restart at 100% dose. On the second occurrence, hold therapy until toxicity reaches grade 0–1 and then restart at 75% dose. Third occurrence, hold therapy until toxicity reaches grade 0–1 and then restart at 50% dose. Fourth occurrence, discontinue therapy.

6.126 **The answer is c.** Allogeneic transplants are indicated for acute myelogenous leukemia, chronic myelogenous leukemia, and acute lymphocytic leukemia. Autologous transplants are indicated for breast cancer predominantly and are used for non-Hodgkin's lymphoma and multiple myeloma.

6.127 **The answer is d.** Growth factors, made through recombinant DNA processes, stimulate pluripotent stem cells to differentiate and mature. These products are administered in transplantation and cause the body to overproduce pluripotent stem cells beyond the body's required needs and also induce cell differentiation and maturation. The administration of HGFs takes place right before pheresis so that more cells are available for collection from the circulation. This process is referred to as mobilization.

6.128   **The answer is b.** Venoocclusive disease is almost exclusive to bone marrow transplantation and is the most common nonrelapse life-threatening complication of preparative regimen–related toxicity for bone marrow transplantation.

6.129   **The answer is a.** Risk factors for late chronic GVHD include, among others, mismatched donor and recipient, female-to-male transplants, positive herpes simplex and cytomegalovirus, patient age over 18 years, prior grade 2–3 acute GVHD, and chronic myelogenous leukemia recipients who received methotrexate and cyclosporine as chronic GVHD prophylaxis.

6.130   **The answer is b.** TBI is given before marrow infusion to prevent graft rejection by the patient's immune system. It offers optimal tumor cell kill because it penetrates the central nervous system and other privileged sites. It is usually given in fractionated doses to reduce toxicities, and it can be given as a booster to patients with bulky disease.

6.131   **The answer is b.** One advantage to using peripheral PPSCs and progenitor cells obtained from peripheral blood is the more rapid recovery of neutrophils and platelets when progenitor cells are used. This is because the committed progenitors collected for blood cell transplant are farther along the differentiation pathway than are the PPSCs harvested from the bone marrow. Another advantage is that no anesthesia is required for blood cell transplant, so there is less risk of complications and fewer medical contraindications than with bone marrow harvest.

6.132   **The answer is a.** The advantages of autologous BMT over allogeneic BMT are the absence of GVHD and fewer toxicities. Autologous BMT is less toxic because there is no venoocclusive disease or GVHD. However, there is a potential risk of tumor contamination in the autologous marrow, and there is no benefit of the GVL effect, which can reduce the risk of relapse.

6.133   **The answer is d.** Homeopathy is based upon the theory of similars, which holds that a drug that causes symptoms at full strength will cure those symptoms if it is diluted.

6.134   **The answer is d.** The mind–body approach can be divided into two different approaches, the use of the mind to overcome dysfunction (i.e., hypnosis) or the use of the psychic energy of the body to overcome problems. The latter approach is embodied in techniques such as healing touch, reiki therapy, and polarity therapy.

6.135   **The answer is c.** The therapeutic dose may be significantly lower in cancer patients and tricyclic antidepressants should be taken as scheduled and should not be withdrawn or stopped suddenly. Doing so may risk cholinergic rebound, including nausea and vomiting, headache, diaphoresis, and chills.

6.136   **The answer is c.** Phytoestrogens are nonsteroidal compounds derived from plants. Soy, a product of the soy plant, is a popular source of phytoestrogens. It contains proteins called isoflavons that are bioactive compounds with a chemical structure similar to estradiol. Isoflavons share many properties with endogenous estrogens and compete for the estrogen receptor in human cells. Black cohosh does not contain phytoestrogens.

CHAPTER 7

Health Promotion

EPIDEMIOLOGY

7.1 Incidence of bone cancer is most common in people with
a. A family tendency for bone cancer
b. Prior high-dose radiation cancer therapy
c. Preexisting bone conditions
d. All of the above

7.2 Which of the following statements regarding the incidence of breast cancer is true?
a. Seventy percent of breast cancer occurs in women who are 50 years of age or older.
b. The incidence of breast cancer has increased, but the mortality rate—especially among African-Americans and Hispanics—has decreased.
c. The incidence of breast cancer is approximately one of every four women.
d. The incidence of breast cancer has increased to epidemic proportions among pre-menopausal women.

7.3 The highest overall incidence of cancer occurs among
a. Young adult Asian/Pacific Islanders
b. Native Americans on reservations in the northwest
c. African-American men
d. None of the above

7.4 For breast cancer the average annual rate per 100,000 individuals has been highest among which females?
a. Japanese
b. White
c. Hawaiian
d. Black

7.5   In the United States the highest incidence of esophageal cancer is found among
       a.   Women aged 29–39 years
       b.   African-American men
       c.   Perimenopausal women
       d.   Men aged 30–40 years

7.6   Incidence of cervical cancer is highest in women who are
       a.   Nulliparous
       b.   Lifetime celibate
       c.   Lifetime monogamous
       d.   Multiparous

7.7   Which of the following has *not* been found to be associated with an increased incidence of
       primary brain tumors?
       a.   Inhaled steroids
       b.   AIDS
       c.   Genetic disorders
       d.   Radiation to the head and neck area

7.8   Jana's research team has identified the relative risk and the frequency of a suspected etiologic
       factor in an entire defined population. A case-control study is conducted. What is the study
       most likely to be seeking to establish?
       a.   Causation
       b.   Attributable risk
       c.   A survival risk
       d.   Prevalence

7.9   Jana's research project is an epidemiologic study of workers in asbestos mines who are free
       of any cancer. Subjects are to be followed over a 10-year period, and the incidence rates of
       certain types of cancers are to be determined. This design is an example of a
       a.   Prospective study
       b.   Retrospective study
       c.   Historical prospective study
       d.   Historical retrospective study

7.10   Eric is a member of a research team that conducts an epidemiologic study. They determine
       that in a given year approximately 1 of every 12,000 American men has prostate cancer. This
       figure represents
       a.   An incidence rate
       b.   A mortality rate
       c.   A prevalence rate
       d.   A survival rate

7.11   The country with the highest incidence of gastric cancer is
       a.   Japan
       b.   China
       c.   England
       d.   The United States

7.12   A fellow nurse remarks that there seems to be an epidemic of breast cancer among young women. Which of the following would be an accurate response to this nurse?
   a.   It is true; the prevalence of breast cancer is increased in this population.
   b.   It seems that breast cancer is occurring more in younger women only because early detection measures such as mammography are detecting breast cancer sooner.
   c.   Breast cancer is being detected earlier when the tumors are smaller because women are more aware of the need to practice early detection measures.
   d.   b or c

7.13   Which of the following statements regarding genetic predisposition to cancer is *not* correct?
   a.   The *BRCA1* gene is associated with increased susceptibility to both breast and ovarian cancer.
   b.   The *BRCA2* gene is associated with an increase in the incidence of breast cancer.
   c.   The genes are involved in approximately 30% of breast cancer cases.
   d.   The genes appear to be more strongly associated with breast cancer diagnosed before the age of 50.

7.14   The overall smoking prevalence is decreasing in the United States. However, the decrease in smoking prevalence is not uniform among all groups. Which of the following statements regarding the prevalence patterns for smoking is *false*?
   a.   Overall smoking prevalence in women has declined more slowly than in men.
   b.   Smoking prevalence has declined more in black than in white adolescents.
   c.   The lung cancer mortality rate for white men in the United States has peaked, but the projected peak for mortality rates in women will not occur until the year 2010.
   d.   With the predicted declines in mortality rates, the absolute number of lung cancer deaths will also decline.

PREVENTION

Risk Factors

7.15   Your patient has lung cancer but never smoked cigarettes. You encourage him to have his first-degree relatives and children discuss their risk for cancer with their physician. Which of the following statements provides rationale for your recommendation?
   a.   Someone in the house is probably a smoker, which is how your patient was exposed, and that person could have lung cancer.
   b.   First-degree relatives of never-smoker lung cancer patients have a 25% increased risk of developing any type of cancer in their lifetime.
   c.   The offspring of never-smoker lung cancer patients have a twofold increased risk of developing cancer.
   d.   b and c

7.16   Liver cancer is often associated with
   a.   A long smoking history
   b.   Obesity
   c.   Cirrhosis
   d.   A bacterial infection

7.17 Mr. Holden quits smoking. He is very anxious about his risk for lung cancer and asks, "How much will my risk be affected?" You explain that the rate of decline in his risk of developing lung cancer is determined by the cumulative smoking exposure before cessation, the age when smoking began, and the
   a. Degree of inhalation
   b. Amount of passive smoke previously exposed to
   c. Brand of cigarettes smoked
   d. Amount of time that has passed since quitting

7.18 Mr. Jantzen's wife wants him to eat more fiber because his brother had colon cancer. Which of the following sources of fiber has been shown to provide the *most* protection against colon cancer?
   a. Cereals
   b. Vegetables
   c. Fruits
   d. Bread

7.19 Which of the following life-style factors increases the risk of oral cancer?
   a. Poor oral hygiene and overuse of harsh mouthwash solutions
   b. Habitual use of alcohol and tobacco
   c. Vitamin A deficiency
   d. All of the above

7.20 Your patient says he just cannot believe that the number of cigarettes he smokes "makes any difference. Either you're a smoker or you're not," he says. You explain that the risk of developing _____ is directly correlated with the number of cigarettes smoked.
   a. Brain cancer
   b. Pancreatic cancer
   c. Oropharyngeal cancer
   d. Skin cancer

7.21 Your brother-in-law tells you that he is tired of "all the negative talk about smoking. There's more prejudice against it than there is real danger." What percentage of lung cancer deaths are caused by cigarette smoking?
   a. 45–50%
   b. 50–60%
   c. 75–85%
   d. 80–90%

7.22 Individuals with esophageal cancer typically have a history of
   a. Occupational exposure to radiation
   b. Obesity
   c. Oral contraceptive use
   d. Heavy alcohol intake

7.23 Which of the following are risk factors for cervical carcinoma?
   a. Herpes simplex virus 2
   b. Human papillomavirus
   c. Women exposed to diethylstilbestrol in utero
   d. All of the above

7.24   Which of the following factors may increase a woman's risk of cervical carcinoma?
    a. Barrier-type contraception
    b. Limiting the number of sexual partners
    c. Vitamin A, beta-carotene, vitamin C
    d. None of the above

7.25   Ms. Ellis tells you that her adult daughter is pressuring her to give up suntanning. "I've had a good tan for over 20 years," she says. "I like it. Is my daughter being a little hysterical?" You explain that long-term exposure to the sun has been associated with skin cancer and also with
    a. Colorectal cancer
    b. Breast cancer
    c. Cancer of the lip
    d. Uterine cancer

7.26   Although the exact etiology of multiple myeloma is not known, certain factors increase the risk. Which of the following has been associated with an increased incidence of multiple myeloma?
    a. Chronic low-level exposure to radiation
    b. Chronic antigenic stimulation
    c. Chronic high-dose vitamin intake
    d. a and b

7.27   Which of the following has been associated with an increased incidence of breast cancer in women?
    a. Living near high-energy electromagnetic wires
    b. Radiation to chest
    c. Exposure to chemicals used in hair dye
    d. All of the above

7.28   Which of the following risk factors is associated with an increased incidence of thyroid cancer?
    a. Exposure to nuclear fallout
    b. Previous radiation to the neck
    c. History of goiter
    d. All of the above

7.29   Esophageal cancer is associated with which of the following risk factors?
    a. Dietary deficiencies of selenium
    b. Nitrosamines in food
    c. Gastroesophageal reflux disorder
    d. All of the above

7.30   Gastric cancer is associated with which of the following risk factors?
    a. Tobacco use
    b. Alcohol consumption
    c. High intake of smoked or salted meats and fish
    d. Vitamin B_{12} deficiency

7.31   Which of the following factors are associated with a higher incidence of ovarian cancer?
a.   Industrialized nations
b.   Higher education and socioeconomic levels
c.   Lower education and socioeconomic levels
d.   a and b

7.32   Which of the following are risk factors for vulvar carcinoma?
a.   Herpes simplex virus type 2, human papillomavirus, and condylomata
b.   Herpes simplex virus type 1 and HIV
c.   Cervical carcinoma in situ, HIV, and human papillomavirus
d.   Number of sex partners, herpes simplex virus type 2, and condylomata

7.33   Mr. Buck's cancer is reportedly related to his years of exposure to asbestos when he was working in construction. Mr. Buck is 67, worked in construction for 50 years, drinks beer occasionally, and smoked "off and on over the years." From this you can infer that Mr. Buck *most likely* has
a.   Bladder cancer
b.   Mesothelioma or bronchogenic cancer
c.   Gastrointestinal cancer
d.   Oral carcinoma

7.34   In addition to cigarette smoking and occupational exposure, heavy use of which category of drugs has been shown to increase the risk of cancer of the renal pelvis?
a.   Antipsychotics
b.   Nonnarcotic analgesics
c.   Narcotics
d.   Hypnotics

7.35   During his physical examination Mr. Pederson, a coal miner, asks you about his relative risk of developing lung cancer. The best response to his question would be to
a.   Tell him that his risk is due to his exposure to coal
b.   Ask him about his family history of lung cancer and explain that multiple factors cause the disease
c.   Get his demographic information, and ask him about his exposure to tobacco smoke
d.   Ask him about his diet and his smoking history

7.36   Mr. Frank's cancer has been associated with occupational exposure to a carcinogen. He works as a chemical dye manufacturer. Of the following choices, which type is he most likely to have based on this small clue?
a.   Bladder cancer
b.   Colorectal cancer
c.   Testicular cancer
d.   Esophageal cancer

7.37   For individuals that prepare cytotoxic agents, exposure occurs primarily through which of the following routes?
a.   Inhalation
b.   Ingestion
c.   Absorption
d.   All of the above

7.38   The etiology of bladder cancer can be linked to certain risk factors. Which of the following risk factors has been associated with an increased incidence of bladder cancer?
    a. Smoking
    b. Occupational exposure to chemicals used in textile and dye industry
    c. Exposure to *S. haemotobium*
    d. All of the above

7.39   Although the cause has not been established, certain occupations increase an individual's risk of developing a glioma or a meningioma, including
    a. Exposure to wood dust
    b. Exposure to aniline dyes
    c. Exposure to chemicals in pesticides, herbicides, and fertilizers
    d. Exposure to nickel

7.40   Mr. Allen has been exposed to asbestos in the workplace for most of his adult life (he is now 75); Mr. Eliot, 64, has smoked since he was 17; Ms. Frank, 43, calls herself "a dedicated sun-tanner." Which patient is probably at greatest risk for cancer mortality?
    a. Mr. Allen
    b. Mr. Eliot
    c. Ms. Frank
    d. a and b

Prevention Strategies

7.41   There are 44.5 million adult smokers in the United States; 70% want to quit and 40% make a serious attempt to quit each year. How many of these 40% actually succeed?
    a. 30%
    b. 20%
    c. 10%
    d. 5%

7.42   Alexis, 27, brings her mother Margie, 48, in for a breast exam. Both women have avoided regular medical care because they fear the discovery of problems. During the course of the interview, you discover that neither is familiar with the rationale behind regular breast self-examinations (BSEs) or mammography. As part of your patient education plan, you tell them which of the following?
    a. Alexis should have a breast exam every year but should perform BSE monthly; her mother should do both every 6 months.
    b. Alexis should begin getting mammograms annually. Her mother should get one every 2 years.
    c. Margie is the only one who should be getting BSEs at this time; Alexis will, too, at 30 years of age.
    d. Alexis should have a breast exam every 3 years; Margie, every year.

7.43   One of the early signs of ovarian cancer is
    a. Frequent urinary tract infections
    b. Thin bloody vaginal discharge
    c. Heavy and painful menstruation
    d. None of the above; there are usually no early signs of ovarian cancer.

7.44   Physical recognition of cutaneous melanoma by practitioners and those at risk can be initiated by using the ABCDE rule. In this rule *C* stands for
a.   Change in symmetry
b.   Crusting or bleeding
c.   Color variation or dark black color
d.   Cause

7.45   A Baltimore study group focuses on smoking cessation among a specific target population. This group's research is focusing on _____ prevention.
a.   Primary
b.   Secondary
c.   Tertiary
d.   Integrated

7.46   After her father's death from colon cancer, Ellen takes the initiative in preventing colon cancer for herself by eating less fat and more fruits and vegetables and by taking up running. She is engaged in
a.   Illness behavior
b.   Sick role behavior
c.   Health protective behavior
d.   Information-seeking behavior

7.47   Which of the following statements about primary prevention of skin cancers is *false*?
a.   Ultraviolet radiation is strongest during the mid-part of the day.
b.   For most people sunscreen is not required on overcast days.
c.   Certain medications (e.g., oral contraceptives) can make individuals photosensitive.
d.   Surfaces such as sand and water can reflect more than one-half of the ultraviolet radiation onto the skin.

7.48   Which of the following are effective primary preventive strategies for smoking cessation as it relates to head and neck carcinoma?
a.   Increase public awareness of the dangers of smoking
b.   Promote the negative image of smoking in the media
c.   Promote the "Great American Smokeout" program
d.   All of the above

EARLY DETECTION

Health History

7.49   Which of the following statements about dysplastic nevi (DN) is *not* correct?
a.   DN may be familial or nonfamilial.
b.   Most persons affected by DN have about 25–75 abnormal nevi.
c.   DN develop from precursor lesions of cutaneous melanoma, known as congenital nevi.
d.   A distinctive feature of DN is a "fried egg" appearance with a deeply pigmented papular area surrounded by an area of lighter pigmentation.

7.50   Primary risk factors for breast cancer include
a.   Age in the 30- to 45-year group
b.   Family history of breast cancer
c.   Two or more heterosexual relationships
d.   Lower socioeconomic status

7.51   Which of the following statements regarding the *BRCA2* gene is *true*?
   a.   This gene mutation is associated with postmenopausal breast cancer.
   b.   This gene is related to breast cancer in men.
   c.   This gene is associated with early-onset female breast cancer.
   d.   b and c

7.52   A patient arrives at a clinic for cancer risk assessment. The most significant risk factors for the patient are listed below. Based on this information, you determine that one risk factor is specific to the individual yet outside the individual's control. This patient's risk factor is
   a.   Cigarette smoking
   b.   Exposure to asbestos
   c.   Air pollution
   d.   Familial polyposis

7.53   One of the factors that seems to place a woman at higher risk for the development of ovarian cancer is
   a.   Occupational exposure
   b.   Many sexual partners
   c.   Diethylstilbestrol use by the mother
   d.   A history of breast cancer

7.54   Which of the following statements regarding involuntary inhalation of tobacco smoke is *not* accurate?
   a.   There is an increased risk of lung cancer and heart disease among individuals who have never smoked but are living with a spouse who smokes cigarettes.
   b.   There is no evidence to support the idea that involuntary inhalation of tobacco smoke increases the risk of lung cancer in nonsmokers.
   c.   Approximately 17% of lung cancers among nonsmokers can be attributed to high levels of exposure to cigarette smoke during childhood and adolescence.
   d.   Long-term exposure to environmental tobacco smoke increases the risk of lung cancer in women who have never smoked.

7.55   Which of the following statements regarding ovarian cancer risk in families is *not* correct?
   a.   Women who have two or more first-degree relatives with a history of ovarian cancer have a significantly increased risk for ovarian cancer.
   b.   Ovarian cancer is an autosomal dominant mode of inheritance with variable penetrance.
   c.   A woman who has one first-degree relative with ovarian cancer has an overall risk that is two to four times the average risk of having ovarian cancer.
   d.   Ovarian cancer tends to be common among lower income groups, especially African-American, Hispanic, and Native American women.

7.56   Which of the following statements regarding breast cancer risk is *not* accurate?
   a.   Only 5–7% of all breast cancers are due to tumor-suppressor genes *BRCA1* and *BRCA2*.
   b.   As many as 30% of women diagnosed with breast cancer under the age of 35 have inherited susceptibility.
   c.   Most women (70%) who develop breast cancer have no known risk factors.
   d.   A woman with a strong family history of breast cancer has a 70% chance that her cancer is caused by an inherited mutation in the *BRCA1* gene.

7.57   Your patient has prostate cancer and is undergoing leuprolide therapy. He recently began to complain of pain in his hip. He underwent a bone scan and was found to have an isolated lesion that was thought to be malignant. Biopsy was done, and a sarcoma was confirmed. This finding represents which of the following?
a.   This is most likely a metastases from his prostate cancer.
b.   This is histologically dissimilar from a prostate cancer and is therefore considered to be a second primary cancer and potentially curable.
c.   This is most likely a benign condition because he is receiving treatment for cancer.
d.   This finding represents a guarded prognosis because his immune system obviously is failing.

7.58   Mr. Svensen has had treatment for a primary kidney tumor, which was completely eradicated. Now, however, the surgeon discovers a biopsy proven metastatic lesion in the lung. The metastatic site seems to be solitary, and Mr. Svensen is very healthy otherwise. Given these limited clues, what method of treatment will be used for his metastatic lesion?
a.   Chemotherapy to provide systemic control of metastasis
b.   Cytoreductive surgery to reduce the mass so combination therapy will be effective
c.   Combination radiation and chemotherapy
d.   Surgical resection

7.59   The most common second malignant neoplasms following radiation therapy are
a.   Breast carcinomas and gynecologic tumors
b.   Cancers of the gastrointestinal tract
c.   Sarcomas of the bone and soft tissue
d.   Tumors of the bladder and lung

7.60   Your patient is a 5-year survivor of Hodgkin's disease. Your annual workup is conducted with the knowledge that she is most at risk for developing which of the following second primary cancers?
a.   Breast cancer
b.   Leukemia
c.   Lung cancer
d.   Non-Hodgkin's lymphoma

7.61   Mr. Allen, a heavy smoker for 20 years, has lung cancer and has completed his radiation and chemotherapy. He is instructed to return for checkups frequently because he is also at risk for which cancer?
a.   Bladder cancer
b.   Melanoma
c.   Sarcoma
d.   Leukemia

7.62   Tony was treated for bilateral retinoblastoma as a child. His mother comments that he has recently complained of joint pain. You are concerned and order an x-ray of the joint. Your concern is based on which of the following?
a.   Patients with retinoblastoma have a high incidence of metastatic disease to the bone.
b.   Long-term effects of chemotherapy cause joint degeneration.
c.   Radiation causes osteomalacia.
d.   Children with a genetic form of retinoblastoma have a higher incidence of sarcoma.

7.63   Judith had Hodgkin's disease as a child and received mantle radiation therapy. It has been more than 20 years since her treatment. Which of the following statements is *not* correct concerning her follow-up care?
  a.   She needs to continue her annual physical exams and mammograms because she is most at risk for second malignancies at this time.
  b.   She can relax more because her risk for second malignancies decreases every year.
  c.   Her highest risk for second malignancies is breast cancer and lung cancer.
  d.   Second malignancies are most likely to occur in the field of radiation.

7.64   Late effects involving the central nervous system are *most likely* to occur in which of the following individuals?
  a.   A child treated for Hodgkin's disease
  b.   A child treated for bone sarcoma
  c.   An adult treated for small cell carcinoma of the lung
  d.   An adult treated for primary hypothyroidism

7.65   Which of the following statements about the late effects of cancer treatment is *incorrect*?
  a.   Late effects are believed to progress over time.
  b.   Late effects are believed to involve different mechanisms from those of the acute side effects of chemotherapy and radiation.
  c.   Late effects are severe and clinically subtle.
  d.   Late effects are the consequence of biologic cure.

7.66   The risk of developing a second malignant neoplasm after treatment for a primary malignancy depends on several factors, including all of the following *except*
  a.   The type and dose of treatment received (e.g., radiation and alkylating agents)
  b.   A common underlying etiologic factor (e.g., smoking)
  c.   Genetic susceptibility (e.g., genetic retinoblastoma)
  d.   The timing of withdrawal of chemotherapeutic agents (e.g., MOPP latency)

7.67   Four years ago Ms. Smith successfully completed treatment for breast cancer. Now she is diagnosed with acute myelogenous leukemia (AML). Which is *most likely* to have contributed to Ms. Smith's AML?
  a.   Alkylating agents
  b.   Anthracyclines
  c.   Vinca alkaloids
  d.   Antimetabolites

7.68   Mantle radiation for Hodgkin's disease is associated with an increased risk of which of the following cancers?
  a.   Breast cancer, especially in those irradiated before the age of 30
  b.   Lung cancer
  c.   Liver cancer
  d.   None of the above

7.69 Mrs. Ana has breast cancer and has been taking tamoxifen for 4 years. She complains of inter-mittent vaginal bleeding and believes she might be menopausal but is concerned. Your most appropriate advice and rationale would include which of the following?
a. She should not be concerned; she is probably experiencing menopause due to the tamox-ifen and the bleeding should improve over time.
b. Her bleeding is probably due to the hormonal changes caused by the tamoxifen, and she should have follicle-stimulating hormone and luteinizing hormone testing to determine whether she is menopausal.
c. Tamoxifen can cause endometrial changes and even cancer. She needs to see her gyne-cologist for an exam and possibly an endometrial biopsy.
d. Ovarian cancer is common in women who have breast cancer, and she should be exam-ined by her gynecologist.

Physical Exam

7.70 One way that basal cell carcinoma (BCC) is distinguished from squamous cell carcinoma (SCC) is by its
a. Common occurrence on the head and hands
b. Lower incidence
c. Slower growth rate
d. Less well-demarcated margins

7.71 Which of the following is the *most likely* presenting symptom in a patient with lymphoma?
a. Edema in the upper part of the body
b. Enlarged cervical lymph nodes
c. A palpable mass in the axillary or inguinal lymph nodes
d. An upper respiratory infection

7.72 Ms. Allison notices a "funny discoloration" on her arm and comes in for an examination. She tells you that her brother died at age 38 from a common skin cancer. Ms. Allison's brother most likely had and you should be suspicious for
a. Squamous cell carcinoma
b. Basal cell carcinoma
c. Melanoma
d. Leukoplakia

7.73 Mr. Eliot, 64 and a smoker for 17 years, has an undifferentiated neoplasm arising in the prox-imal right bronchus. Which symptom most typically reflects this?
a. Barrel chest
b. Bulges on the thorax
c. Breathlessness
d. Superior vena cava obstruction

7.74 Mrs. Johns is pregnant and discovers a mass in the upper outer quadrant of her left breast. Following her physical exam the physician is *most likely* to order which of the following tests?
a. Ultrasound
b. Fine-needle aspiration
c. Mammogram (diagnostic)
d. a or b

7.75 Mrs. Blase has carcinoma of the oral cavity. Although her main complaint initially concerned a painless lesion that she believed she had had for some time, she has recently begun to report a referred pain in her jaw and increased difficulty chewing and swallowing. This kind of referred pain can indicate
a. Induration
b. Ulceration
c. Pressure affecting adjacent nerves
d. Any of the above

7.76 The most common presenting symptom of testicular cancer is
a. A small hard mass in the scrotum
b. A dragging sensation
c. Swelling
d. Dull aching or pain in the scrotal area

Screening Methods and Recommendations

7.77 Testing for the human papillomavirus (HPV) in addition to the Pap test in women over age 30 is recommended for which of the following reasons?
a. Women who test negative for both tests may not need to be rescreened for up to 3 years.
b. Women with atypical squamous cells of uncertain significance (ASCUS) who test positive for high-risk HPV are candidates for immediate colposcopy.
c. Women with ASCUS who test negative for high-risk HPV are rescreened at a later date.
d. All of the above

7.78 Which of the following statements is *not true* regarding prostate-specific antigen (PSA)?
a. PSA is elevated only in men who have prostate cancer.
b. When tumor destroys the natural tissue barrier, PSA enters the bloodstream.
c. PSA levels are used as a screening test for prostate cancer.
d. Procedures such as biopsies can cause false PSA levels.

7.79 Which of the following tests is recommended by the American Cancer Society and the National Cancer Institute to screen for colorectal cancer?
a. Flexible sigmoidoscopy
b. Digital rectal examination
c. Hemoccult test
d. All of the above

7.80 Early detection of gastric cancer is unlikely because
a. The cancer metastasizes readily
b. People tend to self-medicate themselves for gastrointestinal distress
c. Risk factors for the disease have not yet been identified
d. None of the diagnostic tests or procedures currently available accurately detect gastric cancer in its early stages

7.81 The American Cancer Society recommends that all women who are sexually active or who are 18 years of age or older have a Pap smear performed
a. Every 3 years
b. Every 2 years
c. Annually
d. Biannually

ANSWER EXPLANATIONS

7.1   **The answer is d.** All three factors play some role in the development of bone cancer: familial tendency, prior cancer therapy in the form of high-dose irradiation, and some preexisting bone conditions such as Paget's disease.

7.2   **The answer is a.** Seventy percent of breast cancer occurs in women who are 50 years of age or older.

7.3   **The answer is c.** The highest overall cancer incidence rates occur among African-American men.

7.4   **The answer is b.** For breast cancer the average annual rate per 100,000 individuals has been highest among white females.

7.5   **The answer is b.** In the United States African-American men have a significantly higher incidence of esophageal cancer than white men; similarly, African-American women have a higher incidence of the disease than white women. This type of cancer also seems to develop at a younger age in African-Americans than it does in whites.

7.6   **The answer is d.** Cervical carcinoma is infrequent in women who are nulliparous and those who are celibate or monogamous throughout their lives. Multiparity is a risk factor.

7.7   **The answer is a.** Increased incidence of primary brain tumors is associated with all these choices *except* inhaled steroids.

7.8   **The answer is b.** Attributable risk is the difference in the incidence or death rates between the group exposed to some factor and unexposed groups. It is used to evaluate the magnitude of change in an outcome (e.g., respiratory cancer) with the removal of the suspect antecedent factor (e.g., smoking). Provided that the relative risk and the frequency of the suspect factor in the entire defined population are known, attributable risk can be estimated from a case-control study. Otherwise, it must be calculated directly from a prospective study.

7.9   **The answer is a.** In this prospective study subjects (miners) are being selected with varying degrees of exposure to the suspected factor (asbestos). They have not experienced the outcome thought to be associated with the factor (lung cancer or some other cancer). They are then being followed over time to see whether the outcome (e.g., a type of cancer) occurs.

7.10   **The answer is c.** The prevalence rate is the total number of cases—new and existing—in a given population during a specific time period, in this case 1 year. It is a function of both incidence and duration. In other words, the higher the survival rate (duration) for a type of cancer, the higher its prevalence rate will be.

7.11   **The answer is a.** Japan has the highest incidence of gastric cancer in the world, and stomach cancer is the major cause of death in that country. The incidence of gastric cancer is low in the United States. The dramatic differences in geographic distribution of the disease remain an enigma to epidemiologists.

7.12   **The answer is d.** Because women are now more aware of breast cancer and early detection methods, cancer of the breast is being found when tumors are small and the woman is younger. So it is not that breast cancer is occurring more in younger women, it is that it is being discovered before the tumor is large and the woman is older.

7.13   **The answer is c.** The genes are involved in less than 15% of breast cancer cases.

7.14   **The answer is d.** Even with the predicted declines in mortality rates, the absolute number of lung cancer deaths will continue to rise because of the increasing size of the population.

7.15   **The answer is d.** Young-onset cancers (cancer diagnosed before the age of 50) are increased by 44% among first-degree relatives of never-smoker lung cancer patients compared to control subjects. Male first-degree relatives of lung cancer patients who never smoked have a 36% increased risk of developing cancer within their lifetime and an 89% increased risk of developing young-onset cancer. Approximately 13% of patients with lung cancer are never-smokers.

7.16   **The answer is c.** Hepatocellular carcinomas are associated with environmental and hereditary factors, hepatitis B and hepatitis C viruses, and cirrhosis. Alcoholic cirrhosis is a common risk factor for liver cancer in the United States.

7.17   **The answer is a.** There is a gradual decrease in the former smoker's risk of dying from lung cancer; eventually the risk is almost equivalent to that of a nonsmoker. The rate of decline of risk after cessation of smoking is determined by the cumulative smoking exposure before cessation, the age when smoking began, and the degree of inhalation.

7.18   **The answer is b.** Most studies of differing epidemiologic designs support the hypothesis that high fiber intake is protective against colon cancer, although not all studies are supportive. In studies in which the source of fiber has been examined, fiber from vegetables appears protective against colon cancer, whereas the data for cereal fibers are less supportive of a protective effect.

7.19   **The answer is d.** The synergistic use of both alcohol and tobacco has long been implicated in the etiology of oral cavity malignancies. Insufficient oral hygiene and frequent overuse of harsh mouthwash solutions have been linked to primary cancers of the oral cavity. Deficiencies in vitamin A and regular use of marijuana have also been connected to the development of oral cavity tumors.

7.20   **The answer is c.** Active tobacco use has been linked to many cancer types (lung, oropharyngeal, bladder, and esophagus), and a clear linear relationship exists between the number of cigarettes smoked and the risk of lung and oropharyngeal cancers.

7.21   **The answer is d.** Eighty to 90% of lung cancer deaths are estimated to be caused by cigarette smoking.

7.22   **The answer is d.** Esophageal cancer appears to be associated with heavy alcohol intake, heavy tobacco use, and poor nutrition; cirrhosis, vitamin deficiency, anemia, and poor oral hygiene may be contributing factors.

7.23   **The answer is d.** Females exposed to diethylstilbestrol in utero have a higher incidence of clear cell adenocarcinoma of the cervix and vagina. Human papillomaviruses (HPV) are members of the family of DNA tumor viruses that can cause cellular hyperproliferation and a variety of warty infections. HPV 18 is the most common papillomavirus found in women with adenocarcinoma of the cervix, and HPV 16 is more commonly associated with squamous carcinoma. Herpes simplex virus type 2 (HSV-2) has been shown to be carcinogenic in animals. Women with cervical cancer usually have higher HSV-2 specific antibody titers than do controls.

7.24   **The answer is d.** Several factors may lower a woman's risk of developing preinvasive lesions as precursors to invasive cervical cancer. These include barrier-type contraception; vasectomy; recommended daily allowances of vitamin A, beta-carotene, and vitamin C; limiting the number of sexual partners; and initiating sexual activity at a later age.

7.25   **The answer is c.** Long-term exposure to the sun has been associated with cancer of the lip and oral cancer.

7.26   **The answer is d.** Chronic low-level exposure to radiation and chronic antigenic stimulation are associated with an increased incidence of multiple myeloma.

7.27   **The answer is b.** A risk of breast cancer has been associated with exposure of the breast to ionizing radiation therapy for a broad spectrum of health problems, including chronic mastitis, tuberculosis, and thymus disorders. Mantle radiation for Hodgkin's disease is associated with an increased risk relative to age during treatment. Increased risk starts 10 years after exposure and depends on dose and age at exposure.

7.28   **The answer is d.** Thyroid cancer has increased dramatically in children exposed to high levels of radioactive fallout from the nuclear accidents. High rates of follicular and papillary tumors are noted in individuals with a history of goiter or family history of thyroid disease.

7.29   **The answer is d.** Medical conditions of chronic irritation such as hiatal hernia, gastroesophageal reflux disorder, and diverticula have been cited as possible etiologic factors. Dietary deficiencies of selenium are considered risk factors.

7.30   **The answer is c.** High intake of excessive salt such as smoked or salted meats and fish are correlated with increased gastric cancer risk in populations. Neither smoking tobacco nor drinking alcohol has been demonstrated to increase the risk of gastric carcinoma.

7.31   **The answer is d.** With the exception of Japan, industrialized nations have the highest incidence of ovarian cancer. Women with higher educational and socioeconomic levels tend to delay childbearing, have fewer children, and have a higher incidence of ovarian cancer.

7.32   **The answer is a.**

7.33   **The answer is b.** Asbestos, the major carcinogenic fiber, is believed to be related to about 2000 cases of mesothelioma annually in the United States. However, asbestos causes more bronchogenic cancers than mesotheliomas, perhaps 6000, because of its synergism with tobacco smoke. Lung cancer is rare in asbestos workers who do not smoke. Data do not support an association between gastrointestinal cancer and asbestos.

7.34   **The answer is b.** Heavy use of the nonnarcotic analgesics aspirin and/or acetaminophen has been shown to increase the risk of cancer of the renal pelvis. Similarly, an association has been made between analgesics and renal cell cancer, but this association has not as yet been substantiated.

7.35   **The answer is c.** It is misleading to suggest that coal poses the most obvious risk. By asking Mr. Pederson for demographic information, the nurse would be able to assess his exposure to air pollution and possibly his exposure to radon (certain areas have been identified as higher in radon activity than others). Because tobacco has an interactive and synergistic effect on the development of lung cancer when combined with other carcinogens, this would also be a good factor to explore. Genetics and diet have not been shown to have a significant effect on the development of lung cancer.

7.36 **The answer is a.** One of the strongest risk factors for bladder cancer involves occupational exposure to 2-naphthylamine, benzidine, and aniline dyes. Workers exposed to aromatic amines have a fourfold greater risk of bladder cancer.

7.37 **The answer is d.** Direct exposure to cytotoxic agents can occur during admixture, administration, or handling. Exposure occurs through inhalation, ingestion, or absorption.

7.38 **The answer is d.** The risk factors related to bladder cancer are cigarette smoking, occupational exposure to industrial chemicals, age, gender, and exposure to *S. haemotobium*.

7.39 **The answer is c.** Agricultural workers exposed to multiple chemicals in pesticides, herbicides, and fertilizers have had a higher than expected incidence of gliomas.

7.40 **The answer is b.** Mr. Eliot is at greatest risk. Cigarette smoking is the largest single preventable cause of premature death and disability and the major single cause of cancer mortality. Individuals like Mr. Allen who are exposed to high levels of asbestos and other respiratory carcinogens in the workplace also have an increased risk, but it is not the single major cause of cancer mortality. Cancers of the skin—most often caused by excessive sun exposure—are the most common cancers in humans, but they too are not the major single cause of cancer mortality.

7.41 **The answer is d.** There is a need for innovative prevention and cessation strategies to overcome this low rate of success.

7.42 **The answer is d.** All women starting at age 20 should perform BSE monthly. Women in Alexis' age category (20–40 years of age) should have a breast physical exam every 3 years, and women older than 40 years should have a breast physical examination every year.

7.43 **The answer is d.** Ovarian cancer is typically asymptomatic in its early stages. As the disease progresses women may experience vague abdominal discomfort, leading to loss of appetite, flatulence, or urinary frequency; more often than not, these symptoms are no more than annoying and are not taken seriously by the patient and her physician. By the time a diagnosis of ovarian cancer is made, the cancer has spread beyond the ovary in 75% of cases.

7.44 **The answer is c.** Physical recognition of cutaneous melanoma by practitioners and those at risk can be initiated by using the "ABCDE" rule. In this rule, *A* = asymmetry, *B* = border irregularity, *C* = color variation or dark black color, *D* = diameter greater than 0.6 cm, and *E* = elevation.

7.45 **The answer is b.** Primary prevention is the avoidance of exposure to carcinogens; secondary prevention is the prevention of promotion by smoking cessation, changes in diet, and administration of chemopreventive agents presumed to act on promotion. Tertiary prevention consists of arresting, removing, or reversing a premalignant lesion to prevent recurrence or progression to cancer.

7.46 **The answer is c.** Health-protective behavior consists of actions taken by people to protect, promote, or maintain their health.

7.47 **The answer is b.** Sunscreen should always be applied on overcast days because 70–80% of ultraviolet radiation can penetrate cloud cover.

7.48 **The answer is d.** Avoiding the use of tobacco and alcohol is key to the prevention of head and neck cancer. As public awareness of the dangers of tobacco use grows and a negative image of smoking is portrayed in the media, it is anticipated that the incidence of head and neck cancer will decrease. The campaign of "Through With Chew" is primarily directed toward boys aged 11–17 who might use smokeless tobacco.

7.49 **The answer is c.** DN are precursor lesions of cutaneous melanoma (CM) that develop from normal nevi, usually after puberty. It has been reported that 50% of CM evolves from some form of DN. They may be familial or nonfamilial, with the risk of CM in a family member with DN approaching 100% in melanoma-prone families. DN are often larger than 5 mm and can number from 1 to 100, with most affected persons having 25–75 abnormal nevi. They appear typically on sun-exposed areas, especially on the back, but also may be seen on the scalp, breasts, and buttocks. Pigmentation is irregular, with mixtures of tan, brown, and black or red and pink. A distinctive feature is a "fried egg" appearance.

7.50 **The answer is b.** The primary risk factors for breast cancer are increasing age, family history of breast cancer, history of benign breast disease, late age at first live birth, nulliparity, early age at menarche, late age at menopause, higher socioeconomic status, being Jewish, estrogen replacement therapy, exposure of the female breast to ionizing radiation in infancy, mammographic parenchymal patterns that are dense, having complex fibroadenomas, and being single.

7.51 **The answer is d.** *BRCA2* has been identified on the long arm of chromosome 13 (13q12-13). This mutation seems to be associated with male breast cancer and early-onset female breast cancer.

7.52 **The answer is d.** Choice **a** is individual but under the person's control; choice **b** is typically a group risk factor shared by persons from the same occupation; choice **c** is typically a group risk factor shared by persons from the same geographic residence. Only choice **d**, an inherited condition, is both specific to the individual and, at the same time, outside the person's control.

7.53 **The answer is d.** Hormonal factors such as nulliparity, infertility, and estrogen therapy have been connected to the development of ovarian cancer. A family history of breast cancer or colon cancer doubles the risk of ovarian cancer.

7.54 **The answer is b.**

7.55 **The answer is d.** Ovarian cancer tends to be more common among white upper-income groups in highly industrialized countries. Jewish women experience a 40% higher incidence rate than do African-American, Hispanic, and Native American women.

7.56 **The answer is d.** A woman with a strong family history of breast cancer is generally defined as having four or more genetically related women affected with the disease; about 40% of their cancers are caused by an inherited mutation in the *BRCA1* gene and another 40% by *BRCA2*.

7.57 **The answer is b.** A second primary lesion refers to an additional histologically separate malignant neoplasm in the same patient. A general rule is always to biopsy the first recurrence, because it may represent a new, curable, or treatable malignancy.

7.58 **The answer is d.** Surgery may be used to resect a metastatic lesion if the primary tumor is believed to be eradicated, if the metastatic site is solitary, and if the patient can undergo surgery without significant morbidity.

7.59   **The answer is c.** Sarcomas of the bone and soft tissue are the most common second malignant neoplasms following radiation therapy, with the incidence peaking at 15–20 years following radiation. In a large study of survivors of childhood cancer, the risk of bone cancer was highest among children treated for retinoblastoma and Ewing's sarcoma, but also increased significantly in patients treated for rhabdomyosarcoma, Wilms' tumor, and Hodgkin's disease. In addition to sarcomas and leukemia, a variety of solid tumors have been linked to treatment with radiation, including carcinomas of the breast and tumors of the bladder, rectum, and uterus.

7.60   **The answer is b.** In patients with Hodgkin's disease, there is a 77-fold increased risk of the development of leukemia within 4 years of initial treatment.

7.61   **The answer is a.** Patients with lung cancer are at greater risk for the development of bladder cancer because both tumors are associated with smoking.

7.62   **The answer is d.** Genetic susceptibility is an important factor in case finding. Children with the genetic form of retinoblastoma, which is usually bilateral, have a much higher incidence of sarcoma compared to those with the nongenetic form of the disease.

7.63   **The answer is b.** In a study of survivors of Hodgkin's disease, a 17% cumulative risk of second cancers was noted 20 years posttreatment. The most common tumors were lung and breast cancers, with 77% of the tumors occurring in or adjoining the field of radiation.

7.64   **The answer is c.** The late effects of central nervous system treatment, including neuropsychological, neuroanatomic, and neurophysiologic changes, have been observed most commonly in children with acute lymphoblastic leukemia and brain tumors and in adult small cell carcinoma of the lung patients, all of whom received central nervous system treatment for the primary tumor or as prophylaxis against meningeal disease.

7.65   **The answer is c.** The late effects of treatment for biologic cure result from physiologic changes related to particular treatments or to the interactions among the treatment, the individual, and the disease. Unlike the acute side effects of chemotherapy and radiation, however, late effects are believed to progress over time and by different mechanisms. They can appear months to years after treatment; can be mild, severe, or life threatening; and can be clinically obvious, clinically subtle, or subclinical. Their impact appears to depend on the age and development stage of the patient.

7.66   **The answer is d.** Adults and children who have received chemotherapy or radiation therapy, or both, for a primary malignancy are at increased risk for the development of a second malignant neoplasm. Alkylating agents and ionizing radiation are the treatments most closely linked to a second malignant neoplasm. In addition to the type and dose of treatment received, the risk of the development of a secondary cancer depends on several predisposing factors, including choices **b** and **c**.

7.67   **The answer is a.** Alkylating agents have a demonstrated causative relationship to acute myelogenous leukemia (AML). AML is the most frequently reported second cancer following aggressive chemotherapy for Hodgkin's disease, non-Hodgkin's lymphoma, multiple myeloma, ovarian cancer, and breast cancer.

7.68   **The answer is a.** The risk of breast cancer correlates with increased radiation dosage, especially if a woman is exposed to radiation in the period of young adulthood.

7.69   **The answer is c.** Tamoxifen acts as an antiestrogen on breast tissue but has a weak estrogenic effect on endometrial tissue and has been associated with thickening of the endometrium and changes from polyps to hyperplasia and cancer. Ovarian cancer does occur in women with breast cancer, but bleeding is not a symptom associated with ovarian cancer.

7.70   **The answer is c.** BCC is the least aggressive type of skin cancer and has its origins in either the basal layer of the epidermis or in the surrounding dermal structures. It is most commonly found on the nose, eyelids, cheeks, neck, trunk, and extremities. It grows slowly by direct extension and has the capacity to cause major local destruction. Metastasis is rare and most often occurs in the regional lymph nodes. SCC, on the other hand, may arise in any epithelium. It is most commonly found on the head and hands. It is more aggressive than BCC: It has a faster growth rate, less well-demarcated margins, and a greater metastatic potential. Metastatic disease is usually first noted in the regional lymph nodes.

7.71   **The answer is b.** Three-fourths of lymphoma patients present with enlargement of cervical or supraclavicular lymph nodes, but enlarged axillary or inguinal nodes may be the presenting symptoms. Such nodes are characteristically painless, firm, rubbery in consistency, freely movable, and of variable size. Weakness, fatigue, and general malaise may be a part of the presenting picture.

7.72   **The answer is c.** There are three types of skin cancer: basal cell carcinoma, squamous cell carcinoma, and melanoma. However, melanoma is the most common skin cancer to result in death.

7.73   **The answer is d.** Superior vena cava obstruction is a common complication of lung cancer; approximately 80% of these cases are caused by undifferentiated neoplasms arising in proximal right bronchi. Barrel chest is associated with pulmonary emphysema or normal aging. Bulges on the thorax are often a manifestation of a neoplasm on the ribs. Breathlessness is a more generalized indication of obstruction of the lungs.

7.74   **The answer is d.** Sonography is the imaging modality of choice in a young woman, a pregnant woman, or a lactating woman who has not discovered any lumps or other signs of cancer. Fine-needle aspiration is also appropriate.

7.75   **The answer is d.** Referred pain is an important sign that can indicate induration, ulceration, or pressure affecting adjacent nerves. As the lesion increases in size, the individual may experience difficulty chewing foods and swallowing.

7.76   **The answer is a.** The most common sign of testicular cancer is a small hard mass in the scrotum. However, a dragging sensation, swelling, dull aching, or pain in the scrotal area also may be a presenting symptom.

7.77   **The answer is d.** HPV testing may also have a role in initial cervical cancer screening. The combination of HPV testing and Pap testing for screening women over the age of 30 is recommended. The combination is not recommended for screening younger women because most will have HPV infections that will clear without causing precancerous cervical lesions.

7.78   **The answer is a.** Conditions other than prostate cancer can give rise to elevated PSA levels.

7.79   **The answer is d.** All of these tests are recommended in screening for colorectal cancer.

7.80 **The answer is b.** The earliest symptoms of gastric cancer, such as a sense of fullness or heaviness and moderate distention after meals, are usually vague. Home remedies and self-medications are often used successfully for a while until other symptoms appear. Because of the elusive nature of gastric disorders, this type of cancer is usually quite advanced by the time medical attention is sought.

7.81 **The answer is c.** The American Cancer Society currently recommends that all women who are or have been sexually active or who are 18 years of age or older should have annual Pap smears. After a woman has had three negative annual Pap smears, the test may be performed less frequently at the discretion of her physician.

CHAPTER 8

![Professional Performance]

Professional Performance

APPLICATION OF STATEMENT ON THE SCOPE AND STANDARDS OF ONCOLOGY NURSING PRACTICE

8.1   Which of the following statements regarding Oncology Nursing Society certification by the Oncology Nursing Certification Corporation is *inaccurate*?
   a. Registered nurse licensure is the only education requirement for Oncology Certified Nurse (OCN®).
   b. A BSN is the basic entry into practice requirement to be an OCN®.
   c. Master's degree in nursing is required for the Advanced Oncology Certified Nurse (AOCN®).
   d. A minimum of 500 hours of supervised practice in an advance practice role in oncology nursing is required for the AOCN®.

8.2   Which of the following best describes the difference between the eligibility criteria for the advanced oncology nursing certification examination for the Advanced Oncology Certified Nurse (AOCN®) and the Advanced Oncology Certified Nurse Practitioner (AOCNP)?
   a. To qualify to be certified as an AOCNP, the nurse must be at least master's prepared and complete an accredited nurse practitioner program, whereas the AOCN® only requires a master's degree in nursing.
   b. An AOCN® is qualified to be certified as an AOCNP provided he or she completes a minimum of 500 hours of supervised practice as an advanced practice nurse.
   c. If a nurse is in an advanced practice role, he or she is eligible to become certified as an AOCNP if he or she can pass the test.
   d. To be eligible for the AOCNP, the nurse must spend greater than 50% of his or her time delivering direct patient care.

8.3   Professional nurses occasionally question why it is important to be recertified on a regular basis by the Oncology Nursing Certification Corporation. Which of the following would be a valid response to this issue?
   a. Certification further validates that the nurse is qualified to provide competent care.
   b. Certification is a major component of receiving Magnet Hospital status through the American Nurses Credentialing Center.
   c. Many employers recognize certification through pay differentials.
   d. All of the above

8.4   As a nurse, you know that which of the following is part of your caregiving role?
        a. Determining the meaning of your patient's pain
        b. Deriving nursing diagnoses
        c. Assisting in selecting interventions
        d. All of the above

8.5   The Oncology Nursing Society endorses the title advanced practice nurse to designate
        a. Clinical nurse specialist (CNS) and nurse practitioner (NP) roles in oncology nursing
        b. The merger of the CNS and NP roles
        c. Exclusion of other master's-prepared nurses in education, administration, or research roles
        d. All of the above

8.6   Research comparing whether nursing care by oncology certified nurses (OCN®) results in superior patient care outcomes in comparison to care by noncertified nurses found which of the following to be *true*?
        a. Improved patient outcomes have not been correlated to certification and quality nursing care.
        b. Certified nurses reported higher self-esteem and received better performance ratings from their supervisors than did nurses who were not certified.
        c. Nursing care by OCNs® results in superior patient outcomes in comparison to care by noncertified nurses.
        d. a and b

8.7   Within the conceptual framework for cancer nursing education developed in accordance with the Outcome Standards for Cancer Nursing Practice, which of the following concepts is central to oncology nursing practice?
        a. Community environment
        b. Health care system
        c. Individual and family
        d. Health–illness

8.8   Which of the following generally applies to the nurse specialist at an advanced level of nursing education rather than the generalist level?
        a. A baccalaureate degree
        b. A broader scope of practice
        c. Clinical experience
        d. Conceptual knowledge and skills

8.9   The purpose of the Standards of Oncology Nursing Education is to provide guidelines for *all but* which of the following?
        a. Plan and evaluate generalist education
        b. Plan and evaluate continuing education programs
        c. Provide certification for advanced education programs
        d. Plan and evaluate advanced education

8.10   The mission of the Oncology Nursing Certification Corporation is to advance oncology nursing through the certification process. To be eligible for the certification examination, a nurse must have accomplished *all but* which of the following?
        a. A current registered nurse license
        b. A minimum of 50 continuing education units in the area of oncology nursing practice
        c. One year of experience as a registered nurse over the 3-year period before application
        d. At least 1000 hours of oncology nursing practice within 2.5 years of application for a current license

8.11 To be eligible for the Advanced Oncology Nursing Certification examination, the nurse must have accomplished *all but* which of the following?
   a. Certification in oncology nursing at the basic level
   b. A master's degree or higher
   c. Experience in administration, education, practice, or research
   d. A current registered nurse license

APPROPRIATE SOURCES OF DATA FOR EVIDENCE-BASED PRACTICE

8.12 A genetic variant on chromosome 8 was recently discovered and is thought to be useful in accomplishing which of the following?
   a. Identify individuals at risk for lung cancer
   b. Identify men at risk for prostate cancer
   c. Determine susceptibility to chemotherapy
   d. Determine susceptibility to hormonal therapy

8.13 Which of the following statements is *true* concerning the findings of the National Institutes of Health State-of-the-Science Conference on Tobacco Use: Prevention, Cessation and Control?
   a. More people who have ever smoked have quit.
   b. The number of people who have ever smoked and subsequently quit is about equal.
   c. The highest rate of new smokers is people in their twenties.
   d. Twenty percent of smokers quit after receiving a diagnosis of a smoking-related cancer.

8.14 The primary reason that individuals who seriously try to quit smoking over the course of a year fail is which of the following?
   a. Available smoking cessation interventions are ineffective.
   b. Most people try but do not really want to quit because they believe they cannot succeed.
   c. There is a high out-of-pocket expense for interventions.
   d. Most people are in relationships where their partner smokes, and this contributes to failure of both individuals.

8.15 When reviewing a research survey it is important to ensure whether the survey has been validated for reliability. Which of the following is a type of research reliability measure?
   a. Question and answer format
   b. Test–retest format
   c. External consistency reliability
   d. Connect–disconnect analysis

8.16 One of the statistical methods used to determine reliability is Cronbach's coefficient alpha. Which of the following best describes what this statistical measure refers to?
   a. It is a measure of the strength of the internal consistency of a set of survey questions.
   b. It is a measure of the likeness of individuals being surveyed.
   c. It is a predictive measure of the sameness of the findings as they relate to similar research findings.
   d. It is a measure of whether two observers agree.

8.17 Adjuvant therapy with aromatase inhibitors (AIs) such as letrozole or anastrozole is known to provide a survival benefit for women with breast cancer. A troubling side effect of this therapy and one under investigation includes which of the following?
   a. Increased incidence of second malignancy
   b. Progressive gastrointestinal irritation
   c. Significant bone loss
   d. Increased risk of renal insufficiency

8.18 Which of the following agents is *least likely* to result in loss of bone mineral density?
   a. Leuprolide
   b. Tamoxifen
   c. Anastrozole
   d. Cyclophosphamide

8.19 Which of the following preventive behaviors is recommended to prevent osteonecrosis of the jaw (ONJ) associated with intravenous or oral bisphosphonate therapy?
   a. Steroid therapy
   b. Antibiotic flushes
   c. Avoid invasive dental procedures
   d. All of the above

8.20 A phase IV clinical trial is designed
   a. To address the use of drugs, usually in combination, with cure as the goal of therapy
   b. To answer questions regarding various doses and schedules
   c. To offer new information regarding risks and toxicities
   d. All of the above

8.21 The Breast Cancer Prevention Trial tested the ability of which of the following to prevent breast cancer in healthy women at high risk for the disease?
   a. Sulindac
   b. Retinoic acid
   c. Tamoxifen
   d. Beta-carotene

8.22 A major barrier for both patients and institutions to participation in national studies is which of the following?
   a. Trials sponsored by drug companies pose a financial burden for most oncology programs.
   b. The National Cancer Institute rarely is committed to research to prevent cancer because success is fairly limited; thus it only consistently supports research to improve the quality of life for those who develop cancer.
   c. Third-party payers often do not cover experimental treatment, which includes all research trials.
   d. b and c

8.23 The reliability of a measure can be said to depend on
   a. The homogeneity or consistency of the items on the measurement scale
   b. The extent to which the measure produces the same score when applied at two different times or in two different ways
   c. Test–retest or alternative form and interrater repeatability
   d. All of the above

8.24 Content validity
   a. Need not depend on the degree to which the scale superficially appears to measure the construct
   b. Includes the degree to which the items represent the range of significant attributes
   c. Includes statistical evidence to support inferences
   d. Must include the physical and psychological domains but not the social one (which is covered under construct validity)

8.25 The Quality of Life Index (QLI)
   a. Was originally a patient-rated scale of five areas of functioning (activity, daily living, health, support, and outlook)
   b. Can distinguish cancer patients with terminal illness from those with recent disease or active treatment
   c. Is probably the best example of a "cancer-specific" scale that in reality measures generic health concepts
   d. All of the above

8.26 Evelyn uses the Functional Living Index–Cancer (FLIC) scale to assess a group of patients to determine the impact of cancer on daily issues. The degree to which this scale superficially appears to measure the construct in question is referred to as
   a. Face validity
   b. True content validity
   c. Construct validity
   d. Criterion validity

8.27 Pilot studies are useful to
   a. Assess the feasibility of a research design
   b. Pretest an instrument
   c. Evaluate the risk, side effects, and compliance with a new nursing management approach
   d. All of the above

EDUCATION PROCESS

8.28 Factors that influence health behaviors include knowledge and education level, socioeconomic status, race, and
   a. Residential location
   b. Marital status
   c. Age
   d. Employment status

8.29 The *majority* of health behavior is motivated or maintained by
   a. Immediate consequences
   b. Delayed consequences
   c. Anticipated consequences
   d. Outcome consequences

8.30 Karen knows that cessation of smoking will decrease her cancer risks, but she doubts she can do it. This demonstrates that the *most* important prerequisite for behavior change that involves an individual's beliefs is
a. Reactions of others
b. Verbal persuasion
c. Outcome expectation
d. Efficacy expectation

8.31 The Health Belief Model attempts to explain health behavior and is guided by
a. The assumption that an individual's subjective perception of the environment determines behavior
b. The assumption that people expect treatment and care
c. The assumption that people change their behaviors in response to familial pressures and familial patterns of disease
d. The assumption that people behave in a specific way in response to intense education and peer pressure

8.32 Predictors of behaviors are determined by three variables:
a. Belief in self, perceived susceptibility, and support systems
b. Support systems, perceived barriers, and perceived benefits
c. Perceived barriers, perceived benefits, and belief in self
d. Perceived barriers, perceived susceptibility, and perceived benefits

8.33 The Health Belief Model is based on the principle that
a. The individual must perceive a threat
b. One can accomplish the behavior change or action required
c. Benefits of the behavior change outweigh barriers or negative outcomes
d. All of the above

8.34 During follow-up counseling for your 47-year-old patient with hereditary breast cancer, you mention that she should consider genetic counseling even though her cancer is not due to *BRCA1* or *BRCA2*. To clear up her confusion, you explain which of the following?
a. Women younger than age 50 with hereditary breast cancer have a significant risk of developing contralateral breast cancer in the next 20 years.
b. It is just precautionary to ensure she does not develop cancer that is due to *BRCA1* or *BRCA2*.
c. Counseling would help her decide whether or not she is a candidate for adjuvant hormone therapy.
d. a and c

8.35 A patient with metastatic breast cancer to the bone is beginning therapy with the intravenous bisphosphonate, zoledronic acid. Your teaching regarding potential side effects of this drug includes which of the following?
a. Changes in periodontal and mucosal tissue of the mouth
b. Bone pain and/or arthralgias and myalgias
c. Gastrointestinal irritation
d. a and b

8.36 Your patient is scheduled to have intensity-modulated radiation therapy with low-energy nonthermal light-emitting diode (LED) photomodulation following lumpectomy for stage II breast cancer. Which of the following teaching points is *most appropriate* to describe the purpose of LED photomodulation?
   a. Photomodulation promotes skin repair and collagen buildup.
   b. Photomodulation promotes radiation effect on the possible tumor cells.
   c. Photomodulation enhances the skin-saving effects of modern radiation therapy.
   d. Photomodulation enhances oxygen exposure to neighboring tissues.

8.37 In the development of patient education materials and resources, pretesting is used primarily during which phase(s)?
   a. Planning and strategy selection
   b. Implementation
   c. Evaluation
   d. All of the above

8.38 It is important to evaluate the reading grade level of educational materials before giving them to a patient, because it has been shown that over 20% of Americans read at or below which grade level?
   a. Third grade
   b. Fifth grade
   c. Seventh grade
   d. Eighth grade

8.39 To evaluate the reading grade level of a patient education pamphlet or brochure, the nurse would do *all but* which of the following?
   a. Select approximately 30 sentences at the beginning, the middle, and near the end of the teaching text. Quiz a representative group of patients to determine their level of understanding.
   b. Select approximately 30 sentences at the beginning, the middle, and near the end of the teaching text. Circle all the words containing three or more syllables and total the number of words circled and divide by 3. More than 12 polysyllabic words is unacceptable.
   c. Select approximately 30 sentences at the beginning, the middle, and near the end of the teaching text. Circle all the words containing three or more syllables, and total the number of words circled. Estimate the square root of the total number of polysyllabic words counted and add 3. This gives the reading level the person must have to fully understand the text being assessed.
   d. Find the average number of polysyllabic words per sentence and divide by the total number of sentences. The resulting number is the reading level.

8.40 You are asked to set up a program to teach self-care to patients in follow-up care after major cancer treatments, such as bone marrow or peripheral stem cell transplant patients. Which of the following will you include?
   a. Care of venous access lines
   b. Administration of parenteral fluids
   c. Symptom management
   d. All of the above

8.41   In your community seminar, when you explain the proper technique for breast self-examination, you should *not* include which of the following instructions?
a.   For the visual inspection note symmetry, size, and shape of the breasts.
b.   Examine yourself in front of the mirror with your arms relaxed at your sides.
c.   Examine yourself in front of the mirror with your hands pressed on your hips.
d.   Examine yourself in front of the mirror with your arms folded behind your back.

8.42   The purpose of the Cancer Patient Education Network is to
a.   Create a database that is readily accessible to cancer patients through any local or regional American Cancer Society office, with the eventual goal of database access from any clinic or physician's office in the United States
b.   Improve communication among health care professionals on cancer education needs and advances
c.   Provide an outreach program from a variety of local or regional offices to serve as a catalyst for cancer education initiatives in these regions and for providing technical assistance for activities related to those initiatives
d.   a and c

8.43   A student nurse under your supervision is about to perform her first breast examination on a patient with known pathology. You know she is using proper technique when she tells you
a.   "I should palpate the normal breast first."
b.   "It is important to press firmly to detect subtle differences beneath the cutaneous layers."
c.   "After the patient is supine, I will start at the armpit and palpate in increasingly small circles, slowly moving in toward the center and finishing at the nipple area."
d.   "The patient can have the examination in an upright position if she is more comfortable."

8.44   In planning a staff education program, which of the following would *least likely* be considered critical to the principles of adult learning?
a.   Adults are independent learners.
b.   An adult's past experiences may be a hindrance to learning.
c.   An adult's readiness to learn comes from life's developmental stages.
d.   Adult learning is task or problem oriented.

8.45   The *best* teaching approach to enable the cancer nurse to keep up with the changing health care environment, treatment modalities, and the nurse's numerous roles and responsibilities is
a.   Didactic lecture
b.   Hospital training with minimal lecture
c.   Self-directed learning
d.   Structured inflexible course work

LEGAL ISSUES

8.46   Failure mode and effect analysis (FMEA) is a risk analysis technique that is used to examine which of the following?
a.   Root-cause analysis
b.   Pharmacy errors in drug dispensing
c.   Risk analysis technique to examine the chemotherapy administration process
d.   Errors in drug administration as it relates to method of administration

8.47 The major difference between root-cause analysis and failure mode and effect analysis (FMEA) as it relates to chemotherapy administration is which of the following?
   a. They are the same process where root-cause analysis follows FMEA.
   b. FMEA is designed to prevent chemotherapy errors.
   c. Root-cause analysis is a prospective risk analysis.
   d. Both FMEA and root-cause analysis provide a "fail-safe" process in drug administration.

8.48 In instances where the advanced practice nurse (APN) is employed by a physician, the physician is able to bill 100% of the Medicare fee schedule for the services provided by the APN as long as which of the following requirements are met?
   a. Physician must be present in the office at the time of the patient's visit.
   b. The patient is being seen for a preexisting problem.
   c. The physician must countersign the patient's chart.
   d. a and b

8.49 The authority for the advanced practice nurse (APN) to prescribe drugs is regulated at the state level but also involves the Drug Enforcement Administration. Whether the nurse has dependent prescriptive authority or independent prescriptive authority is based primarily on which of the following?
   a. Dependent prescriptive authority requires the APN be under the supervision of a physician when performing this task.
   b. Dependent prescriptive authority permits the APN to prescribe only nonnarcotic medications independent of the physician.
   c. Independent prescriptive authority is given only when the APN is certified at the doctoral level.
   d. Independent prescriptive authority requires the APN to be prepared at the doctoral level, attend pharmacology courses, and to be under the direct supervision of the responsible physician.

8.50 While administering chemotherapy to your patient, she mentions she is worried she might be forced to quit her job because her boss forces her to take vacation days when she comes for therapy. She works for a small business owner but states she can always get one of the other 10 employees to cover for her. Your counsel is based on which of the following facts regarding the Americans with Disabilities Act (ADA)?
   a. Provided she has coverage the employer must make reasonable effort to accommodate her needs during therapy.
   b. The patient is not required to get coverage when she is absent due to treatment.
   c. She is not protected by the ADA because she works for a small business owner.
   d. She should see a lawyer to learn more about her rights because she has a right to sue to keep her job.

8.51 If Ann is guilty of misappropriation in the course of conducting her research, she has *most likely*
   a. Misused the research funds entrusted to her through a grant
   b. Committed plagiarism
   c. Tagged her study onto an existing protocol rather than initiating a new project
   d. Deliberately omitted facts or fabricated data and findings

8.52   Following World War II the Nuremberg Code was established to delineate legal responsibility for patient education in the area of informed consent. Content central to this code includes *all but* which of the following?
   a.   The use of voluntary consent to protect human subjects in experimentation
   b.   The use of coercion as deemed necessary to provide quality care
   c.   The individual is capable of providing consent
   d.   An understanding of the risks and benefits

8.53   Which of the following organizations have developed specific requirements for cancer patient education, with responsibilities assigned to nurses and other health professionals?
   a.   The Joint Commission for the Accreditation of Healthcare Organizations (JCAHO)
   b.   The Centers for Medicare and Medicaid Services
   c.   The Association of Community Cancer Centers
   d.   All of the above

ETHICAL ISSUES

8.54   In a research study four basic elements are required to be included in the informed consent document. Which of the following is *not* one of these essential elements?
   a.   Compensation
   b.   Understanding
   c.   Comprehension
   d.   Competence

8.55   The primary ethical struggle in clinical research is which of the following?
   a.   Accurate documentation
   b.   Patient participation
   c.   Construct and execution of the study
   d.   Institutional Review Boards

8.56   A patient with metastatic cancer is admitted to the unit with uncontrolled pain. The physician has ordered morphine as the primary pain medication. The patient frequently requests more pain medication. You suspect he is a drug abuser and has an addiction problem. The most appropriate nursing action would be to do which of the following?
   a.   Substitute other medications in the place of narcotics.
   b.   Refer him to a drug addiction program.
   c.   Call the physician to increase his pain medication.
   d.   Administer less potent analgesics along with the morphine to stretch the effect of the narcotic.

8.57   One of the four ethical principles guiding clinical practice is nonmaleficence. To what does this term refer?
   a.   Helping the patient to balance the benefits against the risks
   b.   Distributing the resources in a fair and reasonable way
   c.   Helping the patient make decisions that are right for him or her
   d.   Avoiding practices that will do harm to the individual

8.58   Which of the following have been identified by the Oncology Nursing Society Ethics Advisory Council as the two most important ethical issues to be addressed?
a.   Advanced directives and end-of-life care
b.   Assisted suicide and end-of-life decisions
c.   Assisted suicide and pain management
d.   Pain management and end-of-life care

8.59   The *Ethical Workup Guide* states that health caregivers should
a.   Construct an exhaustive list of possibilities and relevant ethical issues
b.   Take a position on ethical theory
c.   Decide on an ethically based course of action for a patient
d.   Make decisions based on more than one ethical value

8.60   Research has demonstrated that when confronted with a life-threatening illness, spirituality helps patients to accomplish which of the following before dying?
a.   Define the role of religion in their lives
b.   Find trust in their caregivers
c.   Find a sense of meaning despite the illness
d.   Confirm their belief in a higher power

8.61   The Ethics Advisory Council of the Oncology Nursing Society (ONS) has identified five core values for applying the American Nurses Association (ANA's) Code for Nurses. Which of the following is *not* among the ONS's five core values for nurses?
a.   Respectful care
b.   Quality of care
c.   End-of-life issues
d.   Fairness

PATIENT ADVOCACY

8.62   Research concerning cognitive changes associated with systemic cancer treatment demonstrates that compared to control subjects and to normative data, people who received systemic cancer treatment demonstrated impairment in which of the following areas?
a.   Information processing
b.   Spatial skill
c.   Verbal memory
d.   Attention deficit

8.63   While teaching your 41-year-old female patient about the side effects of high-dose chemotherapy she asks you about the possibility that she may become menopausal. Your discussion is based on which of the following research findings regarding risk of menopause as it relates to high-dose chemotherapy?
a.   Because the treatment is dose dense, lasting only 9 weeks, she is not likely to experience permanent menopause.
b.   High-dose chemotherapy is associated with a high rate (90%) of ovarian failure.
c.   She has a 55% risk of permanent menopause.
d.   Data are not available to address this issue with certainty.

8.64   Your 36-year-old patient with testes cancer is completing a course of curative chemotherapy and begins to inquire about his ability to father children and whether or not they might have a higher risk of birth defects as a result of his treatment. Your most appropriate response would include which of the following?
a.   Men with azoospermia immediately after chemotherapy will not recover a sperm count.
b.   Chromosomal abnormalities have been observed in survivors and could result in miscarriages or still births, so he should not pursue fathering a child.
c.   It is recommended that men wait at least 6 months after the end of cancer treatment before attempting to conceive children.
d.   It is recommended that men wait at least 2 years after the end of cancer treatment before attempting to conceive children because most recurrences occur in that time period.

8.65   Which of the following *most accurately* describes the National Coalition for Cancer Survivorship (NCCS)?
a.   It provides referral to local support services for patients and families.
b.   It addresses barriers to employment and access to health insurance.
c.   It advocates for changes in health care delivery.
d.   All of the above

8.66   The Patient Self-Determination Act (PSDA) was passed by the U.S. Congress in 1990. This act requires that all health care institutions do which of the following?
a.   Ensure health care to all regardless of ability to pay
b.   Provide all patients with written information regarding informed consent
c.   Provide written information regarding financial obligations
d.   Provide written information about advanced directives

8.67   Which of the following statements concerning advanced directives (AD) is *false*?
a.   An AD is a statement made by a competent person that directs their medical care in the event that they become incompetent.
b.   ADs do not address all possible medical situations, only terminal conditions due to illness or injury.
c.   An AD is a legally binding contract.
d.   A directive may not always be honored due to the inability of medicine to determine the terminality of the patient's condition.

8.68   The primary goal of the Patient Self-Determination Act is to
a.   Facilitate a systematic process of eliciting and honoring patient wishes
b.   Control health care costs in the last 6 months of life
c.   Require health care institutions to notify patients on admission of their rights under the law to execute an advance directive
d.   Facilitate a responsible use of technological intervention

8.69   A patient makes some comments about a living will that leads you to conclude the patient needs more information. You know he understands what a living will is when he says it
a.   Specifies disbursement of assets
b.   Addresses all possible medical situations
c.   May not always be honored and implemented
d.   All of the above

QUALITY ASSURANCE

8.70　According to the revised and broadened definition of palliative care from the World Health Organization the goal is to promote integration of palliative care earlier in the course of illness. As a result of this effort which of the following might also occur?

a.　Patients would enter hospice later rather than earlier.

b.　Patients would feel less abandonment from their caregivers.

c.　Reimbursement for palliative care can be captured under traditional and existing reimbursement coding.

d.　Continuity of care could suffer.

8.71　Which of the following chemotherapeutic agents is lethal if injected intrathecally and to assure patient safety it has special United States Pharmacopeia (USP) labeling and packaging that must be removed before administration?

a.　Cytarabine

b.　Methotrexate

c.　Vincristine

d.　Interferon

8.72　The Joint Commission on Accreditation of Healthcare Organizations National Patient Safety Goals and Recommendations includes all but which of the following?

a.　Improve safety when using oxygen

b.　Improve the effectiveness of alarm systems in patient care areas

c.　Improve safety when using infusion pumps

d.　Improve safety when stocking, ordering, and dispensing medications

8.73　As we increase the quality of any service while maintaining costs, we

a.　Decrease its value

b.　Lose profitability

c.　Increase the value

d.　None of the above

8.74　Critical paths consist of

a.　Emergency oncological care based on triage followed by categorization and individualized treatment plans

b.　Methods used to resolve oncology care problems through critical thinking

c.　A series of interventions designed to attain specific patient outcomes for a defined group of patients within a specific time frame

d.　All of the above

8.75　Guidelines for handling antineoplastic agents in the home are in accordance with those established by

a.　The U.S. Food and Drug Administration

b.　The Occupational Safety and Health Administration

c.　The American Nurses Association

d.　The Health Care Financing Administration

8.76   Accurate and timely documentation is crucial to the solvency of a home care agency because it is required for
a. Reimbursement
b. Continued referrals
c. Medical consultations
d. Access to hospital records

PROFESSIONAL DEVELOPMENT

8.77   The Coalition for Patients' Rights (CPR) was formed in response to efforts by the American Medical Association (AMA) and other physician groups to affect the practice of licensed health care professionals to provide care to millions of patients. The goal of the CPR is to accomplish which of the following?
a. Promote the efforts of the AMA, thereby promoting practice rights of CPR members.
b. Oppose the efforts of the AMA, thereby promoting practice rights of CPR members.
c. Promote research that examines the qualifications of allied health professionals in rural and underserved areas.
d. Encourage the AMA to advise consumers, regulators, policymakers, and insurers on the qualifications of allied health professionals in general.

8.78   The Balanced Budget Act of 1997 was amended in 1999 to provide Medicare Part B reimbursement to advanced practice nurses (APNs). These nurses are reimbursed at what percentage according to what physicians receive for services in the Physician Fee Schedule?
a. 90%
b. 85%
c. 75%
d. 50%

8.79   The nurse practitioner (NP) is a registered nurse who has advanced education and clinical training in a specialty area. The primary difference between an adult, family, pediatric, or acute care (NP) is which of the following?
a. Educational requirements are essentially the same.
b. A family NP is more general and not considered "advanced" compared to the other practitioner roles.
c. A family NP requires a clinical doctorate in nursing.
d. A master's degree is common but not a baseline requirement for an adult NP.

8.80   The four functional roles of the clinical nurse specialist (CNS) are which of the following?
a. Case management, family counseling, education, consultation
b. Managed care advocate, collaboration, research, clinical practice
c. Acute care, education, consultation, management
d. Clinical practice, education, consultation, research

8.81   According to the Oncology Nursing Society (ONS) the primary difference between an oncology clinical nurse specialist (CNS) and a nurse practitioner (NP) is which of the following?
a. There is no significant difference between these terms.
b. NP is a nurse who has completed an NP program at the master's or doctorate level.
c. CNSs deliver direct care to patients, whereas NPs are more like doctor's assistants.
d. All CNSs are NPs, whereas not all NPs are considered CNSs.

8.82 Specialty certification among health care providers has concentrated on *all but* which of the following avenues of inquiry?
a. Identification of characteristics that differentiate certified and noncertified providers
b. Describing variations in practice that are associated with certification
c. Describing the role of labor unions and demands for certification among health care providers
d. Linking provider certification to patient outcomes

8.83 Terrence is an oncology advanced practice nurse (OAPN) who chooses to work as a consultant rather than as a direct care provider. The OAPN in secondary care may be involved in any of the following *except*
a. Discussing the treatment plan and expected outcomes with the patients and family
b. Planning and implementing initiatives aimed at patient and family education and support
c. Pain and symptom management
d. Establishing standards for oncology practice and developing critical pathways

8.84 Faculty consultation in clinical settings, faculty–clinical staff research projects, and faculty–clinical staff manuscript preparation are all examples of efforts to
a. Identify new research topics
b. Maintain faculty clinical competence
c. Increase academic and hospital revenue
d. Recruit students

8.85 Which of the following is *not* required for use of the designation "oncology certified nurse"?
a. A minimum of 1 year experience as a registered nurse within the last 3 years
b. A baccalaureate degree with credits toward a master's degree
c. A minimum of 1000 hours of cancer nursing practice within the last 2.5 years
d. A passing score on the Oncology Nursing Certification Corporation certification examination

MULTIDISCIPLINARY COLLABORATION

8.86 Ambulatory oncology services have increased over the past few years for all of the following reasons *except*
a. Economic pressures
b. Developments in cancer treatment
c. Innovation in cancer technology
d. Decreased patient acuity

8.87 The hospital in your community approaches a number of physicians and meets with them, campaigning to form a contractual relationship to increase the opportunity to obtain managed-care contracts and align the organizational structure with the financial incentives found in capitation. Such an arrangement is referred to as a
a. Physician–hospital organization (PHO)
b. Preferred provider organization (PPO)
c. Health maintenance organization (HMO)
d. None of the above

8.88   A Chicago physician–hospital organization (PHO) is organized into an integrated delivery system that uses different sites in the community to provide a wide variety of services. This is referred to as
a.   Vertical integration
b.   Horizontal integration
c.   Depth of services
d.   None of the above

8.89   Karen is a nurse practitioner (NP) working in a collaborative practice. In general, in a collaborative practice which of the following is considered basic to success?
a.   NPs function independently in caring for a caseload of patients in the ambulatory setting.
b.   NPs function independently in caring for a caseload of patients in the acute care setting.
c.   The skills of the provider are matched with the needs of the patient.
d.   All of the above

8.90   You are working in an oncology center that has just hired unlicensed assistive personnel (UAP). It is your responsibility to determine the basic guidelines for use of UAP. You establish that UAP may provide
a.   Treatment assessment
b.   Direct patient care
c.   Symptom management planning
d.   All of the above

ANSWER EXPLANATIONS

8.1   **The answer is b.** A graduate-level or bachelor's in nursing degree is not required to be an oncology certified nurse (OCN®).

8.2   **The answer is a.** To qualify to be certified as an AOCN® the nurse must be a licensed registered nurse with a minimum of a master's degree in nursing with a minimum of 500 hours of supervised practice in an advanced practice role in oncology nursing. To be eligible for the AOCNP the nurse must be a licensed registered nurse with at least a master's degree in nursing, but, most important, they must have successfully completed an accredited nurse practitioner program and have a minimum of 500 hours of supervised clinical practice as an oncology nurse practitioner.

8.3   **The answer is d.** An increasing number of employers want certified nurses as employees. Although certification does not validate who we are as nurses or as people, certification does validate that nurses have met stringent requirements for knowledge and experience and are qualified to provide competent care. Nurses who are not certified may provide competent care, but earning oncology certification provides strong evidence beyond a person's claim.

8.4   **The answer is d.** All of these are part of the nursing role as defined by the Oncology Nursing Society as well as describing pain, identifying aggravating and relieving factors, determining individuals' definitions of optimal pain relief, and evaluating efficacy of interventions.

8.5   **The answer is a.** The Oncology Nursing Society (ONS) endorses the title *advanced practice nurse* (APN) to designate clinical nurse specialist (CNS) and nurse practitioner (NP) roles in oncology nursing. The ONS notes that the term *advanced practice nurse* neither implies the merger of the CNS and NP roles nor excludes other master's-prepared nurses in education, administration, or research roles.

8.6   **The answer is d.** Specialty certification is the postentry level credential recognized by most health care professions and has been identified as a desirable indication of clinical competence and quality care. Although research has demonstrated that certified nurses have higher self-esteem and receive better performance ratings from their supervisors than do nurses who are not certified, little evidence exists that certification results in superior patient care.

8.7   **The answer is c.** Central to cancer nursing practice is the individual–family concept. The health–illness concept is the adaptation of the individual and family along a continuum. The practice of cancer nursing occurs in the health care system. The community–environment concept provides the resources and support necessary for individuals with cancer.

8.8   **The answer is b.** Cancer nursing is practiced by both nursing generalists and nursing specialists. Nursing generalists have conceptual knowledge and skills acquired through basic nursing education, clinical experience, and professional development and updated through continuing education. They meet the concerns of individuals with cancer and provide care in a variety of health care settings. Nursing specialists have substantial theoretical knowledge gained through preparation for a master's degree. They meet diversified concerns of cancer patients and their families and function in a broader scope of practice.

8.9   **The answer is c.** The purpose of the standards is to provide guidelines to plan and evaluate generalist education, advanced education, and continuing education programs at all levels. Another purpose is to assess individual knowledge of oncology nursing care. The purpose is to provide guidelines for evaluation, but not to certify.

8.10   **The answer is b.** Nurses are not required to have continuing education units to take the exam.

8.11   **The answer is a.** Nurses do not need to be certified in oncology nursing before taking the advanced certification exam.

8.12   **The answer is b.** The genetic variant on chromosome 8 may account for 8% of prostate cancers in the men of European descent and 16% of prostate cancers in African-American men. Tests for this genetic variant could help identify men who would benefit from earlier or more frequent prostate cancer screening.

8.13   **The answer is a.** With 46 million former smokers in the United States today, more people who have ever smoked have quit, an accomplishment worth emphasizing. Currently available tobacco cessation interventions are effective and could double or triple the quit rates compared to smokers quitting on their own, but not nearly enough smokers request or are offered these interventions.

8.14   **The answer is c.** Evidence indicates that interventions such as medications—including nicotine replacement therapy and bupropion—telephone quitlines, and counseling are individually effective and even more effective in combination. The problems include a lack of awareness among smokers about the availability of existing effective treatments; the high out-of-pocket expense for interventions; and the low percentage of health care professionals who counsel their patients, offer interventions, and provide follow-up.

8.15   **The answer is b.** Surveys must be validated for reliability to ensure that the participants understand the questions in the way the researchers intended to the questions to be understood. Types of reliability measures include alternate form, internal consistency, interobserver, intraobserver, and test–retest formats.

8.16   **The answer is a.** Cronbach's coefficient alpha is a statistic that measures the strength of the internal consistency or homogeneity of a set of survey questions. It is an assessment that measures the extent to which items included on a questionnaire focus on a particular domain (e.g., patient satisfaction, well-being).

8.17   **The answer is c.** The large anastrozole, tamoxifen alone or in combination study, known as the ATAC study, compared anastrozole, tamoxifen, and the combination of both drugs as first-line adjuvant therapy in over 9,000 women. There was a significantly higher incidence of fracture with anastrozole compared with tamoxifen. Bone density in AI-treated patients was lower at 1 year relative to baseline and was further decreased after the second year. The lower bone marrow density at longer follow-up suggest that AI-associated bone loss may be progressive over time.

8.18   **The answer is b.** One of the most beneficial aspects of tamoxifen therapy is that it has bone-protective effects. This was demonstrated in the ATAC trial (see answer 8.17 above), where there was less evidence of fractures in the tamoxifen-only group.

8.19   **The answer is c.** Mouth rinses and antibiotics may be used to treat ONJ, but there is no evidence it helps to prevent it. Steroids are contraindicated in patients at risk for ONJ. Patients who need invasive dental work should have it done well in advance of beginning bisphosphonate therapy, and they should be well aware of the risk associated with this treatment.

8.20   **The answer is d.** Postmarketing or phase IV studies are usually designed to answer questions regarding other uses, doses, and schedules as well as new information regarding risks and toxicity of a new treatment.

8.21   **The answer is c.** The Breast Cancer Prevention Trial tested tamoxifen as a chemopreventive agent in a randomized double-blind trial.

8.22   **The answer is c.** A major barrier for both patients and institutions to participation in national studies is that third-party payers often do not cover experimental treatment, which includes all research trials. Trials sponsored by drug companies generally do not pose a financial concern for oncology programs. The National Cancer Institute clearly is committed to research to prevent cancer as well as to improve the quality of life for those who develop cancer.

8.23   **The answer is d.** Two synonyms for reliability are repeatability and consistency. Repeatability is the extent to which a measure, applied two different times (test–retest) or in two different ways (alternative form and interrater), produces the same score. Consistency is the homogeneity of the items of a scale. Reliability is not a fixed property of measure, and it cannot be assumed to be generalizable.

8.24   **The answer is b.** Content validity includes both face validity (the degree to which the scale superficially appears to measure the construct in question) and true content validity (the degree to which the items accurately represent the range of attributes covered by the construct). Content validity does not include statistical evidence to support inferences made from tests, but it should cut across at least three broad domains (e.g., the physical, psychological, and social) to be considered valid from the perspective of item content.

8.25   **The answer is c.** The QLI is probably the best example of a "cancer-specific" scale that in reality measures generic health concepts. It was originally a physician-rated scale of five areas of functioning (activity, daily living, health, support, and outlook). It has been shown to distinguish cancer patients with terminal illness from those with recent disease or active treatment, as was once popularly assumed.

8.26   **The answer is a.** The degree to which a scale superficially appears to measure the construct in question is referred to as face validity. The degree to which the items accurately represent the range of attributes covered by the construct is called true content validity. Criterion validity includes both concurrent and predictive validity. Data collected simultaneously with the scale data provide evidence of concurrent validity; data collected after the scale data provide evidence for predictive validity. Construct validity extends criterion validity to test the scale in question against a theoretical model and adjusts it according to results to help refine theory.

8.27   **The answer is d.** Pilot studies are useful to assess the feasibility of a research design; to pretest an instrument; and to evaluate the risk, side effects, and compliance with a new nursing management approach.

8.28   **The answer is c.** Age has an influence on health behaviors.

8.29   **The answer is c.** Anticipated consequences, rather than immediate consequences, determine most health behaviors.

8.30   **The answer is d.** Efficacy expectations are the most important prerequisite for behavior change, because stronger efficacy expectations produce more active and sustained efforts in the face of adverse conditions.

8.31   **The answer is a.** The Health Belief Model attempts to explain health behavior and is guided by the assumption that an individual's subjective perception of the environment determines behavior.

8.32   **The answer is d.** Perceived barriers, perceived susceptibility, and perceived benefits are strong predictors of behavior; perceived barriers are the most powerful single predictor. Perceived susceptibility is the weakest predictor but appears to be strongly related to sick role behaviors.

8.33   **The answer is d.** The Health Belief Model is based on the principles that the individual must perceive a threat and believes that something can be done about it. This second expectation has three components: that a behavior change or action will reduce either the severity of or the susceptibility to the threat, that one can accomplish the behavior change or action required, and that benefits of the behavior change outweigh barriers or negative outcomes.

8 Professional Performance

8.34 **The answer is d.** After 20 years the probability of developing contralateral breast cancer is approximately 27% among women with hereditary breast cancer compared to 5% among women with breast cancer in the general population. The risk of contralateral breast cancer is highest among women with hereditary breast cancer that is diagnosed before the age of 50. More than 40% of women in this group develop contralateral breast cancer during the 20 years after their initial breast cancer diagnosis. Adjuvant hormone therapy reduces the risk of contralateral breast cancer.

8.35 **The answer is d.** Oral bisphosphonates cause esophagitis and esophageal ulcers or erosions, requiring that patients remain upright for varying periods after taking the medication. Zoledronic acid is associated with osteonecrosis of the jaw (ONJ) slightly more often than those treated with pamidronate. Early symptoms of ONJ include changes in periodontal and mucosal tissues, soft-tissue infection or swelling, oral mucosal lesions that fail to heal, oral or jaw pain or numbness, and loose teeth.

8.36 **The answer is a.** Exposing women to LED photomodulation can significantly reduce painful treatment-interrupting skin reactions. The process consists of LEDs in a specific array that emits a nonthermal low-energy light at a pulsating frequency. It promotes skin repair. Fibroblasts repair themselves to build up the collagen.

8.37 **The answer is a.** In the development of patient education materials and resources, pretesting is used primarily in the following phases: planning and strategy selection, selecting processes and materials, and developing materials and pretests.

8.38 **The answer is b.** One aspect of printed patient educational materials that has received considerable attention in the nursing literature is reading level. It is estimated that 20% of Americans read below the fifth-grade level. A fifth-grade reading level has been identified as the minimum reading level for making good use of basic written material.

8.39 **The answer is c.**

8.40 **The answer is d.** Self-care teaching and written guidelines for patients and families about care of venous access lines, administration of parenteral fluids, and symptom management are critical to effective management of patients in an ambulatory environment.

8.41 **The answer is d.** In a proper breast self-examination, the woman should stand in front of the mirror, noting the size, shape, and symmetry of her breasts. She should examine herself with her arms relaxed at her side, with her hands pressed on her hips, and with her arms overhead, but not with her arms folded behind her.

8.42 **The answer is b.** The purpose of the Cancer Patient Education Network is to improve communication among health care professionals regarding cancer education needs and advances.

8.43 **The answer is a.** The examiner should palpate the normal breast first. It is important to press very lightly (not firmly) and gently to detect subtle differences. When the patient is supine, the examiner starts at the areolar area and palpates in increasingly wider concentric circles. Finally, the patient is to be in a supine position.

8.44 **The answer is b.** Adults' past experiences are resources for learning and should be drawn on to enhance the learning process. Self-images are often defined, at least in part, by adults' past experiences, and they have a deep investment in their value.

8.45 **The answer is c.** Adult learning concepts, including problem-centered approaches to teaching, immediate application of knowledge, recognition of individual experience, flexible scheduling, and self-directed learning, must be incorporated into educational offerings.

8.46 **The answer is c.** Promoting a culture of safety involves a philosophical shift from error measurement to *proactive* assessment of potential harm. Failure mode and effect analysis is a *prospective* risk analysis technique that can be used to examine the chemotherapy administration process. It is a systematic, multidisciplinary, team-based approach to error *prevention*, which is why the other choices are not correct.

8.47 **The answer is b.** FMEA is a prospective risk management approach that allows cancer centers to potentially prevent chemotherapy errors rather than react to them, as is done in root-cause analysis, which is a retrospective process conducted after chemotherapy errors have occurred. The fundamental purpose of FMEA is to recommend and take actions to reduce the likelihood of process errors (failures).

8.48 **The answer is d.** Physicians may bill for 100% of the Medicare fee schedule for the services provided by the APN as long as the following requirements for incident to services are met:
1. The collaborating physician must be present in the same office suite.
2. The patient must have been seen by the physician at least once, and a plan of care must be documented by the physician.
3. The patient must not have a new problem.
4. Services must be of the type commonly provided in a physician's office.
5. The physician need not countersign the patient's chart, but the office schedule must document the physician's presence in the office at the time of the patient's visit.

8.49 **The answer is a.** The level of prescriptive authority varies from independent prescriptive authority including controlled substances to dependent prescriptive authority excluding controlled substances. The dependent authority requires that the APN be under supervision of a physician when performing this task. The task may be prescribing controlled or non-controlled substances. Some states may require documentation of a certain amount of pharmacology coursework, but a doctorate is not required.

8.50 **The answer is c.** The ADA requires employers to make reasonable accommodation for employees with a disability. Cancer is considered a disability under the ADA. Scheduling changes would be considered reasonable, for example, but turning a full-time job into a part-time job is not required. The ADA applies to employers with 15 or more employees, so patients with disabilities who are employed by small businesses are not protected.

8.51 **The answer is b.** Misappropriation refers to an intentional or reckless act of plagiarism or a violation of the confidentiality associated with the review of scientific manuscripts or grants.

8.52 **The answer is b.** Central to this code is the use of voluntary consent to protect human subjects in experimentation. Such consent assumes not only the ability to consent and freedom from coercion, but also that there is an understanding of the risks and benefits and that the subject is giving an informed consent.

8 Professional Performance

8.53 **The answer is d.** In addition to legal obligations for patient education, a variety of accreditation or other certifying standards address specific requirements for patient education, with responsibilities assigned to nurses and other health professionals. In 1993 the JCAHO reorganized its standards for accreditation to bring stronger focus to the area of patient and family education. Other agencies and organizations have joined this call for patient education as an integral part.

8.54 **The answer is a.** Legal, regulatory, medical, and ethical groups have described the process of informed consent to contain four essential elements: understanding, comprehension, voluntariness, and competence.

8.55 **The answer is b.** The primary ethical struggle in clinical research is that comparatively few individuals accept the risk of being research subjects in order to benefit others and society. Ethicists raise the point that asking subjects to bear the risk of harm for the good of others creates the potential for maltreatment or misuse.

8.56 **The answer is c.** Failure of the nurse and her employer to fulfill their obligations and responsibilities could result in increased pain and suffering, leading to emotional and mental anguish. Ethically, regardless of whether the patient is "addicted," the nurse has a responsibility first do no harm and to call the doctor for more pain medication.

8.57 **The answer is d.** The four ethical principles guiding clinical practice are autonomy, nonmaleficence, beneficence, and justice.
- Autonomy—process of helping patients make the decisions that are right for them
- Nonmaleficence—do no harm
- Beneficence —help the patient to balance the benefits against the risk of harm
- Justice—the distribution of resources in a fair and reasonable way

8.58 **The answer is b.** Assisted suicide and end-of-life decisions were identified as the two most important ethical issues by the Oncology Nursing Society Ethics Advisory Council and by 900 nurses surveyed by the American Nurses Association.

8.59 **The answer is c.** The *Ethical Workup Guide* requires caregivers to plan an ethically justifiable course of action for their patient. They can use one or more of the ethical values in their decision.

8.60 **The answer is c.** Spirituality greatly affects a patient's journey through a life-threatening illness and provides a sense of meaning despite the illness. Although the other selections may also be true, they are part of how one finds a sense of meaning through spirituality.

8.61 **The answer is c.** The ONS's five core values of respectful care, quality of life, competence, collegiality, and fairness speak from the shared experience of oncology nurses and provide a context for applying the ANA's Code for Nurses in oncology nursing practice.

8.62 **The answer is c.** Compared to control subjects, individuals who received systemic cancer treatment were impaired in executive functioning, verbal memory, and motor functioning. Information processing was slowed in people with cancer compared to control subjects but not in studies where the comparison was with normative values.

8.63   **The answer is b.** Women older than 40 who develop amenorrhea have the highest risk of experiencing an abrupt permanent menopause. In contrast to standard-dose chemotherapy, high-dose chemotherapy is associated with a high rate of ovarian failure (90%), even in young women. It is the nurse's responsibility to inform patients regarding their risks associated with reproductive and hormonal sequelae of chemotherapy.

8.64   **The answer is c.** The effect of cancer treatment on sperm counts may be temporary or permanent. Some men with azoospermia immediately after cancer treatment eventually recover sperm counts sufficient to conceive children. Studies comparing the offspring of survivors with the offspring of survivors' siblings have demonstrated no increased risk of birth defects among the children of survivors. Because of the uncertainty about treatment-related chromosomal damage, men should wait at least 6 months after the end of cancer treatment before attempting to conceive or to harvest sperm for assisted reproduction.

8.65   **The answer is d.** The NCCS focuses on a wide range of issues related to quality of life for cancer survivors and their families.

8.66   **The answer is d.** PSDA requires that all health care institutions receiving Medicare or Medicaid reimbursement ask the patients they admit if they have an advance directive. If patients do not, the institution is obligated to provide written information about such directives.

8.67   **The answer is c.** An AD is a one-person statement, not a legally binding contract.

8.68   **The answer is c.** The Patient Self-Determination Act may also serve to control health care costs in the last 6 months of life and to facilitate a responsible use of technological intervention. However, these are not the primary goals of the Act. The Act does not necessarily facilitate a systematic process of eliciting and honoring patient wishes.

8.69   **The answer is c.** Patients can become confused about what a living will is. It does not specify disbursement of assets. It does not address all possible medical situations. The words "artificial" and "extraordinary" are often used in an advanced directive (AD); however, these words can be interpreted differently. A directive may not always be honored and implemented. An AD is a one-person statement, not a legally binding contract.

8.70   **The answer is c.** The lack of reimbursement structures is often described as a barrier to palliative care. However, as experts in the field address earlier palliative intervention, reimbursement for these efforts can be captured under traditional and existing reimbursement coding. An easy transition toward appropriate end-of-life (EOL) care would be facilitated rather than impeded. EOL care is being differentiated from palliative care because EOL care implies time-defined care that does not recognize the complex skills of palliative medicine. The use of the phrase *end of life* may promote a discontinuous care model rather than a collaborative model with earlier referral for palliative services.

8.71   **The answer is c.** Errors in the route of administration for vincristine prompted United States Pharmacopeia labeling requirements and standards for vincristine packaging, which include cautionary labeling that states "FATAL IF GIVEN INTRATHECALLY. FOR IV USE ONLY. DO NOT REMOVE COVERING UNTIL MOMENT OF INJECTION." Cytarabine, methotrexate, interferon, and thiotepa have all been given safely intrathecally.

8.72   **The answer is a.** Additional safety goals include improve patient identification procedures, improve communication, perform the correct surgical procedure on the correct patient and correct site, and reduce the risk of health care–acquired infection.

8.73 **The answer is c.** As we increase the quality of any service while maintaining costs, we increase the value.

8.74 **The answer is c.** Critical paths consist of a series of interventions specific to a group of patients with common attributes that are designed to promote the attainment of specific patient outcomes within a specific time frame.

8.75 **The answer is b.** Potential hazards associated with the administration of antineoplastic agents have prompted the Occupational Safety and Health Administration to set guidelines for compounding, transporting, administering, and disposing of toxic chemotherapy agents.

8.76 **The answer is a.** Accurate descriptive documentation of home health nursing care is vital to reimbursement and continuation of home health services. It has been postulated that the rise in health care expenditures, including those for home health care, has led the government and fiscal intermediaries to enact regulations requiring specific documentation and has increased focused review in an effort to decrease costs by denial of payment for services designated by the reviewer as "noncovered."

8.77 **The answer is b.** The CPR was formed to ensure that the growing needs of the American health system can be met and that patients have access to quality health care providers of their choice. The coalition represents more than 3 million licensed professionals who provide affordable health care services. The AMA and other physician groups want to limit the ability of licensed health care professionals such as advanced practice nurses, psychologists, nurse midwives, and chiropractors to provide care to millions of patients.

8.78 **The answer is b.** The Balanced Budget Act of 1997 was amended in 1999 to provide Medicare Part B reimbursement to APNs at 85% of what physicians receive for services in the Physician Fee Schedule. State-specific practice acts determine the extent to which APNs can receive Medicaid reimbursement, if at all. It is important to realize that Medicare is the federal mandate for reimbursement fee structures for APNs regardless of state-specific practice acts.

8.79 **The answer is c.** Except for family NPs, a master's degree is now considered the minimum education required for entry: family NP requires a clinical doctorate in nursing.

8.80 **The answer is d.** The majority of CNSs work within tertiary care centers, primarily in inpatient settings, as staff and patient/family educators and consultants. As economic changes forced efficient use of resources, many CNS roles in tertiary care sites were eliminated. Some CNSs chose case management for managed care organizations as a way to advocate for patients and for quality cost-effectiveness. The roles of the CNS are clinical practice, education, consultation, and research.

8.81 **The answer is b.** ONS recognizes nurses who have become experts in coordinating and providing direct and indirect care to people with cancer through study and precepted clinical practice in oncology at the graduate level as oncology CNSs. The term NP describes the nurse whose educational preparation includes completion of an NP program at the master's or doctorate level. The role of the NP is to provide comprehensive clinical care to individuals, with an emphasis on health promotion, disease prevention, diagnosis, and management of acute and chronic diseases. ONS recognizes NPs who have expertise in the specialty of oncology as oncology NPs.

8.82 **The answer is c.** Few studies have evaluated specialty certification in the health care professions or described links between provider certification and patient outcomes. Three avenues of inquiry have been typical of the research on specialty certification among health care providers. These include identifying characteristics that differentiate certified and noncertified providers, describing variations in practice, and linking provider certification to patient outcomes. Labor unions do not have a role.

8.83 **The answer is a.** As a consultant, the OAPN in secondary care is involved in planning and implementing initiatives aimed at patient and family education and support. The OAPN's expertise is also used in symptom management, and OAPNs are often important members of multidisciplinary pain and symptom management teams. They also may act as consultants to an institution in establishing standards for oncology practice and developing critical pathways.

8.84 **The answer is b.** Faculty need to be prepared in oncology nursing and need to be both knowledgeable in the latest trends and clinically competent. In addition to joint appointments, new and different ways to ensure competence must be explored.

8.85 **The answer is b.** The Oncology Nursing Certification Corporation administers a certification program for cancer nurses. A certification examination is offered twice yearly. Nurses with a registered nurse license, 1 year experience as a registered nurse within the last 3 years, and a minimum of 1000 hours of cancer nursing practice within the last 2.5 years are eligible to take this examination.

8.86 **The answer is d.** Advances in cancer treatment and technology, the influences of economics, and quality-of-life issues have promoted ambulatory services as a method for providing cancer patient and family care. With shortened hospitalizations driven by reimbursement changes, patients are being discharged quicker and sicker; therefore the patient acuity is actually higher.

8.87 **The answer is a.** In a physician–hospital organization (PHO), a contractual relationship between physicians and the hospital accomplishes several goals: it increases the opportunity to obtain managed-care contracts, aligns the organizational structure with the financial incentives found in capitation, and measures quality of care through outcomes.

8.88 **The answer is b.** Horizontal integration occurs when a PHO is organized into an integrated delivery system that uses different sites in the community to provide a wide variety of services. With vertical integration these services are capable of being provided within the same system. Vertical integration is sometimes referred to as depth of services and horizontal integration as breadth of services.

8.89 **The answer is d.** In a collaborative practice NPs function independently in caring for a caseload of patients, whether in the ambulatory or the acute care setting. Care is provided based on competence: The skills of the provider are matched with the needs of the patient.

8.90 **The answer is b.** UAP may provide direct patient care. They should not be used in those situations in which the patient's disease or response is unpredictable or in which specialized knowledge or skills are needed, such as chemotherapy, pain management, symptom management plans, toxicity grading, and unstable patient assessment.

STUDY NOTES

STUDY NOTES